T0227313

Social and Economic Dimensions of Sleep Disorders

Editor

ANA C. KRIEGER

SLEEP MEDICINE CLINICS

www.sleep.theclinics.com

Consulting Editor
TEOFILO LEE-CHIONG Jr

March 2017 • Volume 12 • Number 1

ELSEVIER

1600 John F. Kennedy Boulevard • Suite 1800 • Philadelphia, Pennsylvania, 19103-2899

http://www.theclinics.com

SLEEP MEDICINE CLINICS Volume 12, Number 1
March 2017, ISSN 1556-407X, ISBN-13: 978-0-323-50987-9

Editor: Katie Pfaff
Developmental Editor: Donald Mumford

© **2017 Elsevier Inc. All rights reserved.**

This periodical and the individual contributions contained in it are protected under copyright by Elsevier, and the following terms and conditions apply to their use:

Photocopying
Single photocopies of single articles may be made for personal use as allowed by national copyright laws. Permission of the Publisher and payment of a fee is required for all other photocopying, including multiple or systematic copying, copying for advertising or promotional purposes, resale, and all forms of document delivery. Special rates are available for educational institutions that wish to make photocopies for non-profit educational classroom use. For information on how to seek permission visit www.elsevier.com/permissions or call: (+44) 1865 843830 (UK)/(+1) 215 239 3804 (USA).

Derivative Works
Subscribers may reproduce tables of contents or prepare lists of articles including abstracts for internal circulation within their institutions. Permission of the Publisher is required for resale or distribution outside the institution. Permission of the Publisher is required for all other derivative works, including compilations and translations (please consult www.elsevier.com/permissions).

Electronic Storage or Usage
Permission of the Publisher is required to store or use electronically any material contained in this periodical, including any article or part of an article (please consult www.elsevier.com/permissions). Except as outlined above, no part of this publication may be reproduced, stored in a retrieval system or transmitted in any form or by any means, electronic, mechanical, photocopying, recording or otherwise, without prior written permission of the Publisher.

Notice
No responsibility is assumed by the Publisher for any injury and/or damage to persons or property as a matter of products liability, negligence or otherwise, or from any use or operation of any methods, products, instructions or ideas contained in the material herein. Because of rapid advances in the medical sciences, in particular, independent verification of diagnoses and drug dosages should be made. Although all advertising material is expected to conform to ethical (medical) standards, inclusion in this publication does not constitute a guarantee or endorsement of the quality or value of such product or of the claims made of it by its manufacturer.

Sleep Medicine Clinics (ISSN 1556-407X) is published quarterly by Elsevier Inc., 360 Park Avenue South, New York, NY 10010-1710. Months of issue are March, June, September and December. Business and Editorial Offices: 1600 John F. Kennedy Blvd., Ste. 1800, Philadelphia, PA 19103-2899. Customer Service Office: 3251 Riverport Lane, Maryland Heights, MO 63043. Periodicals postage paid at New York, NY and additional mailing offices. Subscription prices are $203.00 per year (US individuals), $100.00 (US students), $476.00 (US institutions), $244.00 (Canadian and international individuals), $135.00 (Canadian and international students), $540.00 (Canadian institutions) and $529.00 (International institutions). Foreign air speed delivery is included in all *Clinics* subscription prices. All prices are subject to change without notice. **POSTMASTER:** Send change of address to *Sleep Medicine Clinics*, Elsevier Health Sciences Division, Subscription Customer Service, 3251 Riverport Lane, Maryland Heights, MO 63043. Customer Service: **Tel: 1-800-654-2452 (U.S. and Canada); 314-447-8871 (outside U.S. and Canada). Fax: 314-447-8029. E-mail: journalscustomerservice-usa@elsevier.com (for print support); journalsonline support-usa@elsevier.com (for online support).**

Reprints. For copies of 100 or more of articles in this publication, please contact the Commercial Reprints Department, Elsevier Inc., 360 Park Avenue South, New York, NY 10010-1710. Tel.: 212-633-3874; Fax: 212-633-3820; E-mail: reprints@elsevier.com.

Sleep Medicine Clinics is covered in *MEDLINE/PubMed (Index Medicus)*.

SLEEP MEDICINE CLINICS

THE CLINICS ARE AVAILABLE ONLINE!
Access your subscription at:
www.theclinics.com

PROGRAM OBJECTIVE
The goal of *Sleep Clinics of North America* is to keep practicing physicians up to date with current clinical practice by providing timely articles reviewing the state of the art in patient care.

TARGET AUDIENCE
All practicing physicians and other healthcare professionals.

LEARNING OBJECTIVES
Upon completion of this activity, participants will be able to:
1. Review the clinical, socio-economic, and cost-benefit analysis of sleep disorders.
2. Discuss the diagnosis and management of sleep disorders.
3. Recognize the benefits of screening for sleep disorders in populations with conditions such as heart failure and atrial fibrillation.

ACCREDITATION
The Elsevier Office of Continuing Medical Education (EOCME) is accredited by the Accreditation Council for Continuing Medical Education (ACCME) to provide continuing medical education for physicians.

The EOCME designates this enduring material for a maximum of 15 *AMA PRA Category 1 Credit*(s) ™. Physicians should claim only the credit commensurate with the extent of their participation in the activity.

All other health care professionals requesting continuing education credit for this enduring material will be issued a certificate of participation.

DISCLOSURE OF CONFLICTS OF INTEREST
The EOCME assesses conflict of interest with its instructors, faculty, planners, and other individuals who are in a position to control the content of CME activities. All relevant conflicts of interest that are identified are thoroughly vetted by EOCME for fair balance, scientific objectivity, and patient care recommendations. EOCME is committed to providing its learners with CME activities that promote improvements or quality in healthcare and not a specific proprietary business or a commercial interest.

The planning committee, staff, authors and editors listed below have identified no financial relationships or relationships to products or devices they or their spouse/life partner have with commercial interest related to the content of this CME activity:
Dianne M. Augelli, MD; Daniel A. Barone, MD; Frances Chung, MBBS, FRCPC; Nancy A. Collop, MD, FAASM; Lourdes M. DelRossi, MD, FAASM; Luciano F. Drager, MD, PhD; Anjali Fortna; Pedro R. Genta, MD, PhD; Michael A. Grandner, PhD, MTR, CBSM; Romy Hoque, MD, FAASM; Ana C. Krieger, MD, MPH, FAASM, FCCP; Meir H. Kryger, MD, FRCP(C); Vaishnavi Kundel, MD; Brienne Miner, MD, MHS; Anne Marie Morse, MD; Mahesh Nagappa, MD, DNB; Rafael Pelayo, MD; Katie Pfaff; Kannan Ramar, MD; Sarah A. Reynolds, NP; Prabhjyot Saini, MSPH; Bernardo J. Selim, MD; Neomi Shah, MD, MPH; Yamini Subramani, MD; Michael Thorpy, MD; Rajakumar Venkatesan; Saiprakash B. Venkateshiah, MD; Amy Williams; Jean Wong, MD, FRCPC; Kin M. Yuen, MD, MS.

The planning committee, staff, authors and editors listed below have identified financial relationships or relationships to products or devices they or their spouse/life partner have with commercial interest related to the content of this CME activity:
Sudansu Chokroverty, MD receives royalties/patents from Elsevier, Springer International Publishing AG, & Oxford University Press.
Matthew R. Ebben, PhD receives royalties/patents from Weill Cornell Medicine.
Teofilo Lee-Chiong Jr, MD is a consultant/advisor for Elsevier and CareCore International, has stock ownsership in and an employment affiliation with Elsevier, and receieves royalties/patents from Lippincott; Oxford University Press; CreateSpace; and Wiley.
David B. Rye, MD, PhD is a consultant/advisor for Flamel Technologies SA; Jazz Pharmaceuticals; UCB, Inc; and XenoPort, Inc, and receives royalties/patents from Balance Therapeutics.

UNAPPROVED/OFF-LABEL USE DISCLOSURE
The EOCME requires CME faculty to disclose to the participants:
1. When products or procedures being discussed are off-label, unlabelled, experimental, and/or investigational (not US Food and Drug Administration [FDA] approved); and
2. Any limitations on the information presented, such as data that are preliminary or that represent ongoing research, interim analyses, and/or unsupported opinions. Faculty may discuss information about pharmaceutical agents that is outside of FDA-approved labelling. This information is intended solely for CME and is not intended to promote off-label use of these medications. If you have any questions, contact the medical affairs department of the manufacturer for the most recent prescribing information.

TO ENROLL

To enroll in the Sleep Medicines Clinic Continuing Medical Education program, call customer service at 1-800-654-2452 or sign up online at http://www.theclinics.com/home/cme. The CME program is available to subscribers for an additional annual fee of USD $140.

METHOD OF PARTICIPATION

In order to claim credit, participants must complete the following:

1. Complete enrolment as indicated above.
2. Read the activity.
3. Complete the CME Test and Evaluation. Participants must achieve a score of 70% on the test. All CME Tests and Evaluations must be completed online.

CME INQUIRIES/SPECIAL NEEDS

For all CME inquiries or special needs, please contact elsevierCME@elsevier.com.

Contributors

CONSULTING EDITOR

TEOFILO LEE-CHIONG Jr, MD
Professor of Medicine, National Jewish Health,
School of Medicine, University of Colorado
Denver, Denver, Colorado; Chief Medical
Liaison, Philips Respironics, Pennsylvania

EDITOR

ANA C. KRIEGER, MD, MPH, FAASM, FCCP
Medical Director, Center for Sleep Medicine,
Weill Cornell Medicine/New York–Presbyterian
Hospital; Associate Professor of Medicine,
Departments of Medicine, Neurology and
Genetic Medicine, Weill Cornell Medical
College, Cornell University, New York,
New York

AUTHORS

DIANNE M. AUGELLI, MD
Assistant Professor, Department of Medicine,
Center for Sleep Medicine, Weill Cornell Medical
College, Cornell University, New York, New York

DANIEL A. BARONE, MD
Assistant Professor of Neurology, Center for
Sleep Medicine, Weill Cornell Medical College,
New York, New York

SUDANSU CHOKROVERTY, MD
JFK Neuroscience Institute/Seton Hall
University, Edison, New Jersey

FRANCES CHUNG, MBBS, FRCPC
Professor, Department of Anesthesiology,
Toronto Western Hospital, University Health
Network, University of Toronto, Toronto,
Ontario, Canada

NANCY A. COLLOP, MD, FAASM
Director, Emory Sleep Center; Professor of
Medicine and Neurology, Division of
Pulmonary, Critical Care and Sleep Medicine,
Department of Medicine, Emory University
School of Medicine, Atlanta, Georgia

LOURDES M. DELROSSO, MD, FAASM
Assistant Professor, Department of Pediatrics,
University of California San Francisco, UCSF
Benioff Children's Hospital Oakland, Oakland,
California

LUCIANO F. DRAGER, MD, PhD
Associate Professor of Medicine, Hypertension
Unit of the Renal Division and Heart Institute
(InCor), Hospital das Clínicas, University of São
Paulo School of Medicine, São Paulo,
São Paulo, Brasil

MATTHEW R. EBBEN, PhD
Center for Sleep Medicine, Weill Cornell
Medical College, New York, New York

PEDRO R. GENTA, MD, PhD
Assistant Professor of Medicine, Pulmonary
Division, Heart Institute (InCor), Hospital das
Clínicas, University of São Paulo School of
Medicine, São Paulo, São Paulo, Brasil

MICHAEL A. GRANDNER, PhD, MTR, CBSM
Director, Sleep and Health Research Program, Department of Psychiatry; Assistant Professor, Departments of Medicine and Psychology, College of Medicine; Director, Behavioral Sleep Medicine Clinic, Banner-University Medical Center, Member, Sarver Heart Center, University of Arizona, Tucson, Arizona

ROMY HOQUE, MD, FAASM
Assistant Professor, Department of Neurology, Emory Sleep Center, Emory University School of Medicine, Atlanta, Georgia

ANA C. KRIEGER, MD, MPH, FAASM, FCCP
Medical Director, Center for Sleep Medicine, Weill Cornell Medicine/New York–Presbyterian Hospital; Associate Professor of Medicine, Departments of Medicine, Neurology and Genetic Medicine, Weill Cornell Medical College, Cornell University, New York, New York

MEIR H. KRYGER, MD, FRCP(C)
Professor, Pulmonary, Critical Care, and Sleep Medicine, Department of Internal Medicine, Yale School of Medicine, New Haven, Connecticut; VA Connecticut Healthcare System, West Haven, Connecticut

VAISHNAVI KUNDEL, MD
Postdoctoral Fellow, Division of Pulmonary, Critical Care, and Sleep Medicine, Icahn School of Medicine at Mount Sinai, New York, New York

GERALDO LORENZI FILHO, MD, PhD
Associate Professor of Medicine, Pulmonary Division, Heart Institute (InCor), Hospital das Clínicas, University of São Paulo School of Medicine, São Paulo, São Paulo, Brasil

BRIENNE MINER, MD, MHS
Geriatric and Sleep Medicine Fellow, Department of Internal Medicine, Yale School of Medicine, New Haven, Connecticut

ANNE MARIE MORSE, MD
Sleep-Wake Disorders Center, Montefiore Medical Center, and Albert Einstein College of Medicine, Bronx, New York

MAHESH NAGAPPA, MD, DNB
Assistant Professor, Department of Anesthesia and Perioperative Medicine, London Health Science Centre and St. Joseph Health Care, Schulich School of Medicine and Dentistry, Western University, London, Ontario, Canada

RAFAEL PELAYO, MD
Clinical Professor, Stanford Sleep Disorders Clinic, Stanford University School of Medicine, Redwood City, California

KANNAN RAMAR, MD
Associate Professor in Medicine, Division of Pulmonary and Critical Care Medicine, Mayo Clinic Center for Sleep Medicine, Mayo Clinic, Rochester, Minnesota

SARAH A. REYNOLDS, NP
Center for Sleep Medicine, Weill Cornell Medical College, New York, New York

DAVID B. RYE, MD, PhD
Professor, Department of Neurology and Program in Sleep, Emory University School of Medicine, Atlanta, Georgia

PRABHJYOT SAINI, MSPH
Senior Associate, Department of Neurology, Emory University School of Medicine, Atlanta, Georgia

BERNARDO J. SELIM, MD
Assistant Professor of Medicine, Division of Pulmonary and Critical Care Medicine, Mayo Clinic Center for Sleep Medicine, Mayo Clinic, Rochester, Minnesota

NEOMI SHAH, MD, MPH
Director, Sleep Medicine Fellowship, Division of Pulmonary, Critical Care, and Sleep Medicine, Icahn School of Medicine at Mount Sinai, New York, New York; Department of Epidemiology and Population Health, Albert Einstein College of Medicine, Bronx, New York

YAMINI SUBRAMANI, MD
Clinical Fellow, Department of Anesthesiology, Toronto Western Hospital, University Health Network, University of Toronto, Toronto, Ontario, Canada

MICHAEL THORPY, MD
Sleep-Wake Disorders Center, Montefiore
Medical Center, and Albert Einstein College of
Medicine, Bronx, New York

SAIPRAKASH B. VENKATESHIAH, MD
Assistant Professor, Division of Pulmonary,
Critical Care and Sleep Medicine, Department
of Medicine, Emory University School of
Medicine, Atlanta, Georgia

JEAN WONG, MD, FRCPC
Associate Professor, Department of
Anesthesiology, Toronto Western Hospital,
University Health Network, University of
Toronto, Toronto, Ontario, Canada

KIN M. YUEN, MD, MS
Adjunct Faculty, Stanford Sleep Disorders
Clinic, Stanford University School of Medicine,
Redwood City, California

Contents

Biological needs for sleep are met by engaging in behaviors that are largely influenced by the environment, social norms and demands, and societal influences and pressures. Insufficient sleep duration and sleep disorders such as insomnia and sleep apnea are highly prevalent in the US population. This article outlines some of these downstream factors, including cardiovascular and metabolic disease risk, neurocognitive dysfunction, and mortality, as well as societal factors such as age, sex, race/ethnicity, and socioeconomics. This review also discusses societal factors related to sleep, such as globalization, health disparities, public policy, public safety, and changing patterns of use of technology.

Pediatric disorders tend to affect the immediate support unit, adults and children. High costs for direct consumption of medical care are offset by early diagnosis and treatment of pediatric sleep disorders. Pediatric sleep disorders are underdiagnosed and undertreated. Attention-deficit/hyperactivity disorder may result from insufficient or fragmented sleep. Delaying school start time resulted in decreased car crashes in teen drivers and improved mood.

There are normal changes to sleep architecture throughout the lifespan. There is not, however, a decreased need for sleep and sleep disturbance is not an inherent part of the aging process. Sleep disturbance is common in older adults because aging is associated with an increasing prevalence of multimorbidity, polypharmacy, psychosocial factors affecting sleep, and certain primary sleep disorders. It is also associated with morbidity and mortality. Because many older adults have several factors from different domains affecting their sleep, these complaints are best approached as a multifactorial geriatric health condition, necessitating a multifaceted treatment approach.

Insomnia is a highly prevalent, often chronic condition, which is left untreated or not treated according to recommended guidelines in most cases. This results in high health and financial burdens to society. The cost of untreated insomnia and the prevailing reliance on sedative-hypnotic use as a first-line treatment are evaluated in this article. The cost-benefit potential of cognitive behavioral therapy for insomnia is also assessed.

Most central disorders of hypersomnolence are conditions with poorly understood pathophysiologies, making their identification, treatment, and management challenging for sleep clinicians. The most challenging to diagnose and treat is idiopathic hypersomnia. There are no FDA-approved treatments, and off-label usage of narcolepsy treatments seldom provide benefit. Patients are largely left on their own to alleviate the compound effects of this disorder on their quality of life. This review covers the major points regarding clinical features and diagnosis of idiopathic hypersomnia, reviews current evidence supporting the available treatment options, and discusses the psychosocial impact and effects of idiopathic hypersomnia.

The burden of narcolepsy is likely the result of 2 main aspects: the clinical difficulties and disability incurred as a direct effect of the disorder and the socioeconomic burden. The clinical burden includes the symptoms, diagnosis, comorbidities, treatment, and even mortality that can be associated with narcolepsy. Lifelong therapy is necessary for these patients. Effective treatment results in long-term benefits from both patient and societal perspectives by improving clinical outcomes, potentially enabling improved education and increased employment and work productivity, and quality of life. Thus, reducing the time to appropriate management results in improved outcomes in these patients.

Sleep disorders and neurologic illness are common and burdensome in their own right; when combined, they can have tremendous negative impact at an individual level as well as societally. The socioeconomic burden of sleep disorders and neurologic illness can be identified, but the real cost of these conditions lies far beyond the financial realm. There is an urgent need for comprehensive care and support systems to help with the burden of disease. Further research in improving patient outcomes in those who suffer with these conditions will help patients and their families, and society in general.

Hypoventilation during sleep is often an early indicator of the development of respiratory failure. Alterations in ventilation are more pronounced during sleep and often present before the onset of daytime symptoms. This article discusses the most common sleep-related hypoventilatory disorders and recommended treatment approaches for obesity hypoventilation, chronic obstructive pulmonary disease, and neuromuscular disorders. Accurate diagnosis and appropriate treatment is of paramount importance because of the impact on individual health outcomes and overall cost of health care delivery. Appropriate treatment is successful at reducing hospitalizations and health care costs as well as improving quality of life and individual economic burden.

Obstructive sleep apnea (OSA) and atrial fibrillation (AF) are common conditions in the adult population and independently associated with increased morbidity and mortality. There is evidence, although not definitive, that OSA independently contributes to AF incidence and recurrence. Full polysomnography is expensive and may not be readily available to diagnose all patients with OSA and AF. Several patients with OSA do not present the classical signs and symptoms of OSA, impairing the accuracy of screening questionnaires for OSA. In this context, a home sleep test is a promising alternative to screen and diagnose OSA in AF patients. However, the cost-effectiveness of such an approach needs to be studied.

Central sleep apnea (CSA) and obstructive sleep apnea (OSA) are prevalent in heart failure (HF) and associated with a worse prognosis. Nocturnal oxygen therapy may decrease CSA events, sympathetic tone, and improve left ventricular ejection fraction, although mortality benefit is unknown. Although treatment of OSA in patients with HF is recommended, therapy for CSA remains controversial. Continuous positive airway pressure use in HF-CSA may improve respiratory events, hemodynamics, and exercise capacity, but not mortality. Adaptive servo ventilation is contraindicated in patients with symptomatic HF with predominant central sleep-disordered events. The role of phrenic nerve stimulation in CSA therapy is promising.

Obstructive sleep apnea (OSA) is a chronic disease affecting millions of people worldwide. Untreated OSA can lead to about a 2-fold increase in medical expenses, mainly because of cardiovascular morbidity. OSA is highly prevalent in the surgical population, with an increased risk of perioperative complications. This article describes the perioperative and long-term social and economic benefits of preoperative screening for OSA. Screening patients to identify high-risk OSA is important to decrease the adverse outcomes and associated health care costs in the perioperative period. Screening for OSA is particularly relevant because most patients are undiagnosed at the time of surgery.

This article provides the current state of evidence on the socioeconomic impact of portable testing (PT) for sleep apnea. It seems the traditional in-laboratory polysomnography and the newer home-based PT model for sleep apnea diagnosis both have places in a sleep medicine diagnostic algorithm. PT would be cost-effective in a selected group of patients as long as certain criteria, discussed in this article, are carefully considered.

Sleep disorders may interact with the law, making awareness important. Insufficient sleep and obstructive sleep apnea (OSA) are prevalent and associated with excessive sleepiness. Patients with excessive sleepiness may have civil or criminal liability if they fall asleep and cause a motor vehicle accident. Awareness of screening and treatment of OSA is increasing in certain industries. Parasomnia associated sleep-related violence represents a challenge to clinicians, who may be called on to consider parasomnia as a contributing, mitigating, or exculpatory factor in criminal proceedings. Improving access to sleep medicine care is an important aspect in reducing the consequences of sleep disorders.

Preface
The Costly Face of Sleep Disorders

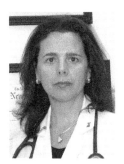

Ana C. Krieger, MD, MPH, FAASM, FCCP
Editor

Welcome to the March 2017 issue of the *Sleep Medicine Clinics*. This issue is dedicated to reviewing the social and economic impacts of sleep disorders. The importance of sleep has become a topic of frequent discussion in the literature. The progress experienced over the past century, including an increased availability of artificial light, easy access to processed and manufactured foods, improved communication, and transcontinental travel, has fundamentally altered our daily activities and clearly impacted sleep physiology. Modern societies are now facing challenges in achieving adequate sleep and experiencing a multitude of sleep disturbances.

Technological advances have been, nonetheless, key to scientific knowledge expansion and research development. Since the discovery of electroencephalography almost a century ago, the field of Sleep Medicine has grown exponentially, moving from obscurity to a well-known multidisciplinary medical specialty. Sleep disorders have become more easily identified, and new treatment approaches have been developed. With an estimated prevalence of more than 30% of the adult US population, sleep disturbances are associated with an increased burden to the health care and financial systems, carrying intrinsic costs to the individual and society in general.

In this issue of *Sleep Medicine Clinics*, an outstanding group of collaborators was gathered to discuss the socioeconomic implications of disrupted sleep. The topics presented include a review of the current state of sleep health, the impact of pediatric and geriatric sleep disturbances, as well as the costs associated with insomnia, hypersomnia syndromes, and narcolepsy in our society. The reader will also find articles on the impact of specific neurologic, cardiac, and respiratory disorders in sleep, and on the application of perioperative screening and portable testing, closing with an overview of the legal and regulatory framework in sleep medicine.

Thank you for your interest in this publication. We hope the information shared will help to better understand the implications of sleep disturbances, and the pressing need to improve sleep for all.

I would like to express my gratitude to the dedicated colleagues that contributed to this issue, and I wish you all a healthy journey toward optimal sleep.

Ana C. Krieger, MD, MPH, FAASM, FCCP
Weill Cornell Medicine/
New York–Presbyterian Hospital
Departments of Medicine, Neurology
and Genetic Medicine
Weill Cornell Medical College
Cornell University
425 East 61st Street–5th Floor
New York, NY 10065, USA

E-mail address:
ack2003@med.cornell.edu

Sleep Med Clin 12 (2017) xv
http://dx.doi.org/10.1016/j.jsmc.2016.12.001
1556-407X/17/© 2016 Published by Elsevier Inc.

Sleep, Health, and Society

Michael A. Grandner, PhD, MTR, CBSM

KEYWORDS

- Sleep • Sleep disorders • Epidemiology • Social factors • Health • Disparities • Society

KEY POINTS

- Insufficient sleep and sleep disorders are highly prevalent in the population and are associated with significant morbidity and mortality.
- Adverse outcomes of insufficient sleep and/or sleep disorders are weight gain and obesity, cardiovascular disease, diabetes, accidents and injuries, stress, pain, neurocognitive dysfunction, psychiatric symptoms, and mortality.
- Exposure to sleep difficulties varies by age, sex, race/ethnicity, and socioeconomic status; significant sleep health disparities exist in the population.
- Societal influences, such as globalization, technology, and public policy, affect sleep at a population level.

CONCEPTUALIZING SLEEP IN A SOCIAL CONTEXT

Sleep represents an emergent set of many physiologic processes under primarily neurobiological regulation that impact many physiologic systems. As such, many advances have been made over the past several decades that have shed light on these neurobiologic mechanisms of sleep-wake,[1–4] with especially exciting work in the area of functional genetics/genomics[5,6] and molecular mechanisms of sleep-related regulation.[7–9] Still, the phenomenon of sleep exists outside the nucleus and the cell membrane—sleep is experienced phenomenologically. Sleep is a biological requirement for human life, alongside food, water, and air. Like consumption of food and unlike breathing air, achieving this biological need requires the individual to engage in volitional behaviors. Although many of these behaviors are genetically and intrapersonally driven (eg, it is not a coincidence that most people prefer to sleep at night, and that most humans sleep in a stereotypical posturally recumbent manner), there is still much variability in sleep behaviors and practices. Because of this, sleep is also socially driven, dictated by the environment, and subject to interpersonal and societal factors.

Sleep in most humans occupies between 20% and 40% of the day. Even prehistoric evidence suggests the importance of sleep in human life[10]; this is consistent with archaeological and historical accounts of sleep having a prominent and important role in even early human society. Sleep was a universal phenomenon that was inescapable and thus was incorporated in social structures. In this way, sleep became not just a set of physiologic processes, but one represented in sociocultural structures. Thus, the timing, environment, and constraints surrounding sleep across human societies began to differ between rich and poor, powerful and powerless, rural and urban, and so forth. As sociologist, Simon Williams, writes, "Where we sleep, when we sleep, and with whom we sleep are all important markers or indicators of social status, privilege, and prevailing power relations."[11]

Conceptualizing Downstream Consequences

The downstream consequences of insufficient sleep duration and/or inadequate sleep quality

Dr M.A. Grandner is supported by National Heart, Lung, and Blood Institute (K23HL110216).
Department of Psychiatry, College of Medicine, University of Arizona, 1501 North Campbell Avenue, PO Box 245002, BUMC Suite 7326, Tucson, AZ 85724-5002, USA
E-mail address: grandner@email.arizona.edu

Sleep Med Clin 12 (2017) 1–22
http://dx.doi.org/10.1016/j.jsmc.2016.10.012
1556-407X/17/© 2016 Elsevier Inc. All rights reserved.

(including sleep disorders and circadian misalignment of sleep) are varied and impact many physiologic systems. Conceptualizing these is therefore difficult. One way to do so is to acknowledge domains of outcomes and recognize the overlaps and relationships among those domains. The recent position statement from the American Academy of Sleep Medicine and Sleep Research Society[12–15] broadly categorizes effects of insufficient sleep as pertaining to the following categories: general health, cardiovascular health, metabolic health, mental health, immunologic health, human performance, cancer, pain, and mortality.

Conceptualizing Upstream Influences: Social Ecological Models

Upstream social and environmental influences on sleep are also complex and overlapping and implicate many potential pathways. With this in mind, a social-ecological framework may be best suited to describe this relationship. The social-ecological model was originally developed to describe the complex ways that an individual's behavior related to their health is a product of influences at the individual level, but that the individual operates in the context of social structures that they are a member of, but these structures exist outside of the individual.[16] For example, an individual has genetic, psychological, and other reasons for consuming a healthy diet, but social structures that they are a part of but exist outside of that individual (like their neighborhood, which may have healthy food; their job, which may or may not have a cafeteria; their family, which may have other food restrictions, and so forth) play a role in that individual's behavior.

This model may also be appropriate for understanding sleep. At the individual level, factors that influence a person's sleep include that person's genetics, knowledge, beliefs, and attitudes about sleep, their overall health, and so forth. The individual level is embedded, though, within a social level, which includes the home (family, bedroom, and so forth), neighborhood, work/school, socioeconomics, religion, culture, race/ethnicity, and other factors. All of these factors influence sleep through the individual. Still, this social level is embedded within a societal level, which includes social forces that exist outside of things like work, family, and neighborhood, including globalization, geography, technology, public policy. These factors, at this high of a level, filter through the social structures that eventually come to bear on the individual. For example, as society embraced the Internet, it caused changes in jobs and families, which led to individual changes that play a role in sleep (such as social networking in bed or browsing the Internet late at night). **Fig. 1** displays a social-ecological model of sleep, illustrating of sleep duration and quality are influenced by factors at the individual level, which is embedded within a social level, which itself is embedded within a societal level. **Fig. 2** brings these models together, with sleep as the fulcrum (shown in **Fig. 1**) at the interface of upstream social-environmental influences (shown in more detail in **Fig. 3**) and downstream health and functional outcomes (shown in more detail in **Fig. 2**). This model brings all of these concepts

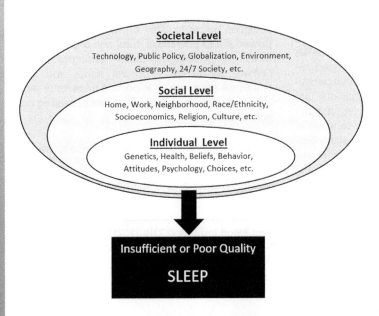

Fig. 1. Social ecological model of sleep.

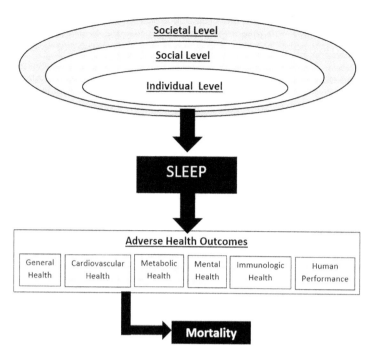

Fig. 2. Social ecological model of sleep and health.

together to describe how sleep is influenced by these societal factors and how those influences, through sleep, may play a role in health. The first version of this model was published in 2010,[17] and it has appeared in several other publications since then.[14,18–20] It may serve as a useful framework for conceptualizing the physiologic processes of sleep in a social context.

POPULATION PREVALENCE OF SLEEP DURATION AND SLEEP DISTURBANCES
Sleep Duration

Population estimates of habitual sleep duration are variable, because few studies used identical methods to derive estimates. The best population-level estimates come from 1 of 3 sources: (1) self-reported time use data, (2) self-reported typical weeknight/work-night sleep, and (3) self-reported average sleep within 24 hours. For US-based data, the primary sources of these estimates come from the American Time Use Survey (ATUS) for time use data, the National Health Interview Survey or National Health and Nutrition Examination Survey (NHANES) for weeknight sleep, and the Behavioral Risk Factor Surveillance System (BRFSS) for 24-hour sleep.

Longitudinal analysis of time-use diaries by Knutson and colleagues[21] found that the proportion of Americans reporting short (<6 hours) sleep was 7.6% in 1975 and 9.3% in 2006. Bin and colleagues[22] examined similar time use data from several countries and showed that, in the United States, sleep duration has generally declined since the 1960s, if only by a small amount. The most comprehensive analysis of time use data related to sleep was recently undertaken by Basner and colleagues.[23] They report that the age group that

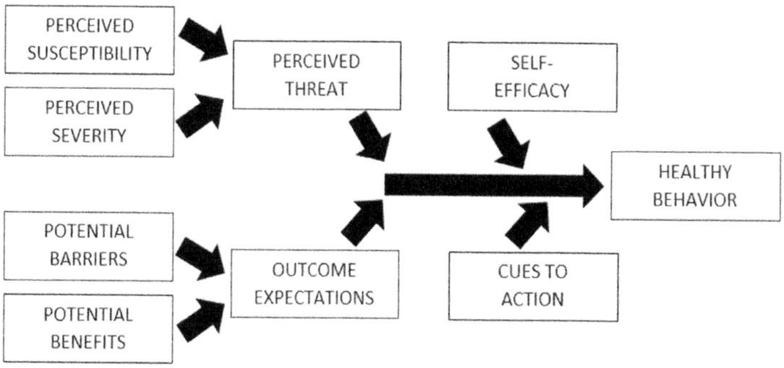

Fig. 3. Health belief model.

receives the most sleep is young adults (8.86 hours on weeknights and 10.02 hours on weekends) and that those aged 25 to 64 report about 0.70 to 0.99 fewer hours on weeknights and 0.62 to 1.16 fewer hours on weekends. Prevalence of sleep duration by hour is not reported, though.

Regarding weekday sleep duration, Grandner and colleagues[24] reported census-weighted estimates of sleep duration using the 2007 to 2008 wave of the NHANES. They report that 6.2% of the population reports less than 5 hours of sleep, 33.78% reports 5 to 6 hours of sleep, 52.68% report 7 to 8 hours of sleep, and 7.38% report at least 9 hours of sleep per typical weeknight. These values from NHANES is similar to values reported from Krueger and Friedman,[25] who assessed similar data from the NHIS using data from 2004 to 2007. They report prevalence of 5 hours or less being 7.8%, 6 hours being 20.5%, 7 hours being 30.8%, 8 hours being 32.5%, and 9 or more hours being 8.5%.

Regarding typical 24-hour sleep, which presumably includes napping, recent data from the Centers for Disease Control and Prevention (CDC) released data from the 2014 BRFSS, which included data from 444,306 American adults. Based on the recently published guidelines,[12,15] the CDC calculated the prevalence of less than 7 hours of sleep duration across all 50 states.[26] The median prevalence of less than 7 hours of sleep was 35.1%, with a range of 28.4% (South Dakota) to 43.9% (Hawaii). This report also documents that the prevalence of 5 hours or less was 11.8%, with prevalence of 6, 7, 8, 9, and 10 or more hours being 23.0%, 29.5%, 27.7%, 4.4%, and 3.6%, respectively.

Taken together, the time diaries generally show more sleep than other retrospective reports, perhaps because they may better capture time in bed but not actual sleep. Indeed, most retrospective sleep reports have this issue,[27] although perhaps it is particularly problematic for time diaries. In general, though, at least one-third of the population seems to be reporting habitual sleep of 6 hours or less. The proportion of those with 6 hours or less is salient, given the risk factors associated with sleep duration described in more detail in later discussion.

Sleep Disturbances

Sleep disturbances are difficult to measure at the population level. Often, population-level assessments of general sleep disturbances subsume insufficient sleep duration and/or sleep disorders that may not expressly fit into this category. The 2006 BRFSS asked the following question to

more than 150,000 residents of 36 US states/territories: "Over the last 2 weeks, how many days have you had trouble falling asleep or staying asleep or sleeping too much?" In an analysis of these responses, values were coded in whole numbers ranging from 0 to 14, but responses aggregated at 0 and 14; therefore, responses were dichotomized as either endorsing or not endorsing "sleep disturbance."[28,29] For men, the prevalence of sleep disturbance ranged from 13.7% (ages 70–74) to 18.1% (ages 18–24), and for women, the prevalence ranged from 17.7% (ages 80 or older) to 25.1% (ages 18–24).[29] Interestingly, reports of sleep disturbance generally declined with age. This finding was recently replicated using data from the 2009 BRFSS, which showed a similar pattern of declining self-report of insufficient sleep with age.[30]

Regarding sleep symptoms, data from the 2007 to 2008 NHANES were examined with regards to prevalence of various sleep symptoms.[31] Long sleep latency (more than 30 minutes) was reported by 18.8% of Americans. Self-reported difficulty falling asleep was reported at a rate of 11.71% for mild symptoms (1–3 times per week) and 7.7% for moderate-severe symptoms (at least half of nights). Similarly, sleep maintenance difficulties were reported by 13.21% endorsing mild and 7.7% endorsing moderate-severe symptoms, and early morning awakenings were reported at a rate of 10.7% for mild and 5.8% for moderate-severe symptoms. Daytime sleepiness and nonrestorative sleep were reported at a rate of 13.0% and 17.8% for mild symptoms, respectively, and 5.8% and 10.9% for moderate-severe symptoms, respectively. Frequent snoring was reported by 31.5% of adults and snorting/gasping during sleep was reported by 6.6% "occasionally" and 5.8% "frequently."

SLEEP EFFECTS ON HEALTH AND LONGEVITY

Because sleep is involved with many physiologic systems, insufficient sleep duration and poor sleep quality have been associated with several adverse health outcomes. Separate literature texts have emerged describing some of the negative effects of insufficient sleep duration, sleep apnea, and insomnia.

Mortality

The first report documenting the relationship between sleep duration and mortality risk was published more than 50 years ago.[32] This first study, an analysis of data from the American Cancer Society's first Cancer Prevention Study of more than one million US adults, found that increased mortality risk was associated with both short (6 hours or less) and long (9 hours or more) sleep duration. Since that time, many other studies have been published, from both large and small cohorts, covering both short and long follow-up periods, from 6 continents. Taken together, this overall pattern of findings, that both short and long sleep are associated with mortality risk, has generally remained consistent across studies, although not all studies found this pattern.[17] Two meta-analyses have been published, using slightly different methods and controls.[33,34] Still, their findings were highly consistent, indicating a 10% to 12% increased risk for short sleep and a 30% to 38% increased risk associated with long sleep duration. Much controversy remains, though, regarding this issue. For example, the precision of measurement of sleep in these studies is often poor.[17,27,35] Self-reported sleep time may better approximate time in bed, and although an actigraphic study found a similar pattern,[36] the cutoffs for short and long sleep indicated an overestimate among self-reports. Also, there is still a lack of clarity on the biological plausibility of the long sleep relationship, although some ideas have been proposed.[37,38] For this reason, most of the attention has been focused on risks associated with short sleep duration, which may be far more prevalent.

Weight Gain and Obesity

Many studies have found associations between sleep duration and adiposity and obesity.[39–41] Although most of these studies are cross-sectional, precluding causality, several other studies have longitudinally examined this relationship, demonstrating that short sleep duration is associated with increased weight gain over time.[42–46] These studies include individuals with otherwise low obesity risk, diverse community samples, and samples where effectiveness of weight loss interventions was mitigated by sleep and circadian factors. Several important caveats seem to be present in this relationship. First, this relationship is dependent on age, with the strongest relationships among younger adults and U-shaped relationships more common in middle-aged adults.[47] Also, this relationship may be moderated by race/ethnicity, with stronger relationships between sleep and obesity among non-Hispanic white and black/African American adults.[24]

Diabetes and Metabolism

Several studies have documented a cross-sectional relationship between insufficient sleep and diabetes risk.[40,48–51] A recent meta-analysis showed that insufficient sleep is associated with a 33% increased risk of incident diabetes.[52] These studies are supported by laboratory findings that show that physiologic sleep loss is associated with diabetes risk factors, including insulin resistance,[53–56] and other diabetes risk factors, such as increased consumption of unhealthy foods.[57–59] Physiologic studies also show that sleep loss can influence metabolism through changes in metabolic hormones,[60,61] adipocyte function,[62] and beta-cell function.[63]

Inflammation

Laboratory studies have shown that physiologic sleep restriction is associated with a proinflammatory state, including elevations in inflammatory cytokines, such as interleukin 1B (IL-1B),[64,65] IL-6,[64,66–68] IL-17,[64,69] tumor necrosis factor-α,[64,68,70–72] and C-reactive protein.[64,69,73–76] Findings at the population level have been more difficult to assess,[64] but similar relationships were found. A recent meta-analysis found no consistent relationship between sleep duration and inflammation,[77] but this may be because it did not include some studies that were more generalizable and with larger samples (eg, Ref.[76]). Also, it is plausible that population-level samples did not optimally measure these markers, because relationships with sleep vary across 24 hours and single time-point blood draws may miss the window of difference.[68]

Cardiovascular Disease

In addition to increased likelihood of obesity, diabetes, and inflammation, insufficient sleep is associated with increased risk of cardiovascular disease. Many studies have found that short sleep duration is associated with hypertension.[24,78–80] Although directionality is difficult to ascertain, several of these studies were longitudinal in nature. A meta-analysis of these longitudinal studies indicated that habitual short-sleep duration is associated with a 20% increased likelihood of hypertension, relative to normal sleep duration.[81] Other studies have supported this association, showing increased 24-hour blood pressure in short sleepers.[82] Other studies have also shown short sleep to be associated with hypercholesterolemia[24,79] and atherosclerosis risk.[83] Regarding cardiovascular endpoints, there is some evidence that habitual short sleep increases likelihood of cardiovascular events,[84] although meta-analyses do not generally show short sleep to be associated with increased cardiovascular mortality.[33,34,85]

Neurocognitive Functioning

Many studies have examined the relationship between laboratory-induced sleep loss and neurocognitive function. The domain that is most often studied is vigilant attention,[86,87] most often operationalized with the psychomotor vigilance task.[87,88] These studies show that as sleep time declines, attentional lapses increase in a somewhat dose-dependent manner.[86,89] Furthermore, these impairments often become cumulative over time[90] and do not seem to level off even after weeks in a laboratory. Other domains of neurocognitive function have also been assessed. For example, reduced sleep duration has been shown to cause impairments in working memory,[91] executive function,[92] processing speed,[93–95] and cognitive throughput.[96] Although some of these effects may be rescued with stimulants such as caffeine, the effects on executive function particularly do not seem to be rescued.[92] Although studies of this phenomenon in the general population are scarce, some studies show that reduced sleep time is associated with drowsy driving[97] and occupational accidents.[98–100]

Mental Health

Many studies have shown that short sleep duration is associated with poor mental health. Sleep disruptions are a common diagnostic feature of many mental health disorders.[101] Patients with mood disorders and anxiety disorders frequently experience short sleep duration. Sleep duration has also been identified as a suicide risk factor.[102] In the general population, overall mental health has been identified as the leading predictor of self-reported insufficient sleep.[30]

BELIEFS AND ATTITUDES ABOUT SLEEP

Real-world sleep may be driven by many of the same factors that drive other health-related behaviors, such as diet and exercise. With this in mind, previous literature from health behavior researchers has identified several models that explain healthy behavior, identifying the roles of beliefs and attitudes.

The Health Belief Model and Application to Sleep

The Health Belief Model was originally developed in the 1960s,[103,104] but has since been used in the study of many health-related behaviors. See **Fig. 3** for a schematic of this model. This model can be applied to sleep behaviors. For example, a person will engage in healthy sleep behaviors (eg, making time for sufficient sleep or adhering to treatment) if they (1) believe that they are susceptible to the adverse effects of insufficient/poor sleep, (2) believe that the adverse effects are severe enough to warrant action, (3) believe that the action will mitigate the adverse effects, (4) believe that barriers to performing the action are sufficiently reduced, (5) are reminded to engage in the action, and (6) believe that performing the action is under their control. According to the health belief model, all of these are required for action. Therefore, just educating patients about the severity of outcomes of inaction, for example, is not sufficient to motivate behavior.

The Integrated Behavioral Model and Application to Sleep

The Integrated Behavioral Model arose from the Theory of Planned Behavior and Theory of Reasoned Action[105] to describe why people engage in behaviors. A schematic for this model is presented in **Fig. 4**. According to this model, attitudes, norms, and agency need to be addressed. Regarding attitudes, this would involve leading individuals to not only endorse helpful beliefs and attitudes about healthy sleep but also associate healthy sleep with positive feelings. Regarding norms, more research is needed to understand how the sleep of a person's (perceived) peers and those to which that individual wishes to conform influences individual sleep behaviors.

Beliefs and Attitudes About Sleep

Across segments of society, sleep practices and beliefs can vary to a great extent. For example, bed-sharing with infants and other family members differentially exists across cultures.[106–111] The cultural impact of dreaming also varies widely across cultures.[112] As globalization and technology penetrate society, sleep-related beliefs and practices can change, including the provision of longer working hours,[113–120] shift work,[121–124] and discouraging otherwise culturally appropriate naps.[125–127] There have been a few studies that examined beliefs and attitudes about sleep. In a sample from Brooklyn, New York, blacks/African Americans who were at high risk of obstructive sleep apnea had higher scores on the Dysfunctional Beliefs and Attitudes about Sleep scale, compared with those who were not at high risk.[128] In a study in the Philadelphia area among older black and white women,[129] participants were administered a questionnaire to evaluate sleep-related beliefs and practices. Black women were more likely to endorse incorrect and unhelpful statements. Sell and colleagues[130] examined sleep knowledge among Mexican Americans in

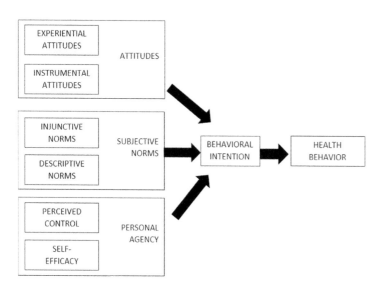

Fig. 4. Integrated behavior model.

San Diego. Non-Hispanic whites were more likely than Mexican Americans to know what sleep apnea was, but when describing the symptoms, both groups had similar knowledge that such a problem existed. Taken together, the role of sleep and health in society is driven by healthy behavior choices. These behavioral decisions, as described in the models above, are largely influenced by beliefs and attitudes about sleep. These beliefs and attitudes, though, are differentially endorsed by racial/ethnic groups, which may underlie sleep difficulties in those populations.

GENDER AND AGE IMPACTS SLEEP IN THE POPULATION
Sleep Changes with Normal Aging in the Population

Physiologic changes in sleep have been well-documented. In a landmark meta-analysis by Ohayon and colleagues,[131] polysomnographic sleep characteristics across the lifespan were examined across 65 studies spanning more than 40 years. This analysis found that with age, polysomnographic total sleep time, sleep efficiency, slow-wave sleep, rapid eye movement (REM) sleep, and REM latency decline, whereas sleep latency, wake after sleep onset, stage 1 sleep, and stage 2 sleep increase. This finding suggests a phenomenon of more disturbed and lighter sleep. In addition to these changes, melatonin secretion declines with age, which may also impact sleep consolidation in older adults.[132] Risk for many sleep disorders also increases with age.[133–135] In particular, sleep disorders, such as insomnia,[136] restless legs syndrome,[137,138] sleep apnea,[139] and REM behavior disorder,[140] include older age

as a risk factor. However, a paradox exists, which was highlighted in a large, international cohort study by Soldatos and colleagues.[141] In this study, older adults were more likely to report difficulties initiating and maintaining sleep. However, they did not endorse a greater level of dissatisfaction with their sleep. A lack of dissatisfaction is similar to results reported in Italy by Zilli and colleagues,[142] who found that younger adults were more likely to report dissatisfaction with sleep than older adults. In the US population, general dissatisfaction with sleep associated with age was examined using the 2006 BRFSS. In a study of more than 150,000 US adults, general sleep disturbance (general difficulties with sleep) was most frequently reported in young adults, and rates generally declined with age.[29] In controlled analyses, no age groups were statistically less likely to report sleep disturbances than the oldest adults, aged 80 or older, although many of the younger groups reported higher levels. These results were replicated using the 2009 BRFSS, which examined self-reported perceived insufficient sleep among greater than 350,000 US adults and found a decline in general sleep insufficiency associated with age.[30] Thus, it appears that sleep objectively worsens with age, but that subjective dissatisfaction with sleep is not associated with normal aging. In fact, this may be a sign of illness or depression.[143]

Population-Level Differences in Sleep Between Men and Women

Differences in sleep between men and women have been widely reported in the literature for decades.[144–149] Overall, in the general population, women report shorter sleep duration,[150] more sleep symptoms,[31] greater rates of insomnia,[151] and lower rates of sleep apnea.[152] In an analysis of sleep disturbances reported in the 2006 BRFSS, it was found that women reported more nighttime sleep disturbances and daytime tiredness than men. Across all age groups, sleep disturbance was reported by between 13.7% and 18.1% of men, depending on age group, and between 17.7% and 25.1% of women.[29] Similarly, for daytime tiredness, rates were 16.4% to 22.9% of men and 20.5% to 29.9% of women, depending on age. In all age groups, women reported nominally more disturbances than men. Statistically, after adjusting for demographics, socioeconomics, health variables, and depression, rates of sleep disturbances were more prevalent among women for all age groups between 25 and 69 years old and rates of daytime tiredness were more common in women for all age groups from 18 to 59 and 75 to 79.

Other issues regarding sleep differences exist between men and women. For example, sleep disturbances are common in pregnancy,[153–155] especially the first and third trimesters. These sleep disturbances can include insomnia, short sleep duration, sleep fragmentation, and gestational sleep apnea. Sleep disturbance in pregnant women can result in adverse outcomes for both the mother and the fetus.[156,157] Sleep in new parents (especially mothers) is also frequently disturbed,[158,159] especially in the first few months after birth. Sleep disturbances among parents of infants are associated with increased postpartum depression,[160–162] increased sleep disturbances among infants, and other adverse outcomes. Women also experience sleep disturbances around menopause. Sleep during the menopausal transition is often characterized by insomnia symptoms and increased sleep fragmentation.[163] Hot flashes are also a common source of sleep disturbance around the menopausal transition.[164]

Some sleep disturbances are disproportionately experienced by men. For example, men are more likely to have obstructive sleep apnea,[139] are more likely to have difficulty adhering to sleep apnea treatment,[165,166] and are more likely to die as a result of complications or consequences of sleep apnea.[167] In addition, men are more likely to be diagnosed with REM Behavior Disorder, which is typically diagnosed among older adults and likely predates neurodegenerative disorders.[168] During the aging process, men are also more likely to demonstrate a steeper decline in slow-wave sleep generation,[131] with lower amounts of slow-wave sleep among older man versus older women.

RACE, ETHNICITY, AND CULTURE ASSOCIATED WITH SLEEP
Insufficient Sleep Associated with Race/ Ethnicity

Many studies have documented a "sleep disparity" in the population,[19,39] such that racial/ethnic minorities, especially in the context of socioeconomic disadvantage, achieve less quality sleep. Most studies in this area have shown that, overall, blacks/African Americans are more likely to experience short sleep duration compared with non-Hispanic whites.[19,39] One nationally representative study found that this pattern is robust even after adjustment for a large number of other demographic and socioeconomic covariates, such that the rate of very short sleep ($\leq$4 hours) was 2.5 times those of non-Hispanic whites and the rate of short (5–6 hours) sleep was about twice as high.[150] A similar pattern was seen for Asians/others, who reported very short sleep at a rate of 4 times that seen in non-Hispanic whites and a short sleep about twice as frequently. Among Hispanics/Latinos, there is less clear evidence of habitual short sleep, especially among Mexican Americans. In addition to epidemiologic studies, some laboratory studies have also examined this issue. For example, blacks/African Americans have been shown to sleep less in the laboratory.[169–171] Also, this group has been shown to demonstrate less slow-wave sleep, compensated by increased stage 2 sleep. Other studies have shown similar patterns for sleep duration in other samples that included minority groups,[172,173] and this topic was the subject of multiple recent reviews.[19,174,175]

Sleep Disturbances Associated with Race/ Ethnicity in the Population

Less work has been done to characterize rates of sleep disturbances in racial/ethnic minorities. One previous study showed that racial/ethnic minorities demonstrated a lower sleep efficiency based on actigraphy.[176] A study in the Philadelphia area found that race differences in poor sleep quality largely depended on socioeconomic status.[177] A nationally representative study found that black/African Americans were 60% more likely than non-Hispanic whites to report sleep latency more than 30 minutes, although they (along with Hispanics/Latinos) were less likely to report "difficulty falling asleep."[31] This discrepancy between self-reported "problems" and computed long sleep latency suggests that symptom reports may vary based on the question asked. Overall, minority groups were less likely to report insomnia symptoms, nonrestorative sleep, and daytime sleepiness, although non-Mexican

Hispanics/Latinos were more likely to endorse sleep apnea symptoms such as snoring.

Several studies have examined the role of racial discrimination as a unique stressor that impacts sleep. A study of residents in Michigan and Wisconsin found that exposure to racial discrimination was associated with sleep disturbances, above the effects of race, sociodemographics, and even depressed mood.[178] This finding, that sleep disturbance is associated with exposure to racism was consistent with other findings that showed that exposure to discrimination was associated with shorter sleep and more sleep difficulties[179] and that these findings are also seen in objective sleep assessments.[169,170] Interestingly, polysomnographic differences in slow-wave sleep between black/African American and non-Hispanic white individuals (ie, reduced slow-wave sleep) were mediated by exposure to discrimination.

Sleep, Acculturation, and Immigration

Few studies have examined sleep related to acculturation. Sell and colleagues[130] found that Mexican Americans who were more acculturated to American lifestyle were more familiar with information about sleep disorders. Also, in a nationally representative sample, speaking only Spanish at home was associated with a decreased likelihood of sleep duration in the short (5–6 hours) and very short (≤4 hours) categories compared with 7 to 8 hours. In this same sample, being born in Mexico (but not any other country) was associated with decreased likelihood of both short and very short sleep duration, but these effects were not significant after adjusting for other demographic and socioeconomic factors, which likely explain this finding.[129]

EMPLOYMENT, NEIGHBORHOOD, AND SOCIOECONOMICS

Although sleep is an important factor in overall health, society has incentivized insufficient sleep. Many of these incentives involve finances and employment. Because of this, there is evidence that one of the strongest societal determinants of sleep is work. The relationship between work and sleep is especially important for safety-sensitive occupations that not only incentivize insufficient sleep but also for which the associated fatigue also jeopardizes the public safety.

Trading Sleep for Work Hours

Replicating and extending prior work in this area, Basner and colleagues[23] examined data from greater than 100,000 Americans over a 9-year period who participated in the ATUS, which is performed annually by the US Bureau of Labor Statistics and uses time diaries to determine work and other activities across 24 hours.[180] In a recent report, Basner and colleagues[23] show that work time, including actual work and other related activities (such as commuting), was the primary determinant of sleep duration. In addition, later start times of school and work were associated with longer sleep, such that each hour of delayed work or training start time was associated with 20 more minutes of sleep. Also, those holding multiple jobs were at greater risk for short sleep duration compared with those only working one job at a time. Although work is a strong determinant of sleep duration, other studies show that employed individuals report the lowest rates of self-reported sleep disturbance.[28] Unemployment, on the other hand, is associated with more sleep problems.[28,30]

Sleep Deprivation and Sleep Disorders in Occupational Settings

Recognition of the role of sleep disorders and sleep deprivation in occupational settings is gaining increased attention. Rosekind and colleagues[181] showed that the typical well-rested worker costs an employer about $1300 per year in lost sleep-related productivity, and this number increases to about $3000 for those with insomnia or insufficient sleep. Furthermore, the loss to productivity permeates many areas of functioning, including time management, mental and interpersonal demands, output demands, and physical job demands. Hui and Grandner[182] show that not only is self-reported poor sleep quality associated with decreased work performance but also worsening sleep longitudinally predicts worsening performance over time. In addition, difficulty sleeping is associated with increased health care costs. Those with difficulty sleeping "often" or "always" were associated with additional health care costs of $3600 to $5200 per person per year more than those who "never" have sleep problems, and these costs increased over time if sleep became worse. Additional analyses from this dataset also showed that poor sleep may motivate employees to make healthy changes as part of a workplace wellness program, but it may also limit those employees' ability to maintain healthy change.[183]

Regarding safety-sensitive occupations such as medicine, law enforcement, and transportation, sleep plays a critical role in safety. For example, sleep apnea occurs at high rates among commercial drivers[184–186] and impairs their ability to drive safely. Accordingly, workplace programs to increase screening and treatment of sleep apnea may have financial benefits for companies.[184] Similar efforts may show effectiveness in rail workers as well.[187,188] Airline pilots face similar challenges, in addition to challenges presented by crossing many time zones. To address these concerns, sleep disorders screening in addition to circadian approaches and scheduled napping have shown effectiveness in improving safety.[189–197] Among law enforcement and first responders, several studies have shown that sleep disturbances are common among police officers[198–203] and firefighters.[204,205] In particular, issues such as sleep apnea, insomnia, and shift work are the most common problems.[206] In a landmark study by Rajaratnam and colleagues,[198] police officers who were at greatest risk of sleep disorders were also more likely to be at risk for job-related problems, such as falling asleep at meetings and using unnecessary violence against citizens. Studies have shown that sleep disturbances in police officers and firefighters are associated with reduced ability to maintain job performance and safety.[198,203,207]

Several studies have been conducted among medical residents and nurses. For nurses, shift work and long work hours have been shown to be related to adverse health outcomes and indicators of reduced functioning.[208–217] Among medical residents, long work hours and shift work have been shown to lead to insufficient sleep duration.[218–221] Furthermore, longer work hours in medical residents have been associated with markers of reduced work performance, although impacts on actual work performance are more inconsistent.[115,222] In a landmark study that compared 2 groups of residency programs, those that gave more time off for sleep did not show measurable changes in work performance.[223] Paradoxically, residents given more time to sleep were more worried about decreases in their quality of work as a result of working less, yet they were more satisfied with the quality of their life and social functioning.

Sleep, Poverty, and Neighborhood Factors

Several studies have shown that poverty is associated with both shorter sleep duration and worse sleep quality.[30] However, once the benefits of income are accounted for (by statistically covarying education, access to health care, and so forth), associations with income are often nonexistent and may go in the opposite direction. For example, in an analysis of data from greater than 350,000 US adults, insufficient sleep was associated with poverty before adjusting for covariates, but after adjustment, the opposite relationship was seen.[30] A positive relationship between income and insufficient sleep after adjusting for covariates suggests that money may not buy sleep, but many of the benefits of income may contribute to healthy sleep. One aspect of this relationship is neighborhood quality. Several studies have investigated the role of the neighborhood in an individual's sleep quality, showing that neighborhoods that are crime-ridden, not socially cohesive, and dirty, are associated with worse sleep quality.[224–227] Furthermore, sleep quality may partially mediate the relationship between neighborhood quality and both mental[227] and physical[225] health. One way that a neighborhood may directly influence sleep would be via the physical environment. There is substantial literature showing that environmental noise[228,229] and light[230–233] can adversely impact sleep and that neighborhoods that are active at night may directly impact sleep through these.

INFLUENCES OF HOME, FAMILY, AND SCHOOL ENVIRONMENT

The home, family, and school environments also likely play important roles in an individual's sleep. For example, household size is negatively associated with sleep, such that more crowded homes are more likely to foster insufficient sleep.[30] Also, as mentioned above, the physical sleep environment can also play a role. Bedrooms that have levels of light, noise, and temperature that are not conducive to sleep may contribute to insufficient sleep.[234–236] Although data on beds and other sleeping surfaces are relatively scarce, an uncomfortable sleeping environment may also reduce sleep ability.[237–239]

Another key issue of the home and family environment on sleep regards the marital relationship. Although most sleep research is performed on individuals sleeping alone in a laboratory, most adults do not sleep alone most nights.[240,241] With this in mind, several studies have explored the important role of marital and relationship quality in sleep quality and how this relates to health. For example, relationship quality has been shown to be an important predictor of sleep health, especially among women, and relationship quality may be an important moderator between sleep quality and health.[241–244]

TECHNOLOGY IN AND OUT OF THE BEDROOM

In 2011, the National Sleep Foundation polled Americans regarding their use of technology in the bedroom. In a report of the findings of this survey, Gradisar and colleagues[245] note that 90% of Americans use some sort of electronic device in the hour before bed. Also, more than two-thirds of adolescents and young adults used a Smartphone in the hour before bed, compared with approximately one-third of middle-aged adults and about one-fifth of older adults. Furthermore, the more engaging the technology application, the more the electronic device use was associated with difficulties falling asleep and nonrestorative sleep. This finding is supported by other work that shows that not only is electronic media use near bedtime prevalent[246] but also the light emitted by the devices[247] as well as the mental engagement[248] can interfere with sleep. Growing awareness of the influence of mobile electronic device use on sleep is a key example of a societal-level change (use of technology) impacting an individual's sleep.

GLOBALIZATION AND 24/7 SOCIETY

Another societal-level factor that impacts sleep is the advent of globalization and a 24/7 society. In the past, social interactions, commercial activities, and work responsibilities were dictated by more local factors. Now, though, the advent of globalization and 24/7 operations often impinge on sleep. Regarding globalization, individuals and organizations are connected across the globe. In combination with a society that institutes shift work and 24-hour operations, entire segments of the population are awake across all hours of the 24-hour day, and access to individuals across time zones is easier than ever. Because of this, social interactions (such as interactions with friends, family, and even online groups), commercial activities (such as eCommerce and availability of entertainment around the clock on demand), and work responsibilities (such as e-mails outside of business hours and business conducted across the globe) can impinge on sleep. The influence of globalization and 24/7 society on sleep behaviors is particularly relevant, because shift work has been repeatedly shown in both laboratory and field studies to be related to adverse health outcomes.

PUBLIC SAFETY AND PUBLIC POLICY

As mentioned above, many safety-sensitive occupations, such as those in transportation, law enforcement, and medicine, require healthy sleep for optimal performance. The problem is that these professions often institute policies that make healthy sleep difficult. As a result, the sleep of an individual in one of those occupations may have ramifications for others in the public. For example, when a large commercial truck crashes, it causes more damage and a greater likelihood of fatal injury.[249,250] For this reason, several policy approaches to sleep

and public safety have been proposed. The Accreditation Council for Graduate Medical Education has already instituted duty hour restrictions on medical residents, based on results from a report by the Institute of Medicine.[218] These restrictions, although controversial,[115,251–253] are likely resulting in increased sleep among medical residents.[222] In the transportation industry, recommendations by the National Highway Transportation and Safety Administration address the need for sleep disorders screening and fatigue mitigation among commercial drivers,[250] although formal regulations have not yet been passed. The Federal Aviation Administration also recently issued guidelines to address sleep issues in pilots.[254] More work is needed in this area, and although regulations to ensure public safety have been proposed, they still have not yet been passed.

Another domain of public safety is drowsy driving. Even among non–commercial drivers, drowsy driving is an important public safety issue. Drowsy driving is prevalent, reported among about 5% of the US population over a 6-month period.[255] Population-level data suggest that short sleep duration is an independent risk factor for drowsy driving, even if respondents believe that they are completely well rested.[97]

Another area of public policy related to sleep involves school start times. Existing evidence suggests that most US schools, especially high schools, start too early for most adolescents.[256–259] Earlier start times not only promote shorter sleep duration among adolescents (who need more sleep than adults) but also do not take into account natural circadian delays that occur in adolescence.[260] It has been proposed that delaying school start times can improve academic performance, improve mental health, and improve overall health in students.[261–266]

Other public policy initiatives have addressed the issue of environmental light and noise in neighborhoods. There are several policies in place, and more being proposed, that limit the brightness of street lights in neighborhoods, increase "quiet time" regulations at night, direct airplanes to avoid some residential areas at night, reduce traffic and train noise at night, and so forth. These approaches are usually regional, and many efforts are ongoing.

One more public policy implication relevant to sleep would be health policy legislation. For example, improving mental health parity laws will do much to intervene on perhaps the most important determinant of sleep health at the population level[30] and will facilitate treatment of insomnia with the most well supported therapy.[267] In addition, health equity legislation may help to address some of the disparities seen in sleep in the population.[20]

These and other future approaches may better promote healthy sleep from a policy standpoint.

IMPORTANT LIMITATIONS OF THE EXISTING LITERATURE

There are several important limitations to the existing literature, which constrain interpretations and generalizations of the data. The most important limitation is that there is a lack of consistency in sleep assessment methods across studies, and this is a problem for several reasons. First, retrospective self-report (eg, survey), prospective self-report (eg, diary), laboratory-based objective (eg, polysomnography), and field-based objective (eg, actigraphy) estimates of sleep tend to disagree with each other, because they capture different elements of sleep well. It is likely that physiologic sleep is substantially less than that which is self-reported.[27] Even among survey methods, there seems to be systematic variation.[35] Second, because there is still no nationally representative dataset that includes any well-validated estimate of sleep duration or quality, generalizability from one dataset to the next is limited. Third, cutoffs and categories used to describe sleep are often inconsistent across studies; for example, the cutoff for the shortest sleep duration category can be as low as 4 hours or less or as high as 7 hours.

Another important limitation is a general lack of physiologic sleep measures at the societal level. Because these measures are typically more expensive and require more infrastructure to implement, they are often infeasible for large studies that require assessment of thousands of people. Until sleep assessment becomes more of a priority, otherwise rich datasets will continue to have just a few nonvalidated survey items measuring sleep. Suboptimal measurement of sleep will make data interpretation difficult, because it is unclear the degree to which associations are referring to physiologic sleep or other factors that become subsumed in self-reported sleep experience.

A third important limitation regards the complexity of social environments. As shown in the Social-Ecological Model, the influences that may play a role in sleep are many, varied, and exist at several levels. Still, most studies do not address the complex nature of social-environmental influences on health. Also, future studies that will examine epigenetic effects will need to better account for gene-environment interactions, and this will require a better operationalization of environmental variables in many cases. An example of one study that brought these methodologies together is cited by Watson and colleagues,[268] who combined geospatial neighborhood analyses with sleep genetic information to characterize a social-environmental influence on sleep duration.

A fourth important limitation to the existing literature is a lack of interventional studies. If, for example, sleep represents a modifiable factor in health disparities, it is plausible that improvements in sleep at the community level could reduce effects of health disparities. However, there is a lack of interventional studies that can demonstrate this; rather, the best examples of investigations in this area use mediational analysis to show that changes in sleep account for changes in health outcomes across groups, such as blood pressure.[269] More sleep interventions at the community level are going to be needed in order to understand the causal role of sleep in these outcomes. Also, there is a general lack of empirically supported interventions for sleep health. Although many interventions exist to promote healthy diet, physical activity, and substance cessation, a lack of standardized sleep health interventions limits knowledge in this area.

FUTURE RESEARCH DIRECTIONS

Several potential future research directions may help advance knowledge in this area. First, expanded epigenetic studies are needed to explore gene-environment interactions. As the science of human sleep genetics develops, more research into how genetic vulnerabilities interact with environmental influences is needed. For example, although it is unlikely that genetics explains racial disparities in sleep, it is plausible that some genetic adaptations to one geographic region may confer risk in another region (eg, less sunlight, different food availability). Also, it may be possible that certain genetic vulnerabilities (eg, airway collapse) may differentially affect groups because body mass indexes increase in the presence of increasing obesity rates due to westernized diets.

Another important direction in research will be to clarify the sleep phenotypes and endophenotypes. Currently, typing of sleep at the community and population level is frequently based on broad sleep duration groups (eg, "short sleepers") or sleep symptoms ("difficulty falling asleep"), although these groups can be highly heterogeneous. Genetic studies are limited by this limited clarity in sleep phenotypes. Short sleepers, for example, may comprise individuals who are "true" short sleepers and need less sleep, those who need more sleep but are able to tolerate less sleep for an extended period of time ("resilient"), and those who are insufficient sleepers. Still, insufficient sleepers may belong to groups that demonstrate neurocognitive and metabolic impairments at variable rates (eg, some individuals may demonstrate more metabolic impairments and some more cognitive). Perhaps more clarity regarding phenotypes will help move forward an agenda of better human sleep genetics.

More intervention studies are also needed at the laboratory, clinical, and community levels that address real-world sleep concerns. As mentioned above, there is a lack of healthy sleep interventions, relative to healthy diet or physical activity recommendations. Without these data, it is difficult to make recommendations in addition to just stating a problem. Also, interventions need to address issues that have generally been ignored yet carry real-world significance For example, despite many adults sleeping between 6 and 7 hours per night, this sleep duration is almost never included in the literature, either because epidemiologic studies categorize at the hour (including them in either 6- or 7-hour groups) or because laboratory studies try to maximize difference between groups (usually comparing 8–6, 5, or 4 hours but not between 6 and 7).[14] These and other real-world issues need to be better captured in intervention studies.

Finally, intervention studies are needed that identify real-world approaches to increasing sleep time among chronically sleep-deprived individuals. Unlike traditional intervention study designs, where changing sleep is the intervention and some health marker is the outcome (which would address the question of whether changing sleep impacts health), study designs are needed whereby changing sleep itself is the outcome. For example, it is known that smoking cessation can positively impact health. However, how does one quit smoking? Just recommending that someone quit is not enough, and literature has emerged that proposes novel ways to achieve this difficult behavioral change. Likewise, changing sleep duration in a real-world setting (with home, work, and other societal pressures) may be difficult, and useful strategies besides simply making recommendations need to be explored.

REFERENCES

1. Cajochen C, Chellappa S, Schmidt C. What keeps us awake?–the role of clocks and hourglasses, light, and melatonin. Int Rev Neurobiol 2010;93: 57–90.
2. Fuller PM, Lu J. Neurobiology of sleep. In: Amlaner CJ, Fuller PM, editors. Basics of sleep guide. 2nd edition. Westchester (IL): Sleep Research Society; 2009. p. 53–62.
3. Mackiewicz M, Naidoo N, Zimmerman JE, et al. Molecular mechanisms of sleep and wakefulness. Ann N Y Acad Sci 2008;1129:335–49.
4. Schwartz JR, Roth T. Neurophysiology of sleep and wakefulness: basic science and clinical implications. Curr Neuropharmacol 2008;6(4):367–78.
5. Franken P. A role for clock genes in sleep homeostasis. Curr Opin Neurobiol 2013;23(5):864–72.
6. Feng D, Lazar MA. Clocks, metabolism, and the epigenome. Mol Cell 2012;47(2):158–67.
7. Gerstner JR, Lenz O, Vanderheyden WM, et al. Amyloid-beta induces sleep fragmentation that is rescued by fatty acid binding proteins in Drosophila. J Neurosci Res 2016. [Epub ahead of print].
8. Xu M, Chung S, Zhang S, et al. Basal forebrain circuit for sleep-wake control. Nat Neurosci 2015; 18(11):1641–7.
9. Cox J, Pinto L, Dan Y. Calcium imaging of sleep-wake related neuronal activity in the dorsal pons. Nat Commun 2016;7:10763.
10. Park DA. The fire within the eye: a historical essay on the nature and meaning of light. Princeton (NJ): Princeton University Press; 1997.
11. Williams S. Sleep and society: sociological ventures into the (Un)known. London: Taylor & Francis; 2005.
12. Watson NF, Badr MS, Belenky G, et al. Recommended amount of sleep for a healthy adult: a joint consensus statement of the American Academy of Sleep Medicine and Sleep Research Society. Sleep 2015;38(6):843–4.
13. Consensus Conference Panel, Watson NF, Badr MS, et al. Joint consensus statement of the American Academy of Sleep Medicine and Sleep Research Society on the recommended amount of sleep for a healthy adult: methodology and discussion. J Clin Sleep Med 2015;11(8):931–52.
14. Consensus Conference Panel, Watson NF, Badr MS, et al. Joint consensus statement of the American Academy of Sleep Medicine and Sleep Research Society on the recommended amount of sleep for a healthy adult: methodology and discussion. Sleep 2015;38(8):1161–83.
15. Consensus Conference Panel, Watson NF, Badr MS, et al. Recommended amount of sleep for a healthy adult: a joint consensus statement of the American Academy of Sleep Medicine and Sleep Research Society. J Clin Sleep Med 2015; 11(6):591–2.
16. Bronfenbrenner U. Toward an experimental ecology of human development. Am Psychol 1977;32: 513–31.
17. Grandner MA, Patel NP, Hale L, et al. Mortality associated with sleep duration: the evidence, the possible mechanisms, and the future. Sleep Med Rev 2010;14:191–203.
18. Grandner MA. Addressing sleep disturbances: an opportunity to prevent cardiometabolic disease? Int Rev Psychiatry 2014;26(2):155–76.

19. Grandner MA, Williams NJ, Knutson KL, et al. Sleep disparity, race/ethnicity, and socioeconomic position. Sleep Med 2016;18:7–18.
20. Grandner MA. Sleep disparities in the American population: prevalence, potential causes, relationships to cardiometabolic health disparities, and future drections for research and policy. In: Kelly R, editor. Health disparities in America. Washington, DC: US Congress; 2015. p. 126–32.
21. Knutson KL, Van Cauter E, Rathouz PJ, et al. Trends in the prevalence of short sleepers in the USA: 1975-2006. Sleep 2010;33(1):37–45.
22. Bin YS, Marshall NS, Glozier N. Secular trends in adult sleep duration: a systematic review. Sleep Med Rev 2012;16(3):223–30.
23. Basner M, Spaeth AM, Dinges DF. Sociodemographic characteristics and waking activities and their role in the timing and duration of sleep. Sleep 2014;37(12):1889–906.
24. Grandner MA, Chakravorty S, Perlis ML, et al. Habitual sleep duration associated with self-reported and objectively determined cardiometabolic risk factors. Sleep Med 2014;15(1):42–50.
25. Krueger PM, Friedman EM. Sleep duration in the United States: a cross-sectional population-based study. Am J Epidemiol 2009;169(9):1052–63.
26. Liu Y, Wheaton AG, Chapman DP, et al. Prevalence of healthy sleep duration among adults –United States, 2014. MMWR Morb Mortal Wkly Rep 2016;65(6):137–41.
27. Kurina LM, McClintock MK, Chen JH, et al. Sleep duration and all-cause mortality: a critical review of measurement and associations. Ann Epidemiol 2013;23(6):361–70.
28. Grandner MA, Patel NP, Gehrman PR, et al. Who gets the best sleep? Ethnic and socioeconomic factors related to sleep disturbance. Sleep Med 2010;11:470–9.
29. Grandner MA, Martin JL, Patel NP, et al. Age and sleep disturbances among American men and women: data from the U.S. Behavioral Risk Factor Surveillance System. Sleep 2012;35(3):395–406.
30. Grandner MA, Jackson NJ, Izci-Balserak B, et al. Social and behavioral determinants of perceived insufficient sleep. Front Neurol 2015;6:112.
31. Grandner MA, Petrov MER, Rattanaumpawan P, et al. Sleep symptoms, race/ethnicity, and socioeconomic position. J Clin Sleep Med 2013;9(9):897–905, 905A–D.
32. Hammond EC. Some preliminary findings on physical complaints from a prospective study of 1,064,004 men and women. Am J Public Health Nations Health 1964;54:11–23.
33. Gallicchio L, Kalesan B. Sleep duration and mortality: a systematic review and meta-analysis. J Sleep Res 2009;18(2):148–58.
34. Cappuccio FP, D'Elia L, Strazzullo P, et al. Sleep duration and all-cause mortality: a systematic review and meta-analysis of prospective studies. Sleep 2010;33(5):585–92.
35. Grandner MA, Patel NP, Gehrman PR, et al. Problems associated with short sleep: bridging the gap between laboratory and epidemiological studies. Sleep Med Rev 2010;14:239–47.
36. Kripke DF, Langer RD, Elliott JA, et al. Mortality related to actigraphic long and short sleep. Sleep Med 2011;12(1):28–33.
37. Youngstedt SD, Kripke DF. Long sleep and mortality: rationale for sleep restriction. Sleep Med Rev 2004;8(3):159–74.
38. Grandner MA, Drummond SP. Who are the long sleepers? Towards an understanding of the mortality relationship. Sleep Med Rev 2007;11(5):341–60.
39. Adenekan B, Pandey A, McKenzie S, et al. Sleep in America: role of racial/ethnic differences. Sleep Med Rev 2013;17(4):255–62.
40. Morselli LL, Guyon A, Spiegel K. Sleep and metabolic function. Pflugers Arch 2012;463(1):139–60.
41. Knutson KL. Does inadequate sleep play a role in vulnerability to obesity? Am J Hum Biol 2012;24(3):361–71.
42. Watanabe M, Kikuchi H, Tanaka K, et al. Association of short sleep duration with weight gain and obesity at 1-year follow-up: a large-scale prospective study. Sleep 2010;33(2):161–7.
43. Chaput JP, Bouchard C, Tremblay A. Change in sleep duration and visceral fat accumulation over 6 years in adults. Obesity (Silver Spring) 2014;22(5):E9–12.
44. Chaput JP, Despres JP, Bouchard C, et al. The association between sleep duration and weight gain in adults: a 6-year prospective study from the Quebec Family Study. Sleep 2008;31(4):517–23.
45. Baron KG, Reid KJ, Kern AS, et al. Role of sleep timing in caloric intake and BMI. Obesity (Silver Spring) 2011;19(7):1374–81.
46. Shechter A, Grandner MA, St-Onge MP. The role of sleep in the control of food intake. Am J Lifestyle Med 2014;8(6):371–4.
47. Grandner MA, Schopfer EA, Sands-Lincoln M, et al. Relationship between sleep duration and body mass index depends on age. Obesity (Silver Spring) 2015;23(12):2491–8.
48. Barone MT, Menna-Barreto L. Diabetes and sleep: a complex cause-and-effect relationship. Diabetes Res Clin Pract 2011;91(2):129–37.
49. Aldabal L, Bahammam AS. Metabolic, endocrine, and immune consequences of sleep deprivation. Open Respir Med J 2011;5:31–43.
50. Bopparaju S, Surani S. Sleep and diabetes. Int J Endocrinol 2010;2010:759509.

51. Zizi F, Jean-Louis G, Brown CD, et al. Sleep duration and the risk of diabetes mellitus: epidemiologic evidence and pathophysiologic insights. Curr Diab Rep 2010;10(1):43–7.

52. Shan Z, Ma H, Xie M, et al. Sleep duration and risk of type 2 diabetes: a meta-analysis of prospective studies. Diabetes Care 2015;38(3):529–37.

53. Buxton OM, Pavlova M, Reid EW, et al. Sleep restriction for 1 week reduces insulin sensitivity in healthy men. Diabetes 2010;59(9):2126–33.

54. Morselli L, Leproult R, Balbo M, et al. Role of sleep duration in the regulation of glucose metabolism and appetite. Best Pract Res Clin Endocrinol Metab 2010;24(5):687–702.

55. Tasali E, Leproult R, Spiegel K. Reduced sleep duration or quality: relationships with insulin resistance and type 2 diabetes. Prog Cardiovasc Dis 2009;51(5):381–91.

56. Spiegel K, Knutson K, Leproult R, et al. Sleep loss: a novel risk factor for insulin resistance and Type 2 diabetes. J Appl Physiol 2005;99(5):2008–19.

57. Spaeth AM, Dinges DF, Goel N. Sex and race differences in caloric intake during sleep restriction in healthy adults. Am J Clin Nutr 2014;100(2):559–66.

58. Kim S, Deroo LA, Sandler DP. Eating patterns and nutritional characteristics associated with sleep duration. Public Health Nutr 2011;14(5):889–95.

59. Nedeltcheva AV, Kilkus JM, Imperial J, et al. Sleep curtailment is accompanied by increased intake of calories from snacks. Am J Clin Nutr 2009;89(1):126–33.

60. Van Cauter E, Spiegel K, Tasali E, et al. Metabolic consequences of sleep and sleep loss. Sleep Med 2008;9(Suppl 1):S23–8.

61. Spiegel K, Tasali E, Penev P, et al. Brief communication: sleep curtailment in healthy young men is associated with decreased leptin levels, elevated ghrelin levels, and increased hunger and appetite. Ann Intern Med 2004;141(11):846–50.

62. Hayes AL, Xu F, Babineau D, et al. Sleep duration and circulating adipokine levels. Sleep 2011;34(2):147–52.

63. Perelis M, Ramsey KM, Marcheva B, et al. Circadian transcription from beta cell function to diabetes pathophysiology. J Biol Rhythms 2016;31(4):323–36.

64. Grandner MA, Sands-Lincoln MR, Pak VM, et al. Sleep duration, cardiovascular disease, and proinflammatory biomarkers. Nat Sci Sleep 2013;5:93–107.

65. Frey DJ, Fleshner M, Wright KP Jr. The effects of 40 hours of total sleep deprivation on inflammatory markers in healthy young adults. Brain Behav Immun 2007;21(8):1050–7.

66. Ferrie JE, Kivimaki M, Akbaraly TN, et al. Associations between change in sleep duration and inflammation: findings on C-reactive protein and interleukin 6 in the Whitehall II Study. Am J Epidemiol 2013;178(6):956–61.

67. Rohleder N, Aringer M, Boentert M. Role of interleukin-6 in stress, sleep, and fatigue. Ann N Y Acad Sci 2012;1261:88–96.

68. Vgontzas AN, Zoumakis E, Bixler EO, et al. Adverse effects of modest sleep restriction on sleepiness, performance, and inflammatory cytokines. J Clin Endocrinol Metab 2004;89(5):2119–26.

69. van Leeuwen WM, Lehto M, Karisola P, et al. Sleep restriction increases the risk of developing cardiovascular diseases by augmenting proinflammatory responses through IL-17 and CRP. PLoS One 2009;4(2):e4589.

70. Chennaoui M, Sauvet F, Drogou C, et al. Effect of one night of sleep loss on changes in tumor necrosis factor alpha (TNF-alpha) levels in healthy men. Cytokine 2011;56(2):318–24.

71. Shearer WT, Reuben JM, Mullington JM, et al. Soluble TNF-alpha receptor 1 and IL-6 plasma levels in humans subjected to the sleep deprivation model of spaceflight. J Allergy Clin Immunol 2001;107(1):165–70.

72. Patel SR, Zhu X, Storfer-Isser A, et al. Sleep duration and biomarkers of inflammation. Sleep 2009;32(2):200–4.

73. Meier-Ewert HK, Ridker PM, Rifai N, et al. Effect of sleep loss on C-reactive protein, an inflammatory marker of cardiovascular risk. J Am Coll Cardiol 2004;43(4):678–83.

74. Miller MA, Kandala NB, Kivimaki M, et al. Gender differences in the cross-sectional relationships between sleep duration and markers of inflammation: Whitehall II study. Sleep 2009;32(7):857–64.

75. Matthews KA, Zheng H, Kravitz HM, et al. Are inflammatory and coagulation biomarkers related to sleep characteristics in mid-life women?: Study of Women's Health across the Nation sleep study. Sleep 2010;33(12):1649–55.

76. Grandner MA, Buxton OM, Jackson N, et al. Extreme sleep durations and increased C-reactive protein: effects of sex and ethnoracial group. Sleep 2013;36(5):769–779E.

77. Irwin MR, Olmstead R, Carroll JE. Sleep disturbance, sleep duration, and inflammation: a systematic review and meta-analysis of cohort studies and experimental sleep deprivation. Biol Psychiatry 2016;80(1):40–52.

78. von Ruesten A, Weikert C, Fietze I, et al. Association of sleep duration with chronic diseases in the European Prospective Investigation into Cancer and Nutrition (EPIC)-Potsdam study. PLoS One 2012;7(1):e30972.

79. Altman NG, Izci-Balserak B, Schopfer E, et al. Sleep duration versus sleep insufficiency as predictors of cardiometabolic health outcomes. Sleep Med 2012;13(10):1261–70.

80. Wang Q, Xi B, Liu M, et al. Short sleep duration is associated with hypertension risk among adults: a

systematic review and meta-analysis. Hypertens Res 2012;35(10):1012–8.

81. Meng L, Zheng Y, Hui R. The relationship of sleep duration and insomnia to risk of hypertension incidence: a meta-analysis of prospective cohort studies. Hypertens Res 2013;36(11):985–95.

82. Mezick EJ, Hall M, Matthews KA. Sleep duration and ambulatory blood pressure in black and white adolescents. Hypertension 2012;59(3):747–52.

83. King CR, Knutson KL, Rathouz PJ, et al. Short sleep duration and incident coronary artery calcification. JAMA 2008;300(24):2859–66.

84. Amagai Y, Ishikawa S, Gotoh T, et al. Sleep duration and incidence of cardiovascular events in a Japanese population: the Jichi Medical School cohort study. J Epidemiol 2010;20(2):106–10.

85. Cappuccio FP, Cooper D, D'Elia L, et al. Sleep duration predicts cardiovascular outcomes: a systematic review and meta-analysis of prospective studies. Eur Heart J 2011;32(12):1484–92.

86. Goel N, Rao H, Durmer JS, et al. Neurocognitive consequences of sleep deprivation. Semin Neurol 2009;29(4):320–39.

87. Lim J, Dinges DF. Sleep deprivation and vigilant attention. Ann N Y Acad Sci 2008;1129:305–22.

88. Dinges DF, Powell JW. Microcomputer analyses of performance on a portable, simple visual RT task during sustained operations. Beh Res Meth Instr Comp 1985;17:652–5.

89. Banks S, Dinges DF. Behavioral and physiological consequences of sleep restriction. J Clin Sleep Med 2007;3(5):519–28.

90. Van Dongen HP, Baynard MD, Maislin G, et al. Systematic interindividual differences in neurobehavioral impairment from sleep loss: evidence of trait-like differential vulnerability. Sleep 2004;27(3):423–33.

91. Verweij IM, Romeijn N, Smit DJ, et al. Sleep deprivation leads to a loss of functional connectivity in frontal brain regions. BMC Neurosci 2014;15:88.

92. Killgore WD, Grugle NL, Balkin TJ. Gambling when sleep deprived: don't bet on stimulants. Chronobiol Int 2012;29(1):43–54.

93. Jackson ML, Croft RJ, Kennedy GA, et al. Cognitive components of simulated driving performance: sleep loss effects and predictors. Accid Anal Prev 2013;50:438–44.

94. Saint Martin M, Sforza E, Barthelemy JC, et al. Does subjective sleep affect cognitive function in healthy elderly subjects? The Proof cohort. Sleep Med 2012;13(9):1146–52.

95. Rupp TL, Wesensten NJ, Balkin TJ. Trait-like vulnerability to total and partial sleep loss. Sleep 2012;35(8):1163–72.

96. Banks S, Van Dongen HP, Maislin G, et al. Neurobehavioral dynamics following chronic sleep restriction: dose-response effects of one night for recovery. Sleep 2010;33(8):1013–26.

97. Maia Q, Grandner MA, Findley J, et al. Short and long sleep duration and risk of drowsy driving and the role of subjective sleep insufficiency. Accid Anal Prev 2013;59:618–22.

98. Chiu HY, Tsai PS. The impact of various work schedules on sleep complaints and minor accidents during work or leisure time: evidence from a national survey. J Occup Environ Med 2013; 55(3):325–30.

99. Lilley R, Day L, Koehncke N, et al. The relationship between fatigue-related factors and work-related injuries in the Saskatchewan Farm Injury Cohort Study. Am J Ind Med 2012;55(4):367–75.

100. Kucharczyk ER, Morgan K, Hall AP. The occupational impact of sleep quality and insomnia symptoms. Sleep Med Rev 2012;16(6):547–59.

101. American Psychiatric Association. Diagnostic and statistical manual of mental disorders. 5th edition. Washington, DC: American Psychiatric Association; 2003. DSM-5.

102. Chakravorty S, Siu HY, Lalley-Chareczko L, et al. Sleep duration and insomnia symptoms as risk factors for suicidal ideation in a nationally representative sample. Prim Care Companion CNS Disord 2015;17(6).

103. Rosenstock IM. Why people use health services. Milbank Mem Fund Q 1966;44(3 Suppl):94–127.

104. Champion VL, Skinner CS. The health belief model. In: Glanz K, Rimer BK, Viswanath K, editors. Health behavior and health education: theory, research, and practice. San Francisco (CA): Jossey-Bass; 2008. p. 45–65.

105. Montano DE, Kasprzyk D. Theory of reasoned action, theory of planned behavior, and the integrated behavioral model. In: Glanz K, Rimer BK, Viswanath K, editors. Health behavior and health education: theory, research, and practice. San Francisco (CA): Jossey-Bass; 2008. p. 68–96.

106. Hooker E, Ball HL, Kelly PJ. Sleeping like a baby: attitudes and experiences of bedsharing in northeast England. Med Anthropol 2001;19(3):203–22.

107. Thoman EB. Co-sleeping, an ancient practice: issues of the past and present, and possibilities for the future. Sleep Med Rev 2006;10(6):407–17.

108. Mindell JA, Sadeh A, Wiegand B, et al. Cross-cultural differences in infant and toddler sleep. Sleep Med 2010;11(3):274–80.

109. Norton PJ, Grellner KW. A retrospective study on infant bed-sharing in a clinical practice population. Matern Child Health J 2011;15(4):507–13.

110. Gettler LT, McKenna JJ. Evolutionary perspectives on mother-infant sleep proximity and breastfeeding in a laboratory setting. Am J Phys Anthropol 2011; 144(3):454–62.

111. Jain S, Romack R, Jain R. Bed sharing in school-age children–clinical and social implications. J Child Adolesc Psychiatr Nurs 2011;24(3):185–9.

112. Shulman D, Strousma GG. Dream cultures: explorations in the comparative history of dreaming. Oxford (United Kingdom): Oxford University Press; 1999.

113. Spurgeon A, Harrington JM, Cooper CL. Health and safety problems associated with long working hours: a review of the current position. Occup Environ Med 1997;54(6):367–75.

114. Goto A, Yasumura S, Nishise Y, et al. Association of health behavior and social role with total mortality among Japanese elders in Okinawa, Japan. Aging Clin Exp Res 2003;15(6):443–50.

115. Lockley SW, Landrigan CP, Barger LK, et al. When policy meets physiology: the challenge of reducing resident work hours. Clin Orthop Relat Res 2006; 449:116–27.

116. Ko GT, Chan JC, Chan AW, et al. Association between sleeping hours, working hours and obesity in Hong Kong Chinese: the 'better health for better Hong Kong' health promotion campaign. Int J Obes (Lond) 2007;31(2):254–60.

117. Basner M, Dinges DF. Dubious bargain: trading sleep for Leno and Letterman. Sleep 2009;32(6): 747–52.

118. Gangwisch JE. All work and no play makes Jack lose sleep. Commentary on Virtanen et al. Long working hours and sleep disturbances: the Whitehall II prospective cohort study. Sleep 2009;32: 737–45. Sleep 2009;32(6):717–8.

119. Virtanen M, Ferrie JE, Gimeno D, et al. Long working hours and sleep disturbances: the Whitehall II prospective cohort study. Sleep 2009;32(6):737–45.

120. Nakata A. Effects of long work hours and poor sleep characteristics on workplace injury among full-time male employees of small- and medium-scale businesses. J Sleep Res 2011;20(4):576–84.

121. Mahan RP, Carvalhais AB, Queen SE. Sleep reduction in night-shift workers: is it sleep deprivation or a sleep disturbance disorder? Percept Mot Skills 1990;70(3 Pt 1):723–30.

122. Rajaratnam SM, Arendt J. Health in a 24-h society. Lancet 2001;358(9286):999–1005.

123. Nag PK, Nag A. Shiftwork in the hot environment. J Hum Ergol (Tokyo) 2001;30(1–2):161–6.

124. Costa G. Shift work and health: current problems and preventive actions. Saf Health Work 2010; 1(2):112–23.

125. Owens J. Sleep in children: cross-cultural perspectives. Sleep Biol Rhythms 2004;2:165–73.

126. Milner CE, Cote KA. Benefits of napping in healthy adults: impact of nap length, time of day, age, and experience with napping. J Sleep Res 2009;18(2): 272–81.

127. Worthman CM, Brown RA. Sleep budgets in a globalizing world: biocultural interactions influence sleep sufficiency among Egyptian families. Soc Sci Med 2013;79:31–9.

128. Pandey A, Gekhman D, Gousse Y, et al. Short sleep and dysfunctional beliefs and attitudes toward sleep among black men. Sleep 2011;34(Abstract Suppl): 261–2.

129. Grandner MA, Patel NP, Jean-Louis G, et al. Sleep-related behaviors and beliefs associated with race/ethnicity in women. J Natl Med Assoc 2013; 105(1):4–15.

130. Sell RE, Bardwell W, Palinkas L, et al. Ethnic differences in sleep-health knowledge. Sleep 2009; 32(Abstract Supplement):A392.

131. Ohayon MM, Carskadon MA, Guilleminault C, et al. Meta-analysis of quantitative sleep parameters from childhood to old age in healthy individuals: developing normative sleep values across the human lifespan. Sleep 2004;27(7):1255–73.

132. Hardeland R. Melatonin in aging and disease -multiple consequences of reduced secretion, options and limits of treatment. Aging Dis 2012;3(2): 194–225.

133. Neikrug AB, Ancoli-Israel S. Sleep disorders in the older adult - a mini-review. Gerontology 2010;56(2): 181–9.

134. Roepke SK, Ancoli-Israel S. Sleep disorders in the elderly. Indian J Med Res 2010;131:302–10.

135. Martin J, Shochat T, Gehrman PR, et al. Sleep in the elderly. Respir Care Clin N Am 1999;5(3): 461–72, ix.

136. Ruiter ME, VanderWal GS, Lichstein KL. Insomnia in the elderly. In: Pandi-Perumal SR, Monti JR, Monjan AA, editors. Principles and practice of geriatric sleep medicine. Cambridge (United Kingdom): Cambridge; 2010. p. 271–9.

137. Yeh P, Walters AS, Tsuang JW. Restless legs syndrome: a comprehensive overview on its epidemiology, risk factors, and treatment. Sleep Breath 2012;16(4):987–1007.

138. Spiegelhalder K, Hornyak M. Movement disorders in the elderly. In: Pandi-Perumal SR, Monti JR, Monjan AA, editors. Principles and practice of geriatric sleep medicine. Cambridge (United Kingdom): Cambridge; 2010. p. 233–40.

139. Peppard PE, Young T, Barnet JH, et al. Increased prevalence of sleep-disordered breathing in adults. Am J Epidemiol 2013;177(9):1006–14.

140. Ferini Strambi L. REM sleep behavior disorder in the elderly. In: Pandi-Perumal SR, Monti JR, Monjan AA, editors. Principles and practice of geriatric sleep medicine. Cambridge (United Kingdom): Cambridge; 2010. p. 241–7.

141. Soldatos CR, Allaert FA, Ohta T, et al. How do individuals sleep around the world? Results from a single-day survey in ten countries. Sleep Med 2005;6(1):5–13.

142. Zilli I, Ficca G, Salzarulo P. Factors involved in sleep satisfaction in the elderly. Sleep Med 2009; 10(2):233–9.

143. Grandner MA, Patel NP, Gooneratne NS. Difficulties sleeping: a natural part of growing older? Aging Health 2012;8(3):219–21.

144. Roehrs T, Kapke A, Roth T, et al. Sex differences in the polysomnographic sleep of young adults: a community-based study. Sleep Med 2006;7(1):49–53.

145. Kimura M. Minireview: gender-specific sleep regulation. Sleep Biol Rhythms 2005;3:75–9.

146. Vitiello MV, Larsen LH, Moe KE. Age-related sleep change: gender and estrogen effects on the subjective-objective sleep quality relationships of healthy, noncomplaining older men and women. J Psychosom Res 2004;56(5):503–10.

147. Voderholzer U, Al-Shajlawi A, Weske G, et al. Are there gender differences in objective and subjective sleep measures? A study of insomniacs and healthy controls. Depress Anxiety 2003;17(3):162–72.

148. Mohsenin V. Gender differences in the expression of sleep-disordered breathing: role of upper airway dimensions. Chest 2001;120(5):1442–7.

149. Armitage R, Hudson A, Trivedi M, et al. Sex differences in the distribution of EEG frequencies during sleep: unipolar depressed outpatients. J Affect Disord 1995;34(2):121–9.

150. Whinnery J, Jackson N, Rattanaumpawan P, et al. Short and long sleep duration associated with race/ethnicity, sociodemographics, and socioeconomic position. Sleep 2014;37(3):601–11.

151. Green MJ, Espie CA, Hunt K, et al. The longitudinal course of insomnia symptoms: inequalities by sex and occupational class among two different age cohorts followed for 20 years in the west of Scotland. Sleep 2012;35(6):815–23.

152. Ye L, Pien GW, Weaver TE. Gender differences in the clinical manifestation of obstructive sleep apnea. Sleep Med 2009;10(10):1075–84.

153. Del Campo F, Zamarron C. Sleep apnea and pregnancy. An association worthy of study. Sleep Breath 2013;17(2):463–4.

154. Ibrahim S, Foldvary-Schaefer N. Sleep disorders in pregnancy: implications, evaluation, and treatment. Neurol Clin 2012;30(3):925–36.

155. Facco FL, Kramer J, Ho KH, et al. Sleep disturbances in pregnancy. Obstet Gynecol 2010;115(1):77–83.

156. Chen YH, Kang JH, Lin CC, et al. Obstructive sleep apnea and the risk of adverse pregnancy outcomes. Am J Obstet Gynecol 2012;206(2):136.e1–5.

157. Okun ML, Luther JF, Wisniewski SR, et al. Disturbed sleep, a novel risk factor for preterm birth? J Womens Health (Larchmt) 2012;21(1):54–60.

158. Moore M, Meltzer LJ, Mindell JA. Bedtime problems and night wakings in children. Sleep Med Clin 2007;2:377–85.

159. Mindell JA, Kuhn B, Lewin DS, et al. Behavioral treatment of bedtime problems and night wakings in infants and young children. Sleep 2006;29(10):1263–76.

160. Okun ML, Luther J, Prather AA, et al. Changes in sleep quality, but not hormones predict time to postpartum depression recurrence. J Affect Disord 2011;130(3):378–84.

161. Chang JJ, Pien GW, Duntley SP, et al. Sleep deprivation during pregnancy and maternal and fetal outcomes: is there a relationship? Sleep Med Rev 2010;14(2):107–14.

162. Pires GN, Andersen ML, Giovenardi M, et al. Sleep impairment during pregnancy: possible implications on mother-infant relationship. Med Hypotheses 2010;75(6):578–82.

163. Ameratunga D, Goldin J, Hickey M. Sleep disturbance in menopause. Intern Med J 2012;42(7):742–7.

164. Regestein QR. Do hot flashes disturb sleep? Menopause 2012;19(7):715–8.

165. Baron KG, Smith TW, Berg CA, et al. Spousal involvement in CPAP adherence among patients with obstructive sleep apnea. Sleep Breath 2011;15(3):525–34.

166. McDowell A. Spousal involvement and CPAP adherence: a two-way street? Sleep Breath 2011;15(3):269–70.

167. Punjabi NM, Caffo BS, Goodwin JL, et al. Sleep-disordered breathing and mortality: a prospective cohort study. PLoS Med 2009;6(8):e1000132.

168. Mahowald MW, Schenck CH. REM sleep behaviour disorder: a marker of synucleinopathy. Lancet Neurol 2013;12(5):417–9.

169. Tomfohr L, Pung MA, Edwards KM, et al. Racial differences in sleep architecture: the role of ethnic discrimination. Biol Psychol 2012;89(1):34–8.

170. Thomas KS, Bardwell WA, Ancoli-Israel S, et al. The toll of ethnic discrimination on sleep architecture and fatigue. Health Psychol 2006;25(5):635–42.

171. Profant J, Ancoli-Israel S, Dimsdale JE. Are there ethnic differences in sleep architecture? Am J Hum Biol 2002;14(3):321–6.

172. Ruiter ME, Decoster J, Jacobs L, et al. Normal sleep in African-Americans and Caucasian-Americans: a meta-analysis. Sleep Med 2011;12(3):209–14.

173. Ruiter ME, DeCoster J, Jacobs L, et al. Sleep disorders in African Americans and Caucasian Americans: a meta-analysis. Behav Sleep Med 2010;8(4):246–59.

174. Grandner MA, Knutson KL, Troxel W, et al. Implications of sleep and energy drink use for health disparities. Nutr Rev 2014;72(Suppl 1):14–22.

175. Knutson KL. Sociodemographic and cultural determinants of sleep deficiency: implications for cardiometabolic disease risk. Soc Sci Med 2013;79:7–15.

176. Mezick EJ, Matthews KA, Hall M, et al. Influence of race and socioeconomic status on sleep: Pittsburgh SleepSCORE project. Psychosom Med 2008;70(4):410–6.

177. Patel NP, Grandner MA, Xie D, et al. "Sleep disparity" in the population: poor sleep quality is strongly associated with poverty and ethnicity. BMC Public Health 2010;10(1):475.

178. Grandner MA, Hale L, Jackson N, et al. Perceived racial discrimination as an independent predictor of sleep disturbance and daytime fatigue. Behav Sleep Med 2012;10(4):235–49.

179. Slopen N, Williams DR. Discrimination, other psychosocial stressors, and self-reported sleep duration and difficulties. Sleep 2014;37(1):147–56.

180. Bureau of Labor Statistics. American time use survey fact sheet. Washington, DC: Bureau of Labor Statistics; 2013.

181. Rosekind MR, Gregory KB, Mallis MM, et al. The cost of poor sleep: workplace productivity loss and associated costs. J Occup Environ Med 2010;52(1):91–8.

182. Hui SK, Grandner MA. Trouble sleeping associated with lower work performance and greater health care costs: longitudinal data from Kansas State Employee Wellness Program. J Occup Environ Med 2015;57(10):1031–8.

183. Hui SK, Grandner MA. Associations between poor sleep quality and stages of change of multiple health behaviors among participants of Employee Wellness Program. Prev Med Rep 2015;2:292–9.

184. Gurubhagavatula I, Nkwuo JE, Maislin G, et al. Estimated cost of crashes in commercial drivers supports screening and treatment of obstructive sleep apnea. Accid Anal Prev 2008;40(1):104–15.

185. Pack AI, Maislin G, Staley B, et al. Impaired performance in commercial drivers: role of sleep apnea and short sleep duration. Am J Respir Crit Care Med 2006;174(4):446–54.

186. Xie W, Chakrabarty S, Levine R, et al. Factors associated with obstructive sleep apnea among commercial motor vehicle drivers. J Occup Environ Med 2011;53(2):169–73.

187. Moore-Ede M, Heitmann A, Guttkuhn R, et al. Circadian alertness simulator for fatigue risk assessment in transportation: application to reduce frequency and severity of truck accidents. Aviat Space Environ Med 2004;75(3 Suppl):A107–18.

188. Paterson JL, Dorrian J, Clarkson L, et al. Beyond working time: factors affecting sleep behaviour in rail safety workers. Accid Anal Prev 2012; 45(Suppl):32–5.

189. Darwent D, Dawson D, Roach GD. Prediction of probabilistic sleep distributions following travel across multiple time zones. Sleep 2010;33(2): 185–95.

190. Dorrian J, Darwent D, Dawson D, et al. Predicting pilot's sleep during layovers using their own behaviour or data from colleagues: implications for biomathematical models. Accid Anal Prev 2012;45(Suppl):17–21.

191. Drury DA, Ferguson SA, Thomas MJ. Restricted sleep and negative affective states in commercial pilots during short haul operations. Accid Anal Prev 2012;45(Suppl):80–4.

192. Gander PH, Signal TL, van den Berg MJ, et al. In-flight sleep, pilot fatigue and Psychomotor Vigilance Task performance on ultra-long range versus long range flights. J Sleep Res 2013;22(6): 697–706.

193. Holmes A, Al-Bayat S, Hilditch C, et al. Sleep and sleepiness during an ultra long-range flight operation between the Middle East and United States. Accid Anal Prev 2012;45(Suppl):27–31.

194. Powell DM, Spencer MB, Petrie KJ. Fatigue in airline pilots after an additional day's layover period. Aviat Space Environ Med 2010;81(11): 1013–7.

195. Roach GD, Darwent D, Dawson D. How well do pilots sleep during long-haul flights? Ergonomics 2010;53(9):1072–5.

196. Roach GD, Petrilli RM, Dawson D, et al. Impact of layover length on sleep, subjective fatigue levels, and sustained attention of long-haul airline pilots. Chronobiol Int 2012;29(5):580–6.

197. Roach GD, Sargent C, Darwent D, et al. Duty periods with early start times restrict the amount of sleep obtained by short-haul airline pilots. Accid Anal Prev 2012;45(Suppl):22–6.

198. Rajaratnam SM, Barger LK, Lockley SW, et al. Sleep disorders, health, and safety in police officers. JAMA 2011;306(23):2567–78.

199. Charles LE, Gu JK, Andrew ME, et al. Sleep duration and biomarkers of metabolic function among police officers. J Occup Environ Med 2011;53(8): 831–7.

200. Fekedulegn D, Burchfiel CM, Hartley TA, et al. Shiftwork and sickness absence among police officers: the BCOPS study. Chronobiol Int 2013;30(7): 930–41.

201. Gu JK, Charles LE, Burchfiel CM, et al. Long work hours and adiposity among police officers in a US northeast city. J Occup Environ Med 2012;54(11): 1374–81.

202. McCanlies EC, Slaven JE, Smith LM, et al. Metabolic syndrome and sleep duration in police officers. Work 2012;43(2):133–9.

203. Neylan TC, Metzler TJ, Henn-Haase C, et al. Prior night sleep duration is associated with psychomotor vigilance in a healthy sample of police academy recruits. Chronobiol Int 2010;27(7):1493–508.

204. Aisbett B, Wolkow A, Sprajcer M, et al. "Awake, smoky, and hot": providing an evidence-base for

managing the risks associated with occupational stressors encountered by wildland firefighters. Appl Ergon 2012;43(5):916–25.

205. Vargas de Barros V, Martins LF, Saitz R, et al. Mental health conditions, individual and job characteristics and sleep disturbances among firefighters. J Health Psychol 2013;18(3):350–8.

206. Grandner MA, Pack AI. Sleep disorders, public health, and public safety. JAMA 2011;306(23):2616–7.

207. Sharwood LN, Elkington J, Meuleners L, et al. Use of caffeinated substances and risk of crashes in long distance drivers of commercial vehicles: case-control study. BMJ 2013;346:f1140.

208. Grundy A, Sanchez M, Richardson H, et al. Light intensity exposure, sleep duration, physical activity, and biomarkers of melatonin among rotating shift nurses. Chronobiol Int 2009;26(7):1443–61.

209. Ruggiero JS, Redeker NS, Fiedler N, et al. Sleep and psychomotor vigilance in female shiftworkers. Biol Res Nurs 2012;14(3):225–35.

210. Chang YS, Wu YH, Hsu CY, et al. Impairment of perceptual and motor abilities at the end of a night shift is greater in nurses working fast rotating shifts. Sleep Med 2011;12(9):866–9.

211. Chung MH, Kuo TB, Hsu N, et al. Recovery after three-shift work: relation to sleep-related cardiac neuronal regulation in nurses. Ind Health 2012;50(1):24–30.

212. Demir Zencirci A, Arslan S. Morning-evening type and burnout level as factors influencing sleep quality of shift nurses: a questionnaire study. Croat Med J 2011;52(4):527–37.

213. Dorrian J, Paterson J, Dawson D, et al. Sleep, stress and compensatory behaviors in Australian nurses and midwives. Rev Saude Publica 2011;45(5):922–30.

214. Eldevik MF, Flo E, Moen BE, et al. Insomnia, excessive sleepiness, excessive fatigue, anxiety, depression and shift work disorder in nurses having less than 11 hours in-between shifts. PLoS One 2013;8(8):e70882.

215. Geiger-Brown J, Rogers VE, Han K, et al. Occupational screening for sleep disorders in 12-h shift nurses using the Berlin Questionnaire. Sleep Breath 2013;17(1):381–8.

216. Geiger-Brown J, Rogers VE, Trinkoff AM, et al. Sleep, sleepiness, fatigue, and performance of 12-hour-shift nurses. Chronobiol Int 2012;29(2):211–9.

217. Geiger-Brown J, Trinkoff A, Rogers VE. The impact of work schedules, home, and work demands on self-reported sleep in registered nurses. J Occup Environ Med 2011;53(3):303–7.

218. Ulmer C, Wolman DM, Johns MME. Institute of Medicine committee on optimizing graduate medical trainee (resident) hours and work schedules to improve patient safety. Resident duty hours: enhancing sleep, supervision, and safety. Washington, DC: National Academies Press; 2009.

219. Amin MM, Graber M, Ahmad K, et al. The effects of a mid-day nap on the neurocognitive performance of first-year medical residents: a controlled interventional pilot study. Acad Med 2012;87(10):1428–33.

220. Arora VM, Georgitis E, Woodruff JN, et al. Improving sleep hygiene of medical interns: can the sleep, alertness, and fatigue education in residency program help? Arch Intern Med 2007;167(16):1738–44.

221. Kim HJ, Kim JH, Park K-D, et al. A survey of sleep deprivation patterns and their effects on cognitive functions of residents and interns in Korea. Sleep Med 2011;12(4):390–6.

222. Reed DA, Fletcher KE, Arora VM. Systematic review: association of shift length, protected sleep time, and night float with patient care, residents' health, and education. Ann Intern Med 2010;153(12):829–42.

223. Bilimoria KY, Chung JW, Hedges LV, et al. National cluster-randomized trial of duty-hour flexibility in surgical training. N Engl J Med 2016;374(8):713–27.

224. Hale L. Do DP. Racial differences in self-reports of sleep duration in a population-based study. Sleep 2007;30(9):1096–103.

225. Hale L, Hill TD, Burdette AM. Does sleep quality mediate the association between neighborhood disorder and self-rated physical health? Prev Med 2010;51(3–4):275–8.

226. Hale L, Hill TD, Friedman E, et al. Perceived neighborhood quality, sleep quality, and health status: evidence from the Survey of the Health of Wisconsin. Soc Sci Med 2013;79:16–22.

227. Hill TD, Burdette AM, Hale L. Neighborhood disorder, sleep quality, and psychological distress: testing a model of structural amplification. Health Place 2009;15(4):1006–13.

228. Pirrera S, De Valck E, Cluydts R. Nocturnal road traffic noise: a review on its assessment and consequences on sleep and health. Environ Int 2010;36(5):492–8.

229. Kawada T. Noise and health: sleep disturbance in adults. J Occup Health 2011;53(6):413–6.

230. Fonken LK, Kitsmiller E, Smale L, et al. Dim nighttime light impairs cognition and provokes depressive-like responses in a diurnal rodent. J Biol Rhythms 2012;27(4):319–27.

231. Hu RF, Jiang XY, Zeng YM, et al. Effects of earplugs and eye masks on nocturnal sleep, melatonin and cortisol in a simulated intensive care unit environment. Crit Care 2010;14(2):R66.

232. Wood B, Rea MS, Plitnick B, et al. Light level and duration of exposure determine the impact of self-luminous tablets on melatonin suppression. Appl Ergon 2013;44(2):237–40.

233. Herljevic M, Middleton B, Thapan K, et al. Light-induced melatonin suppression: age-related reduction in response to short wavelength light. Exp Gerontol 2005;40(3):237–42.

234. Pigeon WR, Grandner MA. Creating an optimal sleep environment. In: Kushida CA, editor. Encyclopedia of sleep. Oxford (United Kingdom): Elsevier; 2013. p. 72–6.

235. Buxton OM, Ellenbogen JM, Wang W, et al. Sleep disruption due to hospital noises: a prospective evaluation. Ann Intern Med 2012;157(3):170–9.

236. Parmeggiani PL. Sleep behaviour and temperature. In: Parmeggiani PL, Velluti RA, editors. The physiologic nature of sleep. London: Imperial College Press; 2005. p. 387–405.

237. McCall WV, Boggs N, Letton A. Changes in sleep and wake in response to different sleeping surfaces: a pilot study. Appl Ergon 2012;43(2):386–91.

238. Shanmugan B, Roux F, Stonestreet C, et al. Lower back pain and sleep: mattresses, sleep quality and daytime symptoms. Sleep Diagn Ther 2007;2(5):36–40.

239. Verhaert V, Haex B, De Wilde T, et al. Ergonomics in bed design: the effect of spinal alignment on sleep parameters. Ergonomics 2011;54(2):169–78.

240. Troxel WM. It's more than sex: exploring the dyadic nature of sleep and implications for health. Psychosom Med 2010;72(6):578–86.

241. Troxel WM, Robles TF, Hall M, et al. Marital quality and the marital bed: examining the covariation between relationship quality and sleep. Sleep Med Rev 2007;11(5):389–404.

242. Troxel WM, Buysse DJ, Hall M, et al. Marital happiness and sleep disturbances in a multi-ethnic sample of middle-aged women. Behav Sleep Med 2009;7(1):2–19.

243. Troxel WM, Buysse DJ, Monk TH, et al. Does social support differentially affect sleep in older adults with versus without insomnia? J Psychosom Res 2010;69(5):459–66.

244. Troxel WM, Cyranowski JM, Hall M, et al. Attachment anxiety, relationship context, and sleep in women with recurrent major depression. Psychosom Med 2007;69(7):692–9.

245. Gradisar M, Wolfson AR, Harvey AG, et al. The sleep and technology use of Americans: findings from the National Sleep Foundation's 2011 Sleep in America poll. J Clin Sleep Med 2013;9(12):1291–9.

246. Orzech K, Grandner MA, Roane BM, et al. Electronic media use within 2 hours of bedtime predicts sleep variables in college students. Sleep 2012;35(Abstract Suppl):A73.

247. Chang AM, Aeschbach D, Duffy JF, et al. Evening use of light-emitting eReaders negatively affects sleep, circadian timing, and next-morning alertness. Proc Natl Acad Sci U S A 2015;112(4):1232–7.

248. Weaver E, Gradisar M, Dohnt H, et al. The effect of presleep video-game playing on adolescent sleep. J Clin Sleep Med 2010;6(2):184–9.

249. NHTSA. Drowsy driving. Wahinton, DC: US Department of Transportation; 2011.

250. Strohl KP, Blatt J, Council F, et al. Drowsy driving and automobile crashes: NCSDR/NHTSA expert panel on driver fatigue and sleepiness. Washington, DC: National Highway Traffic Safety Administration; 1998.

251. Borman KR, Biester TW, Jones AT, et al. Sleep, supervision, education, and service: views of junior and senior residents. J Surg Educ 2011;68(6):495–501.

252. Borman KR, Fuhrman GM. "Resident duty hours: enhancing sleep, supervision, and safety": response of the Association of Program Directors in Surgery to the December 2008 report of the Institute of Medicine. Surgery 2009;146(3):420–7.

253. Sataloff RT. Resident duty hours: concerns and consequences. Ear Nose Throat J 2009;88(3):812–6.

254. Federal Aviation Administration. Fact sheet–sleep apnea in aviation. Washington, DC: FAA; 2015.

255. McKnight-Eily LR, Liu Y, Wheaton AG, et al. Unhealthy sleep-related behaviors—12 States, 2009. MMWR Morb Mortal Wkly Rep 2011;60(8):233–8.

256. Lufi D, Tzischinsky O, Hadar S. Delaying school starting time by one hour: some effects on attention levels in adolescents. J Clin Sleep Med 2011;7(2):137–43.

257. Moore M, Meltzer LJ. The sleepy adolescent: causes and consequences of sleepiness in teens. Paediatr Respir Rev 2008;9(2):114–20 [quiz: 120–1].

258. Wahlstrom K. School start time and sleepy teens. Arch Pediatr Adolesc Med 2010;164(7):676–7.

259. Wolfson AR, Spaulding NL, Dandrow C, et al. Middle school start times: the importance of a good night's sleep for young adolescents. Behav Sleep Med 2007;5(3):194–209.

260. Roenneberg T, Kuehnle T, Pramstaller PP, et al. A marker for the end of adolescence. Curr Biol 2004;14(24):R1038–9.

261. Barnes M, Davis K, Mancini M, et al. Setting adolescents up for success: promoting a policy to delay high school start times. J Sch Health 2016;86(7):552–7.

262. Meltzer LJ, Shaheed K, Ambler D. Start later, sleep later: school start times and adolescent sleep in homeschool versus public/private school students. Behav Sleep Med 2016;14(2):140–54.

263. Millman RP, Boergers J, Owens J. Healthy school start times: can we do a better job in reaching our goals? Sleep 2016;39(2):267–8.

264. Minges KE, Redeker NS. Delayed school start times and adolescent sleep: a systematic review

of the experimental evidence. Sleep Med Rev 2016;28:86–95.

265. Thacher PV, Onyper SV. Longitudinal outcomes of start time delay on sleep, behavior, and achievement in high school. Sleep 2016;39(2): 271–81.

266. Wheaton AG, Chapman DP, Croft JB. School start times, sleep, behavioral, health, and academic outcomes: a review of the Literature. J Sch Health 2016;86(5):363–81.

267. Siebern AT, Manber R. Insomnia and its effective non-pharmacologic treatment. Med Clin North Am 2010;94(3):581–91.

268. Watson NF, Horn E, Duncan GE, et al. Sleep duration and area-level deprivation in twins. Sleep 2016;39(1):67–77.

269. Knutson KL, Van Cauter E, Rathouz PJ, et al. Association between sleep and blood pressure in midlife: the CARDIA sleep study. Arch Intern Med 2009;169(11):1055–61.

Socioeconomic Impact of Pediatric Sleep Disorders

Kin M. Yuen, MD, MS*, Rafael Pelayo, MD

KEYWORDS

- ADD/ADHD • Restless legs/Periodic leg movements in sleep • Pediatric OSA • Parasomnia
- Circadian rhythm disorder • Insomnia • Mood disorder • Guardian/parental effect

KEY POINTS

- Pediatric disorders tend to affect the immediate support unit, adults and children.
- High costs for direct consumption of medical care are offset by early diagnosis and treatment of pediatric sleep disorders.
- Pediatric sleep disorders are underdiagnosed and undertreated.
- Attention deficit hyperactivity disorder may result from insufficient or fragmented sleep.
- Delaying school start time resulted in decreased car crashes in teen drivers and improved mood.

INTRODUCTION

It is difficult to determine the socioeconomic impact of pediatric sleep disorders because one needs to take into account not only the impact over the lifespan of the child but also the impact the disorders can have within the other family members. Within every family unit, sleep disturbance of the young tends to affect every member of that unit. Whether it is a newborn, a new adoptee, a sleepover, or an individual who has taken ill, there is a multiplier effect on everyone's sleep and next day function. This review concentrates on the published data of known pediatric sleep disorders and their economic impacts to date.

DIRECT HEALTH CARE COSTS

There are limited data on prospective health care utilization by children affected by sleep disorders. In 2013,[1] an Australian cross-sectional study that sampled "birth" cohort at ages 0 to 1 year, 2 to 3 years old, and "preschool" cohort at ages 4 to 5 and 6 to 7 reported those that exhibited sleep problems used more health care compared with their peers. Federal Medicare expenditure captured 98% of all children registered in Australia. Longitudinal Study of Australian Children evaluated 5107 children at ages 0 to 1 years in 2004, and 4606 of these children at ages 2 and 3 in 2006. The older group looked at 4983 children ages 4 and 5, and later, at ages 6 to 7. These children were compared with matched controls within randomly selected postal codes. Among all the subjects, 92% had complete sleep and Medicare data. Of children with reported sleep problems, the average additional annual health care costs at age 5 were $141 and for age 7 were $43 (in 2012 Australian dollars). Adjusting for confounders, the increase in health care costs was $98 at age 5 and $18 at age 7. The estimated cost to the Australian government was $27.5 million (95% confidence interval [CI] $9.2 to $46.8 million). This same group also studied the health care costs of children up to age 7 with "special health care needs," with an estimated the additional costs at $161.8 million.[2] It would not be surprising that children with both chronic sleep disorders and additional special health care needs would have higher health care utilization and accompanying costs in any society.[3]

There are no commercial or financial conflicts of interest to declare for K.M. Yuen or R. Pelayo.
Stanford Sleep Disorders Clinic, Stanford University School of Medicine, 450 Broadway Street, 2nd Floor, Redwood City, CA 94063, USA
* Corresponding author.
E-mail address: kin.yuen@stanfordalumni.org

1556-407X/17/© 2016 Elsevier Inc. All rights reserved.

sleep.theclinics.com

The costs that were captured included Medicare Benefit Schedule pays for non–hospital-based medical practitioners, and Pharmaceutical Benefits Schedule that pays for 83% of medication costs.[1] Parent or primary caregiver report of sleep problems and frequency was used as dichotomized variables: no/mild, moderate/severe. The investigators stipulated that subjective perceptions by caregiver of a child having a sleep problem were the "driver" to seek medical care, and more objective measures were not as cost-effective for a large population based–outcome measure. Within the "baby" cohort, the need for "specialized health care" almost doubled the infants that were not reported to have sleep problems: 9.9% as compared with 5.3%. The prekindergarten cohort similarly showed 21.2% usage of specialized health care compared with 12.1% of those without sleep problems. The natures of sleep problems were not reported, however. At age 0, 17.7% of children had "moderate/severe" sleep problems, whereas 7% did at age 7. However, because medical diagnoses were not captured in the analysis, those children with developmental and neurologic challenges might have skewed the usage of benefits and exhibited more sleep problems overall. Nonetheless, assessing overall sleep behavior at birth may help predict those children potentially requiring more medical attention subsequently.

An American study[4] evaluated socioeconomic conditions of sleep for 276 children in 133 girls with a mean age of 9.44 years (SD 0.71). Because of prior reports that children in poorer socioeconomic strata had shorter sleep duration per parental report, parents were interviewed on the telephone regarding their family income level, partner status (single, married), educational level, and whether the child was residing with one or more than one biological parent or other family member who was not a parent. Sleep was estimated using actigraphy on nondominant wrists for 7 consecutive nights. "Lower maternal perceived economic well-being predicted shorter sleep duration and greater variability in sleep onset in children." In addition, when the caregiver had lower educational level, the child had lower sleep efficiency. This study found different results with African American compared with European and American children, suggesting that ethnicity may be a significant moderator in the impact of sleep disorders.

BEHAVIORAL SLEEP PROBLEMS

An estimate of 20% to 30% of infants, toddlers, and preschoolers may present with behavioral challenges in going to sleep and repeated awakenings according to a 2006 review.[5] A report by in 2014 by Meltzer and colleagues[3] showed only 5% of representative samples of pediatric and adolescent patients that reported sleep problems or were diagnosed with a sleep disorder actually received sleep-related treatment recommendation. Only 8% of children diagnosed with sleep disorders and 2% identified with sleep problems received "any type of treatment recommendation." Of 750 children that had well-child visits in urban and suburban primary care settings in Philadelphia, 520 youth (69%) year 1, 490 youth (65%) year 2, and 451 youth (60%) year 3 had documented follow-ups from 2007 through 2010. Of these, 150 were randomly selected, and the average age was 6.21 years (SD 5.4; range 0.28–18 years). More sick visits and calls were incurred among children that had sleep disorders (mean 8.84; 95% CI 7.77–9.90) than those without (mean 6.34; 95% CI 5.56–7.12). Up to one-third of children showed persistence of sleep problems "across time." The families with lower income tended not to have follow-up visits. These results point to how difficult it is to accurately estimate the socioeconomic impact to society of sleep disorders in children.

ATTENTION-DEFICIT/HYPERACTIVITY DISORDER

The socioeconomic impact to society of attention-deficit/hyperactivity disorder (ADHD) in children is large.[6,7] In the US educational system, a student with ADHD incurred an average annual incremental cost to society of $5007 according to a 2011 report.[7] In 2016, the cost of medication was estimated at $1669 per child. Sleep problems in this population are very prevalent.[8–12] The socioeconomic impact of ADHD is not a problem just in the United States; there is a rich international ADHD literature documenting the impact of this condition. Sung and colleagues[13] conducted a cross-sectional study in outpatient clinics of pediatric hospitals, private pediatric practices, and ADHD support groups to evaluate the prevalence of sleep problems among children with ADHD in Victoria, Australia. Among children that were identified to have sleep problems, these children missed or were tardy for school more than their peers without sleep problems. Of 330 families, 239 (74%) completed the survey. Sleep problems were classified as "mild" for 28.5%, and "moderate or severe" for 44.8%. In 2006, caregivers of children between 5 and 18 years completed a survey for the previous 4 weeks with the question, "Has your child's sleep been a problem?" The answers were categorized as "none," "mild," or "moderate/severe." Problems surveyed included "difficulty falling asleep, resisting going to bed, tossing or turning in bed, snoring or difficulty breathing, waking up frequently during the night, difficulty getting up in the morning, and tiredness on waking." Most children were boys: 90.4%, and lived with 2 caregivers (76.6%). Including all sleep problems from mild to moderate/severe, the prevalence was 73%. There was a larger than expected report of difficulty falling asleep: 71% in the mild group, and 84% in the moderate/severe group. Among children with moderate to severe sleep problems and ADHD, the caregivers were 2.7 times more likely to be "clinically depressed, stressed, or anxious" than the families with children without any sleep problems (odds ratio 2.72; 95% CI 1.33–5.54). More importantly, only 45% of caregivers reported being asked about the sleep of their children, and 60% received advice about treatment.

When considering the socioeconomic impact of sleep disorders in the children with ADHD, it is important to point out that treatment of the sleep disorders has been repeatedly shown to improve the ADHD symptoms and would be expected to therefore lower these costs.[14–17] In addition, because ADHD can persist into adulthood, treating sleep problems in children with ADHD should be expected to have long-term societal benefit.

SLEEP DEPRIVATION/RESTRICTION

The most common cause of death among teenagers in the United States is automobile accidents, and sleep deprivation appears to play a role. Martiniuk and colleagues[18] reported in *JAMA Pediatrics* in 2013 that, among 20,822 newly licensed drivers from ages 17 to 24 in Australia, those who slept less than 6 hours per night tended to have more "off the road" crashes (relative risk [RR] 1.21; 95 CI 1.04–1.41), and these accidents occurred more often from 8 PM to 11:59 PM (RR 1.86; 95% CI 1.11–3.13). This prospective study followed provisional drivers for 2 years and documented 19,327 subjects that had full crash reports. For 2015, 27.3% of students reported having 8 or more hours of sleep during school nights. More male students (median 29.3%; range 18.9%–41.5%) than female students (median 23.6%; range 16.2–34.7) had 8 or more hours of sleep.

The results of sleep restriction studies and behavioral correlates were more difficult to define. Fallone and colleagues[19] enrolled 82 subjects (46 boys, 41 girls) ages 8 to 15 years (8.6–15.8 years; mean 11.9, SD 1.6 years) to examine the effects of sleep restriction versus "optimized" sleep and their behavior. After 5 nights of baseline sleep by actigraphy of at least 10 hours' sleep, they were randomly assigned to overnight stay for optimized sleep

(10 hours per night: n = 42; 24 boys and 18 girls) or restricted sleep (4 hours per night: n = 45; 22 boys, 23 girls). Behavior, performance, and sleepiness were assessed the following day. Although sleep restriction was associated with shorter daytime sleep latency by Multiple Sleep Latency Test, increased subjective sleepiness by visual analogue scales, and increased sleepy and inattentive behaviors, it was not associated with increased hyperactive-impulsive behavior or impaired performance on tests of response inhibition and sustained attention. (Assessment tools used included the Child Attention Profile, the Restricted Academic Situation, the Gordon Diagnostic System, and behaviors by trained observers.)

However, a more recent study of Korean high school students by Lee and colleagues[20] found that among 50 students (10 males, 40 females 17.56 ± 0.47 years old) who had "behaviorally induced insufficient sleep," as compared with 51 students (16 males, 35 females, 17.66 ± 0.54 years old) that had adequate nocturnal sleep, the students with less sleep had poorer academic performance, higher degree of impulsivity, and depression.[20] Criteria for "insufficient sleep" group were: (1) sleep duration on weekdays less than or equal to 7 hours; (2) weekend oversleeps greater than or equal to 3 hours; (3) severe daytime sleepiness (Epworth Sleepiness Scale [ESS] ≥10). The "adequate" sleep group contained (1) sleep duration on weekdays greater than or equal to 5 hours; (2) weekend oversleep less than or equal to 2 hours; (3) no significant daytime sleepiness (ESS ≤7); and (4) the absence of significant insomnia. Given these criteria, one can argue that even with sleeping in for non–school days for the "adequate" sleep group, the better performing group itself did not get adequate sleep for their age ranges because the expected total sleep time is 8 to 9 hours per night.

To test the hypothesis that improving students' sleep time will improve their overall performance, a study by Vorona and colleagues[21] looked at the number of crashes in a 2-year follow-up study of adjacent counties after one county had purposely delayed the high school start time by 1 hour.[21] The teens that resided in one county with earlier start time of 7:30 AM (Chesterfield County) had 48.8/1000 crashes per licensed drivers versus the later start time county of 8:30 AM (Henrico County), which had 37.9/1000 (P = .04) for the year 2009 to 2010. For the next year 2010 to 2011, the teens 16 to 17 years residing in the county with the earlier start time again had statistically significant higher crash rate (53.2/1000 vs 42.0/1000), although not for the whole group of ages of 16 to 18 year olds. Meanwhile, the adult crash rates and the traffic congestions did not differ between counties.

Wahlstrom[22] had reported that, by delaying high school start times from 7:30 to 8:30 AM for the fall of 1997 to 2001 9th to 12th grade students in Minneapolis School District got 5 more hours of sleep per week, improved attendance, and had fewer symptoms of depression. There were 467 high school students with 8:30 AM start time, and 169 students with 7:30 AM start time during this comparison. Subjective rated sleepiness in class improved, and days "home sick from school" were statistically significant. Improvements in grades showed a positive trend, but not statistically significant compared with 3 years prior and 3 years after the intervention.

Owens and colleagues[23] also studied the delay in start time from 8 AM to 8:30 AM for 201 high school students for grades 9 to 12 in Rhode Island for an independent school. The students having less than 7 hours of sleep decreased by 79% (from 33.8% to 7.0%); students getting at least 8 hours of sleep increased from 16.4% to 54.7%, but only 11% were getting the recommended 9 or more hours.

Dr Owens and the Adolescent Working Group[24] in its position paper for the American Academy of Pediatrics issued worldwide epidemiologic review of the lack of adequate sleep of teenagers, and the potential role of later start time for high school or secondary schools.[24]

Future prospective studies and sleep tracking devices will likely help provide better data of the extent of sleep loss among youth and the health costs and benefits of adequate sleep time. Changing school start times would be expected to have a significant socioeconomic impact that should improve the quality of life for these children, their families, and communities.

PEDIATRIC OBSTRUCTIVE SLEEP APNEA

It has been estimated that prevalence of pediatric obstructive sleep apnea (OSA) is 1% to 4%. Because children with OSA may become adults with OSA, one can attempt to project the socioeconomic impact of OSA in children by looking at the adult data. A most recent commissioned report for the diagnosis and treatment of OSA conducted by Frost and Sullivan (www.aasmnet.org/sleep-apnea-economic-impact.aspx), and sponsored by the American Academy of Sleep Medicine, surveyed 506 adults online with a diagnosis of OSA. Research also included "100 leading studies on the impact of the condition on everything from heart attack risk to employee absenteeism for the cost benefit analysis." The age ranges of respondents were 3% of 18 to 29 years old, 15% 30 to 49 years old, 56% 50 to 69 years

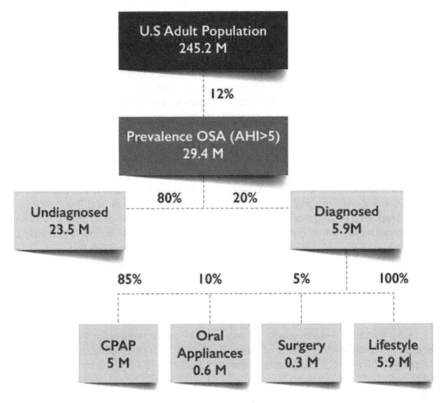

Epidemiology. (© American Academy of Sleep Medicine 2016.)

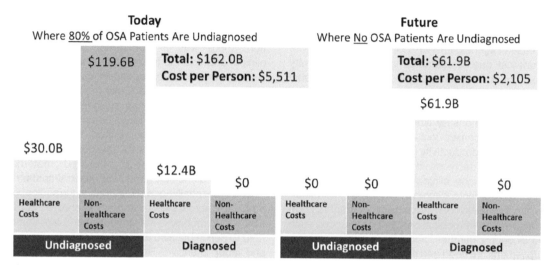

Diagnosing and treating all 29.4 M Americans with OSA could save $100.1 billion. (© American Academy of Sleep Medicine 2016.)

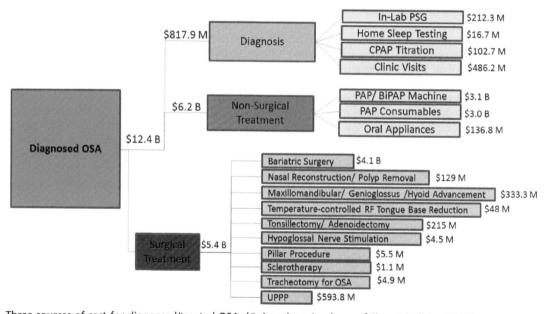

Three sources of cost for diagnosed/treated OSA. (© American Academy of Sleep Medicine 2016.)

old, and 26% 70 to 89 years old. The average age of diagnosis and treatment was 53 years. Only an estimated 12% of the population that has OSA symptoms have been diagnosed. Diagnostic modalities included were in-laboratory polysomnography, home sleep studies, continuous positive airway pressure (CPAP) titration studies as generic for all titration studies (although not separated into in-laboratory or at home), and clinic visits. Modeling treatment options, such as CPAP, oral appliance, surgery, and lifestyle modifications, it found that diagnosing and treating OSA resulted in potentially $100.1 billion savings.[25] Surgical costs included bariatric, nasal "reconstruction,"

"maxillary/genioglossus/hyoid advancement," tongue-base reduction, adenotonsillectomy, hypoglossal nerve stimulation, pillar procedure, sclerotherapy, and tracheostomy.

Economic costs included: (1) direct costs of treatment of comorbid conditions, such as hypertension, diabetes mellitus, obesity, depression, medication and substance use, both as direct utilization of medical care and as undiagnosed and untreated individuals' potential continuation of medical expenses; (2) indirect annual costs for traffic fatalities from drowsiness and commercial truck driver accidents as well as calculated annual costs from undiagnosed OSA drivers; (3) indirect costs of workplace accidents based on data of daylight savings time estimates in 2009 of 5.7% increase in injuries, and 67.6% "increase in days of work lost due to sustained injuries," opportunity costs of absenteeism, and lost wages. Additional cost savings in improvement of mood, productivity, and lessened medical costs were input into costs calculations for workplace savings.

Benefits accrued included quality-of-life measures, gain in productivity (less workplace accidents and injuries, decrease in days out from medical illness and fatigue, clinic visits, disability), decrease in traffic accidents, decreased medical expenditure in direct utilization of medical services, decreases in consumption of medications and substances such as alcohol, cigarettes, and sleeping pills, and improvements in mood and relationship with partners. Insomnia often accompanies OSA patients with sleep fragmentation, and this study included the costs of substance used to treat insomnia into its estimates. Treatment of adults' OSA lessened the number of days absent from 6.3 to 4.5 per year.

Although the risks of hypertension, workplace accidents, and driving accidents are lower for children, the risks of inattention, inopportune naps leading to decreases in learning, and accidents in schoolyard or sports-related injuries have not been yet been fully captured. Data on sleep deprivation and its costs have been reported earlier (see section on attention deficit disorder (ADD)/ADHD). Bariatric surgery data have supported its role in the treatment of older teenagers who are morbidly obese and suffer from OSA and comorbid conditions. Sleep disorders of the young affect the entire family unit. Based solely on direct medical costs alone, the conservative measure of 1% prevalence is considerable.

Because of the current obesity epidemic affecting children and young adults, the prevalence is expected to increase further. The 2015 survey data from the Centers for Disease Control and Prevention estimated 13.9% of American youths are obese.[26] However, further longitudinal studies will help shed light on cardiovascular risks. The health burden of comorbid diabetes has been studied.

INSOMNIA

Owens and colleagues[27] published a national survey for pharmacotherapy for insomnia among child psychiatrists in 2010. The ages of children/adolescents were reported as 6 to 10 years, 10 to 20 years, and greater than 20 years. A surprisingly wide range of medications were being prescribed and recommended with little evidence-based data to support it. The investigators concluded that insomnia is a significant clinical problem in children treated by child psychiatrists for a variety of behavioral, neurodevelopmental, and psychiatric conditions. In addition, there was a worrisome, highly variable clinical approach to insomnia in children.

Improving the sleep of infants can improve the maternal well-being and lower the cost of health care utilization. This was demonstrated in an Australian study that offered behavioral interventions to infants whose mother complained of poor sleep at 7 months of age. Follow-up at 10 and 12 months showed improved maternal mood, overall health, and lower medical costs.[28]

One of the challenges of confronting the socioeconomic impact of sleep disorders in children is the sense that not only is it an immense problem that is hard to define but also the treatments are expensive and labor intensive. However, when it comes to adolescent insomnia that is not true, and perhaps one should not be surprised that technology offers a cost-effective solution. Cognitive behavioral therapy (CBT) is unquestionably the best treatment available for chronic insomnia.[29] A study using online CBT has proven that it can be effective, affordable, and readily available.[30] In this study, teenagers with insomnia were randomized to either face-to-face CBT sessions or Internet-based CBT sessions. Both groups improved when re-evaluated after 1 year, but the Internet group had lower costs. Over time, as the cost of manpower increases and cost to access the Internet decreases, the advantages of Internet-based CBT should be even greater.

RESTLESS LEG SYNDROME

Restless leg syndrome (RLS) is a common but underrecognized condition in children.[31,32] It is a familial disorder, so many of the children may have parents or other family members that are not aware that their episodic discomfort is a neurologic condition with a name and is readily treatable.[33] The authors were unable to locate any publications of the socioeconomic cost of RLS specifically for the pediatric population. However, there have been analyses done of the costs in adults, which can provide a sense of the potential costs in a pediatric population. RLS has a prevalence ranging from approximately 2.5% to 10% and is associated with reductions in quality of life similar to or greater than those seen in patients with other chronic conditions such as type 2 diabetes or osteoarthritis.[34] A study of the direct economic burden of RLS among patients treated with dopamine agonists in a large US managed care system was reported in 2012.[35] The mean all-cause health care costs were $11,485 per patient, "mostly due to multiple medical conditions occurring with RLS." The actual RLS-related costs were only 6.7% of total all-cause costs. The investigators found that the relatively low costs associated with RLS treatment should encourage expanding the coverage of treatment to reduce the suffering and costs associated with RLS.[35]

The socioeconomic impact needs to factor in not only the health care utilization costs but also indirect costs, primarily due to productivity losses, which are as high as 20% in RLS patients.[36] The humanistic burden of RLS with regard to health-related quality of life, work productivity loss, health care resource use, and direct and indirect costs has been studied using a large national survey.[37] RLS patients were matched on demographic and health characteristics to non-RLS. RLS patients had significantly lower health-related quality-of-life scores, including mental component summary, physical component summary, health utilities, and higher levels of work productivity loss in the past 7 days, and overall productivity loss as well as general activity impairment. RLS patients had significantly higher health care resource use in the past 6 months than non-RLS patients: health care provider visits and hospitalizations. Furthermore, the study found that, across outcomes, increasing severity is associated with increased economic and humanistic burden for RLS patients.[37]

Considering how overwhelming the data are on the large socioeconomic impact of RLS in adults, how this affects children must be looked into more closely. RLS may be misdiagnosed as ADHD, which further adds to the socioeconomic impact of this condition in children.[32] Primary care providers, and especially pediatricians, should keep in mind the possibility of RLS being present in any child with behavioral or sleep problems. Accurate diagnosis and successful treatment will undoubtedly improve the socioeconomic burden of this condition.

SUMMARY

Although difficult to quantitate with current available data, the socioeconomic impact of sleep disorders in children is large and will grow unless steps are taken to recognize and treat these disorders sooner. Children with sleep disorders will often grow up to be adults with sleep disorders and may go on to have children of their own, also with sleep disorders. On any given day, a clinician may hear a patient say, "everybody in my family snorers," "my mother would never sleep at night," " my father always woke up feeling tired," " my kids are night owls like me," or " I thought everybody has to rub their legs at night." Sleep disorders are not mere nuisances. The data presented in this review show lost productivity, decreased quality of life, and increased health care utilization are occurring currently in society because of these often readily treatable conditions. Recognizing and treating these conditions in children will lead to a net improvement for all of us.

REFERENCES

1. Quach J, Gold L, Hiscock H, et al. Primary health-care costs associated with sleep problems up to age 7 years: Australian population-based study. BMJ Open 2013;3(5).
2. Quach J, Oberklaid F, Gold L, et al. Primary health-care costs associated with special health care needs up to age 7 years: Australian population-based study. J Paediatr Child Health 2014;50(10):768–74.
3. Meltzer LJ, Plaufcan MR, Thomas JH, et al. Sleep problems and sleep disorders in pediatric primary care: treatment recommendations, persistence, and health care utilization. J Clin Sleep Med 2014;10(4):421–6.
4. El-Sheikh M, Bagley EJ, Keiley M, et al. Economic adversity and children's sleep problems: multiple indicators and moderation of effects. Health Psychol 2013;32(8):849–59.
5. Mindell JA, Kuhn B, Lewin DS, et al. Behavioral treatment of bedtime problems and night wakings in infants and young children. Sleep 2006;29(10):1263–76.
6. Page TF, Pelham WE 3rd, Fabiano GA, et al. Comparative cost analysis of sequential, adaptive, behavioral, pharmacological, and combined treatments for childhood ADHD. J Clin Child Adolesc Psychol 2016;45(4):416–27.
7. Robb JA, Sibley MH, Pelham WE Jr, et al. The estimated annual cost of ADHD to the U.S. Education system. School Ment Health 2011;3(3):169–77.
8. Crabtree VM, Ivanenko A, Gozal D. Clinical and parental assessment of sleep in children with attention-deficit/hyperactivity disorder referred to a pediatric sleep medicine center. Clin Pediatr (Phila) 2003;42(9):807–13.
9. Corkum P, Tannock R, Moldofsky H. Sleep disturbances in children with attention-deficit/hyperactivity disorder. J Am Acad Child Adolesc Psychiatry 1998;37(6):637–46.
10. Gregory AM, Agnew-Blais JC, Matthews T, et al. ADHD and sleep quality: longitudinal analyses from childhood to early adulthood in a twin cohort. J Clin Child Adolesc Psychol 2016;1–11.
11. Lycett K, Mensah FK, Hiscock H, et al. A prospective study of sleep problems in children with ADHD. Sleep Med 2014;15(11):1354–61.
12. Virring A, Lambek R, Thomsen PH, et al. Disturbed sleep in attention-deficit hyperactivity disorder (ADHD) is not a question of psychiatric comorbidity or ADHD presentation. J Sleep Res 2016;25(3):333–40.

13. Sung V, Hiscock H, Sciberras E, et al. Sleep problems in children with attention-deficit/hyperactivity disorder: prevalence and the effect on the child and family. Arch Pediatr Adolesc Med 2008;162(4): 336–42.

14. Papadopoulos N, Sciberras E, Hiscock H, et al. The efficacy of a brief behavioral sleep intervention in school-aged children with ADHD and comorbid autism spectrum disorder. J Atten Disord 2015. [Epub ahead of print].

15. Amiri S, AbdollahiFakhim S, Lotfi A, et al. Effect of adenotonsillectomy on ADHD symptoms of children with adenotonsillar hypertrophy and sleep disordered breathing. Int J Pediatr Otorhinolaryngol 2015;79(8):1213–7.

16. Somuk BT, Bozkurt H, Goktas G, et al. Impact of adenotonsillectomy on ADHD and nocturnal enuresis in children with chronic adenotonsillar hypertrophy. Am J Otol 2016;37(1):27–30.

17. Aksu H, Gunel C, Ozgur BG, et al. Effects of adenoidectomy/adenotonsillectomy on ADHD symptoms and behavioral problems in children. Int J Pediatr Otorhinolaryngol 2015;79(7):1030–3.

18. Martiniuk AL, Senserrick T, Lo S, et al. Sleep-deprived young drivers and the risk for crash: the DRIVE prospective cohort study. JAMA Pediatr 2013;167(7):647–55.

19. Fallone G, Acebo C, Arnedt JT, et al. Effects of acute sleep restriction on behavior, sustained attention, and response inhibition in children. Percept Mot Skills 2001;93(1):213–29.

20. Lee YJ, Park J, Kim S, et al. Academic performance among adolescents with behaviorally induced insufficient sleep syndrome. J Clin Sleep Med 2015; 11(1):61–8.

21. Vorona RD, Szklo-Coxe M, Lamichhane R, et al. Adolescent crash rates and school start times in two central Virginia counties, 2009-2011: a follow-up study to a southeastern Virginia study, 2007-2008. J Clin Sleep Med 2014;10(11):1169–77.

22. Wahlstrom K. Changing times: findings from the first longitudinal study of later high school start times. NASSP Bull 2002;86(633):18.

23. Owens JA, Belon K, Moss P. Impact of delaying school start time on adolescent sleep, mood, and behavior. Arch Pediatr Adolesc Med 2010;164(7): 608–14.

24. Owens J, Adolescent Sleep Working Group, Committee on Adolescence. Insufficient sleep in adolescents and young adults: an update on causes and consequences. Pediatrics 2014;134(3):e921–32.

25. Sullivan Fa. 2016 In an age of constant activity, the solution to improving the nation's health may lie in helping it sleep better. Available at: http://www.aasmnet.org/Resources/pdf/sleep-apnea-patient-experience.pdf.

26. Elkum N, Al-Arouj M, Sharifi M, et al. Prevalence of childhood obesity in the state of Kuwait. Pediatr Obes 2015. [Epub ahead of print].

27. Owens JA, Rosen CL, Mindell JA, et al. Use of pharmacotherapy for insomnia in child psychiatry practice: a national survey. Sleep Med 2010;11(7): 692–700.

28. Hiscock H, Bayer J, Gold L, et al. Improving infant sleep and maternal mental health: a cluster randomised trial. Arch Dis Child 2007;92(11):952–8.

29. Qaseem A, Kansagara D, Forciea MA, et al, Clinical Guidelines Committee of the American College of Physicians. Management of chronic insomnia disorder in adults: a clinical practice guideline from the American College of Physicians. Ann Intern Med 2016;165(2):125–33.

30. De Bruin EJ, van Steensel FJ, Meijer AM. Cost-effectiveness of group and internet cognitive behavioral therapy for insomnia in adolescents: results from a randomized controlled trial. Sleep 2016;39(8): 1571–81.

31. Simakajornboon N, Dye TJ, Walters AS. Restless legs syndrome/Willis-Ekbom disease and growing pains in children and adolescents. Sleep Med Clin 2015;10(3):311–22, xiv.

32. Picchietti MA, Picchietti DL. Restless legs syndrome and periodic limb movement disorder in children and adolescents. Semin Pediatr Neurol 2008;15(2):91–9.

33. Mitterling T, Heidbreder A, Stefani A, et al. Natural course of restless legs syndrome/Willis-Ekbom disease: long-term observation of a large clinical cohort. Sleep Med 2015;16(10):1252–8.

34. Reinhold T, Muller-Riemenschneider F, Willich SN, et al. Economic and human costs of restless legs syndrome. Pharmacoeconomics 2009;27(4):267–79.

35. Meyers J, Candrilli S, Allen R, et al. Health care resource utilization and costs associated with restless legs syndrome among managed care enrollees treated with dopamine agonists. Manag Care 2012; 21(10):44–51.

36. Salas RE, Kwan AB. The real burden of restless legs syndrome: clinical and economic outcomes. Am J Manag Care 2012;18(9 Suppl):S207–12.

37. Durgin T, Witt EA, Fishman J. The humanistic and economic burden of restless legs syndrome. PLoS One 2015;10(10):e0140632.

Sleep in the Aging Population

Brienne Miner, MD, MHS[a],*, Meir H. Kryger, MD, FRCP(C)[a,b]

KEYWORDS

- Aging • Insomnia • Sleep disorders • Multimorbidity • Polypharmacy • Geriatric syndromes

KEY POINTS

- Changes to sleep architecture with normal aging include decreases in total sleep time, sleep efficiency, slow wave sleep, and REM sleep, and an increase in wake after sleep onset.
- Although sleep disturbance is common with aging, it is not an inherent part of the aging process; medical, psychiatric, and psychosocial factors overshadow age as risk factors.
- Sleep disturbance in older adults is associated with increased morbidity and mortality.
- The evaluation and management of sleep disturbances in older adults is best approached as a multifactorial geriatric health condition, arising from impairments in multiple domains.

INTRODUCTION

Sleep is an important component for health and wellness across the lifespan. The number of people in the United States who are 65 years or older is steadily increasing, and is expected to double over the next 25 years to about 72 million. By 2030, roughly 1 in 5 people in this country will be over the age of 65.[1] Sleep complaints are common among older adults, and as this segment of the population grows, so too will the prevalence of sleep disturbances. However, sleep problems are not an inherent part of the aging process. There are changes to sleep architecture over the lifespan that are not, in themselves, pathologic, but can be viewed as making older adults more vulnerable to sleep disturbances.[2] It is the consequences of aging, in the form of medical and psychiatric comorbidity, medication and substance use, psychosocial factors, and primary sleep disorders that put older adults at risk for sleep disturbance. The increasing prevalence of multimorbidity (ie, having at least 2 concurrent diseases in the same individual)[3] among older adults means that sleep disorders might arise from multiple different domains. Thus, sleep disturbance in this age group should be considered a multifactorial geriatric health condition (previously referred to as a geriatric syndrome),[4] requiring consideration of multiple risk factors and a comprehensive treatment approach.

NORMAL AGE-RELATED CHANGES TO SLEEP–WAKE PHYSIOLOGY

Physicians addressing sleep complaints in older adults are commonly asked about how much sleep is enough. The National Sleep Foundation recommends 7 to 8 hours of sleep for adults aged 65 and older.[5] This recommendation is supported by evidence that older adults sleeping anywhere from 6 to 9 hours have better cognition, mental

Funding Sources: Dr B. Miner is supported by T32AG1934, the John A. Hartford Center of Excellence at Yale and the Yale Claude D. Pepper Older Americans Independence Center (P30AG021342).
Disclosure Statement: Drs B. Miner and M.H. Kryger have no commercial or financial conflicts of interest to disclose.
a Department of Internal Medicine, Yale School of Medicine, 333 Cedar Street, New Haven, CT 06520, USA;
b VA Connecticut Healthcare System, 950 Campbell Avenue, West Haven, CT 06516, USA
* Corresponding author.
E-mail address: brienne.miner@yale.edu

1556-407X/17/© 2016 Elsevier Inc. All rights reserved.

and physical health, and quality of life compared with older adults with shorter or longer sleep durations. Thus, the need for sleep is not reduced in older adults, but the ability to get the required sleep may be decreased owing to normal changes in sleep architecture through the lifespan.[6]

Age-related changes in sleep physiology have been well-documented using polysomnography (**Table 1**). Most age-dependent changes in sleep parameters occur by age 60 years,[7] with the exception of sleep efficiency. Sleep efficiency (percentage of time spent asleep while in bed), in contrast, continues to show an age-dependent decrease beyond age 90 years. Older adults also have a decrease in total sleep time, with corresponding decreases in the percentage of time in slow wave sleep and REM sleep.[7] Slow wave sleep and REM sleep are thought to promote metabolic and cognitive recovery, and to enhance learning and memory, respectively.[2] Older adults also have an increase in time awake after sleep onset.[7] Although the number of arousals from sleep increases in healthy older adults, evidence suggests they do not have greater difficulty falling back to sleep.[8] There is an increase in sleep latency (the time it takes to fall asleep) up to age 60, with no clear age effect beyond that point.[7]

Circadian rhythms also change over the lifespan. These rhythms are 24-hour intrinsic physiologic cycles that are involved in control of sleep-wake and many other physiologic processes (eg, blood pressure, bone remodeling, release of certain hormones).[9] Aging is associated with a phase advance, resulting in an earlier onset of sleepiness in the evening and earlier morning awakening.[10] Daytime wakefulness is affected by phase advance, with older adults being more alert in the morning and more somnolent in the evening. Although napping is common in older adults, results with regard to the benefit or harm of this practice are mixed. Some studies show beneficial and potentially protective effects of napping in later life, whereas others show it to be a risk factor for morbidity and mortality.[11] There is some evidence to suggest that naps are protective for mortality if nighttime sleep duration is short, but are associated with increased mortality risk if nighttime sleep duration is longer than 9 hours.[12]

SLEEP COMPLAINTS IN OLDER ADULTS
Epidemiology

Major sleep complaints include insomnia and drowsiness. Symptoms of insomnia consist of difficulties with initiating or maintaining sleep (including early morning awakening).[13] Drowsiness has to do with the propensity for sleep and is often established by napping behavior.[14] Many large studies documenting the epidemiology of sleep complaints in older adults have shown that insomnia symptoms and drowsiness are common in this age group. The Established Populations for Epidemiologic Studies of the Elderly included 9282 community-dwelling adults aged 65 and older, and found that 43% of participants reported difficulty with sleep onset or maintenance, and 25% reported napping.[15] The National Sleep Foundation's 2003 Sleep in America Poll confirmed the prevalence of these symptoms, stating that 46% of community-dwelling adults aged 65 to 74 reported insomnia symptoms, and 39% of people in this age group reported napping. These prevalence rates increased to 50% and 46%, respectively, in participants aged 75 to 84 years.[16] It is estimated that 40% to 70% of older adults have chronic sleep problems, and up to 50% of cases are undiagnosed.[6]

The major sleep complaint depends on the cause of the sleep disturbance. Symptoms of insomnia are common in people using activating medications or substances, in those with comorbid medical or psychiatric illness, or in those with restless leg syndrome (RLS). Daytime drowsiness can result from sedating medications, chronic medical illness, or obstructive sleep apnea (OSA). With respect to OSA, whereas drowsiness and snoring are the most common complaints, older adults may also complain of choking or gasping on awakening, observed apneas, morning headache, nocturia, wandering, or confusion.[17,18]

Consequences of Poor Sleep

Sleep complaints, whether related to insomnia symptoms or drowsiness, have important consequences in older adults. Beyond being distressing for the subject, these symptoms predict poor physical and mental health-related quality of life.[19] In longitudinal studies, insomnia complaints

Table 1		
Age-related changes in sleep architecture		
	Decreased	**Increased**
Sleep parameter	• Total sleep time • Sleep efficiency • Slow wave sleep • Rapid eye movement sleep	• Time awake after sleep onset • Number of arousals from sleep • Sleep latency

have been associated with many different detrimental outcomes, including poor self-reported health status, cognitive decline, depression, disability in basic activities of daily living, poorer quality of life, and a greater risk of institutionalization.[2,17] Insomnia is also associated with impaired physical function and an increased risk for falls.[11,17] Daytime drowsiness has also been associated with harmful outcomes in longitudinal studies, including cardiovascular disease, falls, and death.[2] Healthy older adults who have sleep latencies of greater than 30 minutes, sleep efficiencies of less than 80%, or REM sleep percentage of less than 16% or greater than 25% of total sleep are at increased mortality risk, even after controlling for age, gender, and baseline medical burden.[20]

PATHOLOGIC AND PSYCHOSOCIAL FACTORS AFFECTING SLEEP IN THE AGING POPULATION
Pathologic Factors

Although aging per se does not lead to sleep pathology, the aging process is associated commonly with multiple pathologic problems that can affect sleep. Older adults commonly suffer from pain syndromes, arthritis, digestive disease, heart disease, lung disease, renal and urologic diseases, and cancer, all of which can contribute to sleep disturbance through specific symptoms or because of complications or anxiety associated with these diseases.[21] Psychiatric illness is as important as medical comorbidity in its effect on sleep, and has long been recognized to significantly and independently increase the risk for insomnia in older adults.[21,22] Sleep disruption features prominently in many psychiatric conditions, including depression and anxiety, which are common in older adults.[21] Sleep disturbance and depression are intertwined, as insomnia may be a result of depression but also increases the risk of developing depression in older adults.[23]

More so than the impact that a single condition has on sleep problems, one of the major issues leading to a higher risk of sleep problems in older adults is the accumulation of comorbidities. More than 1 in 4 Americans is living with 2 or more chronic conditions, and the prevalence of multiple chronic conditions increases with age.[24] A recent report of fee-for-service Medicare beneficiaries found that the rate of 2 or more chronic conditions was 62% for those aged 65 to 74 years and increased to 82% for those aged 85 years and older.[25] In fact, this situation has become so common that there has been a shift from looking at comorbidity (which focuses on the effect of a single

cooccurring disease with respect to an index disease) to multimorbidity. Multimorbidity refers to the coexistence of 2 or more chronic medical conditions in the same person.[25] However, a more nuanced definition takes into account the both number and the severity of conditions, and considers the link between multimorbidity and cognitive and physical dysfunction, as well as psychosocial factors.[3]

With an increasing number of health problems, the likelihood of sleep complaints increases. This was demonstrated in the 2003 National Sleep Foundation survey, which showed that, among people aged 65 years and older without comorbid illness, 36% reported a sleep problem. This percentage increased to 52% among people with 1 to 3 comorbid conditions, and to 69% among people with 4 or more comorbid conditions.[16] The cumulative effects of multiple chronic conditions on sleep complaints is not surprising, considering that single diseases are known to affect sleep quality in older adults; if one is bad, more than one is likely to be worse.

Medications and Substance Use

Medication use is another factor that may increase risk for sleep disturbances in older adults. The use of prescription medications, over-the-counter medications, and dietary supplements is increasing in this age group. A recent study of a nationally representative sample of community-dwelling adults aged 62 to 85 years found that 88% used at least 1 prescription medication, 38% used over-the-counter medications, and 64% used dietary supplements.[26]

Different classes of medications commonly used in older adults can impact sleep directly through multiple mechanisms. One such effect is increased daytime drowsiness, as can be seen with antihistamines, anticholinergic and anticonvulsant medications, and opiates. Medications can be activating or stimulating, as is the case with pseudoephedrine, beta agonists, corticosteroids, certain antidepressants, methylphenidate, or selegiline. Other medications can exacerbate primary sleep disorders or directly influence sleep architecture. For example, RLS and periodic limb movements of sleep (PLMS) can worsen with the use of certain antidepressants, and sleep disordered breathing can worsen with the use of opiates or benzodiazepines.[21] With respect to sleep architecture, certain beta-blockers have been shown to suppress melatonin secretion and increase sleep fragmentation. Others can worsen parasomnias, induce REM sleep behavior disorder (RBD), or change the amount of time spent in REM sleep.[21] A final factor to consider is whether a medication might be interfering with sleep by worsening other conditions or causing sleep-disruptive symptoms. Several examples of such effects include medications that worsen heart failure, have diuretic effects, create bothersome coughing, or cause nocturnal hypoglycemia.

Polypharmacy may also contribute to heightened risk for sleep disturbance in older adults. Although it is generally defined as the use of multiple medications, there is no consensus definition about the number of medications that constitutes polypharmacy.[27] In epidemiologic studies, polypharmacy is frequently defined as taking 5 or more medications. A 2003 survey of Medicare beneficiaries found that 46% of those surveyed met this definition for polypharmacy.[28] This condition is increasingly common as age-related comorbidities increase, putting older adults at risk for drug–drug and drug–disease interactions.[26,29] Polypharmacy may be compounded by the cascade effect, which refers to the use of medications to treat side effects caused by other medications.[21]

Substance use merits consideration in the older adult with sleep disruption, especially with respect to alcohol, caffeine, and tobacco consumption. Although acute consumption of alcohol may decrease sleep latency, it can increase arousal, leading to sleep that is of poorer quality and shorter duration. Alcohol can also exacerbate sleep-disordered breathing by decreasing pharyngeal muscle tone.[21] The stimulating effects of caffeine can increase sleep latency and number of arousals, leading to a shorter sleep duration.[21] Tobacco consumption has been associated with insomnia in several studies. Nicotine is a potential mediator of this effect, because it may promote wakefulness via an effect on acetylcholine transmission in the central nervous system.[21] However, a causal relationship has not been established.[30]

Psychosocial Factors

Psychosocial factors can impact sleep in older adults in multiple ways. Particularly relevant are the effects of caregiving, social isolation, loss of physical function, and bereavement.

Caregiving is common to the process of aging. Recent evidence from the National Alliance for Caregiving indicates that 43.5 million adults in the United States provided unpaid care to an adult or child in the prior year, and that approximately 1 in 5 of these caregivers was 65 years of age or older.[31] Providing intensive assistance can result in psychological stress, physical strain,

and erratic schedules, all of which may contribute to diminished sleep quality and disruptions in normal sleep patterns. In addition, caregiving is associated with depressed mood as well as erosion of physical health in the caregiver, further increasing the risk for sleep disturbance.[31,32] This can be a vicious cycle, because poor sleep can further erode physical health. Poor overnight sleep in caregivers has also been associated with reduced quality of life and increased inflammatory markers,[32] and is one of the strongest factors leading to institutionalization of a care recipient with dementia.[33]

Rates of social isolation increase after retirement and because 28.3% of adults aged 65 and older live alone.[34] Isolation can impact sleep through its effect on sleep hygiene and zeitgebers (see below). Sleep hygiene refers to a set of behavioral and environmental recommendations that are intended to promote sleep. These recommendations include avoiding caffeine or alcohol, getting regular exercise, and maintaining a regular sleep schedule while avoiding daytime naps.[35] However, the loss of a regular schedule and decreased social contact can lead to loneliness, inactivity, and boredom, potentially promoting behaviors like napping and irregular bedtimes that are counter to the promotion of healthy sleep. Zeitgebers are cues from the environment that entrain circadian rhythms to a 24-hour cycle length, promoting normal sleep–wake habits. Zeitgebers may be light based, but also include exercise, scheduled meals, and other social cues.[36] For socially isolated older adults, there may be inadequate exposure to zeitgebers, leading to irregular sleep–wake patterns. Previous evidence has shown that reports of insomnia and drowsiness were greater in older adults who felt socially isolated,[16] whereas activity and satisfaction with social life protected those aged 65 and older against insomnia symptoms.[37]

Loss of physical function is common among older adults. In 2009, 30% of Medicare enrollees aged 65 and older reported needing assistance with basic activities of daily living.[38] Although this loss has many implications for the health of older adults, it also affects their level of activity and exposure to zeitgebers. Thus, its effects on sleep are similar to those described for social isolation. In a National Sleep Foundation survey, older adults with decreased physical function (defined as difficulty walking one-half mile without help and/or difficulty walking a flight of stairs without help) were more likely to report insomnia symptoms (66% vs 44%) and daytime sleepiness (28% vs 12%).[16] Loss of physical function has also been associated significantly with the development of insomnia symptoms.[15]

Bereavement, the experience of losing a loved one to death,[39] is another factor that may contribute to sleep disturbance in older adults. A recent study found that more than 70% of older adults experienced bereavement over a 2.5-year period.[40] Bereavement is experienced more often in older adults because the loss of a spouse, siblings, or friends is common in this age group.[40,41] The grief experienced from such a loss has been associated with worsening health and functional impairment in older adults,[41] as well as an increased risk for the development of mood and anxiety disorders and substance abuse.[39] Importantly, bereavement in older adults has also been associated with increased loneliness and social isolation.[41] Thus, as with the other psychosocial factors mentioned, worsening health, psychiatric illness, and social isolation play a role in increasing the risk for sleep disturbance in bereavement. Multiple studies have shown an association between bereavement and sleep disturbance.[15,42,43] Older adults are at higher risk for complicated grief after bereavement, a condition in which grief symptoms are more severe and prolonged. The physical and mental health consequences of complicated grief are more severe than those associated with acute grief, and sleep impairment may be worse in these individuals.[41]

SLEEP DISORDERS IN OLDER ADULTS
Insomnia

A diagnosis of insomnia disorder is made clinically via a complaint of dissatisfaction with sleep quality and/or quantity, difficulty initiating or maintaining sleep, waking up too early, and/or nonrestorative or poor sleep, with a negative impact on daytime functioning and occurring at least 3 nights a week for more than 3 months.[44] The majority of insomnia diagnoses in older adults result from "comorbid insomnia."[45] This designation emphasizes the coexistence of insomnia with other medical and psychiatric comorbidities, and acknowledges that it may not be possible to determine whether insomnia is a cause or consequence of coexisting illnesses. As described, multimorbidity, polypharmacy and substance use, and psychosocial factors are common with the aging process and put older adults at risk for a diagnosis of insomnia.

The epidemiology of insomnia in older adults has been the subject of many studies, but summarizing the results is difficult because insomnia is defined differently in these studies. Some look only at insomnia symptoms (eg, difficulty initiating or maintaining sleep, complaints of nonrestorative sleep) with or without inclusion of criteria on frequency or severity of symptoms, whereas others

look at insomnia diagnosis but use different diagnostic criteria. It is widely accepted that insomnia symptoms increase with advancing age, with prevalence rates approaching 50% in adults aged 65 and older.[13] The annual incidence rates for insomnia symptoms have been estimated to be 3% to 5%,[15,22] and remission rates may be as high as 50% over 3 years.[15] With respect to an insomnia diagnosis, the prevalence has been estimated to be around 5%.[46] It is thought that prevalence of insomnia diagnosis increases after 45 years of age, but may remain the same in individuals after 65 years of age.[13] There are different theories about why the discrepancy between insomnia symptoms and diagnosis exists. Some authors have postulated that insomnia symptoms may be better tolerated or the daily demands less for older adults.[47] Others point to a "paradox of well-being" bias in questionnaires, in which older adults are less likely to report dissatisfaction or distress because their actual state of health exceeds the expected level.[11,48]

Obstructive Sleep Apnea

OSA increases with advancing age, with prevalence estimates differing depending on the definition used. Using a definition of 10 or more apneas and/or hypopneas per hour of sleep, OSA prevalence estimates in older adults may be as high as 70% in men and 56% in women. This is in contrast with prevalence estimates in the general adult population of 15% in men and 5% in women.[17] Although it is more common, this condition frequently goes undiagnosed because the phenotype of OSA can look very different in older adults. After the age of 60, the prevalence of OSA is equivalent in males and females, obesity is no longer a significant risk factor, and witnessed apneas and snoring are not reported as frequently.[49] Older adults are also more likely to present with more sleep-related complaints, including daytime sleepiness and nocturia.[50]

Older adults are at risk for OSA for several reasons. With aging, there is loss of tissue elasticity as well as sarcopenic muscle wasting.[11,49] There are also structural changes to the upper airway, including lengthening of soft palate and upper airway fat pad deposition.[11] These age-related changes increase the tendency for oropharyngeal collapse. In addition, ventilatory control instability may predispose older adults to apneic events.[11]

The negative consequences of OSA in older adults include excessive daytime sleepiness, decreased quality of life, neurocognitive impairment, nocturia, and worsening of cardiovascular disease, particularly hypertension, heart failure, and stroke. Diabetes mellitus and depression have also been found to be more common in older adults with OSA. The impact of untreated OSA in older adults on mortality is not clear.[17] However, older adults have similar adherence rates to treatment,[17,49] so there is no clear reason not to treat older adults with OSA.

Restless Leg Syndrome and Periodic Limb Movements of Sleep

RLS and PLMS increase in prevalence and severity with advancing age and have the potential to cause sleep complaints. RLS is a sensorimotor disorder characterized by unpleasant sensations in the limbs that cause an urge to move, especially in the evening. PLMS is a disorder characterized by repetitive episodes of stereotypic limb movements caused by muscle contractions during sleep.[17] In epidemiologic studies, the prevalence of RLS in older adults ranges from 9% to 20%, and PLMS is estimated to be present in 4% to 11% of older adults.[51] Of persons with RLS, 80% will have PLMS. However, PLMS occurs in the absence of RLS approximately 70% of the time.[2] These disorders can contribute to insomnia complaints through disruption of sleep onset or maintenance, as well as contributing to daytime drowsiness.

REM Sleep Behavior Disorder

RBD is a disorder resulting from a lack of the normal atonia seen in REM sleep. As a result, subjects with RBD are able to act out dreams in a way that can be violent and injurious. The majority of cases occur in older adults in the sixth or seventh decades of life, and the disorder is more common in men.[17] Although it may be idiopathic, RBD is associated with a neurodegenerative disorder in 48% to 73% of cases. Subjects with RBD may complain of sleep disruption or vivid dreams.[52]

TREATMENT OF SLEEP DISTURBANCES IN OLDER ADULTS

As we have seen in this article, sleep disturbance is highly pervasive among older adults owing to multiple factors common to the aging process. These include medical and psychiatric comorbidity, polypharmacy and substance use, psychosocial factors (such as caregiving, social isolation, and loss of physical function), and sleep disorders. With rates of multimorbidity increasing in older adults, it is likely that multiple processes in different domains are contributing to their sleep disturbance. Thus, sleep disturbance in this age group should be approached as a multifactorial

geriatric health condition.[2,4] The implication of this designation is that evaluation of sleep disturbance requires consideration of multiple risk factors and a multifaceted treatment approach. Similar approaches have been used in other multifactorial geriatric health conditions, including falls and delirium, and have successfully decreased occurrence of these events.[53,54]

SUMMARY

There are normal changes to sleep architecture throughout the lifespan. There is not, however, a decreased need for sleep and sleep disturbance is not an inherent part of the aging process. Sleep disturbance is common in older adults because aging is associated with an increasing prevalence of multimorbidity, polypharmacy, psychosocial factors affecting sleep, and certain primary sleep disorders. It is also associated with morbidity and mortality, making evaluation and management of sleep disturbance in older adults an important focus. Because many older adults will have several factors from different domains affecting their sleep, these complaints are best approached as a multifactorial geriatric health condition, necessitating a multifaceted treatment approach.

REFERENCES

1. Centers for Disease Control and Prevention. The state of aging and health in America 2013. Atlanta (GA): Centers for Disease Control and Prevention; 2013.
2. Vaz Fragoso CA, Gill TM. Sleep complaints in community-living older persons: a multifactorial geriatric syndrome. J Am Geriatr Soc 2007;55(11): 1853–66.
3. Marengoni A, Angleman S, Melis R, et al. Aging with multimorbidity: a systematic review of the literature. Ageing Res Rev 2011;10(4):430–9.
4. Inouye SK, Studenski S, Tinetti ME, et al. Geriatric syndromes: clinical, research, and policy implications of a core geriatric concept. J Am Geriatr Soc 2007;55(5):780–91.
5. Hirshkowitz M, Whiton K, Albert SM, et al. National Sleep Foundation's sleep time duration recommendations: methodology and results summary. Sleep Health 2015;1(1):40–3.
6. Avidan AY. Normal sleep in humans. In: Kryger MH, Avidan AY, Berry RB, editors. Atlas of clinical sleep medicine. 2nd edition. Philadelphia: Saunders; 2014. p. 65–97.
7. Ohayon MM, Carskadon MA, Guilleminault C, et al. Meta-analysis of quantitative sleep parameters from childhood to old age in healthy individuals: developing normative sleep values across the human lifespan. Sleep 2004;27(7):1255–73.

8. Klerman EB, Davis JB, Duffy JF, et al. Older people awaken more frequently but fall back asleep at the same rate as younger people. Sleep 2004;27(4):793–8.

9. Tranah G, Stone K, Ancoli-Israel S. Circadian rhythms in older adults. In: Kryger MH, Roth T, Dement WC, editors. Principles and practice of sleep medicine. 6th edition. Philadelphia: Elsevier; 2016. p. 1510–5.

10. Monk TH. Aging human circadian rhythms: conventional wisdom may not always be right. J Biol Rhythms 2005;20(4):366–74.

11. Bliwise DL. Normal aging. In: Kryger MH, Roth T, Dement WC, editors. Principles and practice of sleep medicine. 6th edition. Philadelphia: Elsevier; 2016. p. 25–38.

12. Cohen-Mansfield J, Perach R. Sleep duration, nap habits, and mortality in older persons. Sleep 2012;35(7):1003–9.

13. Ohayon MM. Epidemiology of insomnia: what we know and what we still need to learn. Sleep Med Rev 2002;6(2):97–111.

14. Johns MW. Sleepiness in different situations measured by the Epworth Sleepiness Scale. Sleep 1994;17(8):703–10.

15. Foley DJ, Monjan A, Simonsick EM, et al. Incidence and remission of insomnia among elderly adults: an epidemiologic study of 6,800 persons over three years. Sleep 1999;22(Suppl 2):S366–72.

16. National Sleep Foundation. Sleep in America Poll. 2003. Available at: https://sleepfoundation.org/sites/default/files/2003SleepPollExecSumm.pdf. Accessed July 13, 2016.

17. Bloom HG, Ahmed I, Alessi CA, et al. Evidence-based recommendations for the assessment and management of sleep disorders in older persons. J Am Geriatr Soc 2009;57(5):761–89.

18. Ancoli-Israel S, Kripke DF, Klauber MR, et al. Sleep-disordered breathing in community-dwelling elderly. Sleep 1991;14(6):486–95.

19. Reid KJ, Martinovich Z, Finkel S, et al. Sleep: a marker of physical and mental health in the elderly. Am J Geriatr Psychiatry 2006;14(10):860–6.

20. Dew MA, Hoch CC, Buysse DJ, et al. Healthy older adults' sleep predicts all-cause mortality at 4 to 19 years of follow-up. Psychosom Med 2003;65(1):63–73.

21. Barczi SR, Teodorescu MC. Psychiatric and medical comorbidities and effects of medications in older adults. In: Kryger MH, Roth T, Dement WC, editors. Principles and practices of sleep medicine. 6th edition. Philadelphia: Elsevier; 2016. p. 1484–95.

22. Morgan K, Clarke D. Risk factors for late-life insomnia in a representative general practice sample. Br J Gen Pract 1997;47(416):166–9.

23. Livingston G, Blizard B, Mann A. Does sleep disturbance predict depression in elderly people? A study in inner London. Br J Gen Pract 1993;43(376):445–8.

24. U.S. Department of Health and Human Services. Multiple chronic conditions - a strategic framework: optimum health and quality of life for individuals with multiple chronic conditions. Washington, DC: 2010. Available at: http://www.hhs.gov/sites/default/files/ash/initiatives/mcc/mcc_framework.pdf. Accessed November 14, 2016.

25. Salive ME. Multimorbidity in older adults. Epidemiol Rev 2013;35:75–83.

26. Qato DM, Wilder J, Schumm L, et al. Changes in prescription and over-the-counter medication and dietary supplement use among older adults in the United States, 2005 vs 2011. JAMA Intern Med 2016;176(4):473–82.

27. Fried TR, O'Leary J, Towle V, et al. Health outcomes associated with polypharmacy in community-dwelling older adults: a systematic review. J Am Geriatr Soc 2014;62(12):2261–72.

28. Safran DG, Neuman P, Schoen C, et al. Prescription drug coverage and seniors: findings from a 2003 national survey. Health Aff (Millwood) 2005;Suppl Web Exclusives:W5-152. W5-166.

29. Hines LE, Murphy JE. Potentially harmful drug–drug interactions in the elderly: a review. Am J Geriatr Pharmacother 2011;9(6):364–77.

30. Wetter DW, Young TB. The relation between cigarette smoking and sleep disturbance. Prev Med 1994;23(3):328–34.

31. AARP, National Alliance for Caregiving. Caregiving in the US. 2015. Available at: http://www.aarp.org/content/dam/aarp/ppi/2015/caregiving-in-the-united-states-2015-report-revised.pdf. Accessed July 13, 2016.

32. Peng HL, Chang YP. Sleep disturbance in family caregivers of individuals with dementia: a review of the literature. Perspect Psychiatr Care 2013;49(2):135–46.

33. Hope T, Keene J, Gedling K, et al. Predictors of institutionalization for people with dementia living at home with a carer. Int J Geriatr Psychiatry 1998;13(10):682–90.

34. West LA, Cole S, Goodkind D, et al. 65+ in the United States: 2010. Washington, DC: United States Census Bureau; 2014.

35. Irish LA, Kline CE, Gunn HE, et al. The role of sleep hygiene in promoting public health: a review of empirical evidence. Sleep Med Rev 2015;22:23–36.

36. Gabehart RJ, Van Dongen, Hans PA. Circadian rhythms in sleepiness, alertness, and performance. In: Kryger MH, Roth T, Dement WC, editors. Principles and practice of sleep medicine. 6th edition. Philadelphia: Elsevier; 2016. p. 388–95.

37. Ohayon MM, Zulley J, Guilleminault C, et al. How age and daytime activities are related to insomnia in the general population: consequences for older people. J Am Geriatr Soc 2001;49(4):360–6.

38. Federal Interagency Forum on Aging Statistics. Older Americans 2012: key indicators of well-being.

Available at: http://www.agingstats.gov/main_site/data/2012_documents/docs/entirechartbook.pdf. Accessed June 26, 2016.

39. Shear MK. Clinical practice. Complicated grief. N Engl J Med 2015;372(2):153–60.

40. Williams BR, Sawyer Baker P, Allman RM, et al. Bereavement among African American and white older adults. J Aging Health 2007;19(2):313–33.

41. Shear MK, Ghesquiere A, Glickman K. Bereavement and complicated grief. Curr Psychiatry Rep 2013; 15(11):406.

42. Boelen PA, Lancee J. Sleep difficulties are correlated with emotional problems following loss and residual symptoms of effective prolonged grief disorder treatment. Depress Res Treat 2013;2013: 739804.

43. Byrne GJ, Raphael B. The psychological symptoms of conjugal bereavement in elderly men over the first 13 months. Int J Geriatr Psychiatry 1997;12(2):241–51.

44. American Psychiatric Association. Diagnostic and statistical manual of mental disorders. 5th edition. Arlington (VA): American Psychiatric Publishing; 2013.

45. National Institutes of Health. National Institutes of Health State of the Science Conference statement on Manifestations and management of chronic insomnia in adults, June 13-15, 2005. Sleep 2005; 28(9):1049–57.

46. Gooneratne NS, Vitiello MV. Sleep in older adults: normative changes, sleep disorders, and treatment options. Clin Geriatr Med 2014;30(3):591–627.

47. Roth T, Coulouvrat C, Hajak G, et al. Prevalence and perceived health associated with insomnia based on DSM-IV-TR; International Statistical Classification of diseases and related health problems, Tenth Revision; and Research Diagnostic Criteria/International Classification of Sleep Disorders, Second Edition criteria: results from the America Insomnia Survey. Biol Psychiatry 2011; 69(6):592–600.

48. Levy BR. Mind matters: cognitive and physical effects of aging self-stereotypes. J Gerontol B Psychol Sci Soc Sci 2003;58(4):P203–11.

49. Phillips B. Obstructive sleep apnea in the elderly. In: Kryger MH, Roth T, Dement WC, editors. Principles and practices of sleep medicine. 6th edition. Philadelphia: Elsevier; 2016. p. 1496–502.

50. Endeshaw Y. Clinical characteristics of obstructive sleep apnea in community-dwelling older adults. J Am Geriatr Soc 2006;54(11):1740–4.

51. Hornyak M, Trenkwalder C. Restless legs syndrome and periodic limb movement disorder in the elderly. J Psychosom Res 2004;56(5):543–8.

52. Schenck CH, Mahowald MW. REM sleep behavior disorder: clinical, developmental, and neuroscience perspectives 16 years after its formal identification in SLEEP. Sleep 2002;25(2):120–38.

53. Inouye SK, Bogardus ST Jr, Charpentier PA, et al. A multicomponent intervention to prevent delirium in hospitalized older patients. N Engl J Med 1999; 340(9):669–76.

54. Tinetti ME, Baker DI, McAvay G, et al. A multifactorial intervention to reduce the risk of falling among elderly people living in the community. N Engl J Med 1994; 331(13):821–7.

The Cost of Insomnia and the Benefit of Increased Access to Evidence-Based Treatment

Cognitive Behavioral Therapy for Insomnia

Sarah A. Reynolds, NP*, Matthew R. Ebben, PhD

KEYWORDS

- Insomnia • Prevalence • Cost • Pharmacology • CBT-I • Patient access

KEY POINTS

- Insomnia is a costly condition associated with direct and indirect costs estimated at more than $150 billion in the US annually.
- Most insomnia-related expenses are indirect costs. Given that insomnia is inexpensive to treat, increased access to treatment has the potential to generate substantial cost savings.
- Behavioral treatments for insomnia are favorable because they address the underlying problem and do not have many of the health risks associated with sedative-hypnotic use.
- CBT-I is a nonpharmacologic intervention that safely and cost-effectively treats insomnia.
- In the interest of minimizing cost and the lack of CBT-I providers, self-administered, group, and stepped care delivery of this intervention have been developed.

PREVALENCE AND COST OF INSOMNIA

The prevalence of insomnia is high, between 4.7% and 22.1% depending on the diagnostic criteria used.[1–4] Insomnia is associated with decreased quality of life, accidents, increased psychiatric and somatic comorbidities, and problems with work performance.[5] There is also a large financial cost associated with insomnia, although it is difficult to estimate because most of the expense is from indirect costs, and the criteria for insomnia-related expenses vary between studies. The cost of direct insomnia treatment has been estimated to account for only 4% to 16.7% of the total cost.[6,7]

Stoller's[7] 1994 analysis remains one of the most frequently cited estimates of annual costs associated with insomnia in US dollars. Based on her calculations, the annual cost associated with insomnia in the United States has been estimated to be $92.45 to $107.53 billion. To achieve this figure, Stoller[7] combines the estimated expenses of direct medical costs, lost productivity, insomnia-related depression and alcohol abuse, and accidents. The main critique of this estimate is that it may have overestimated costs based on the high prevalence rate used for the calculations. However, it must be noted that estimated indirect costs associated with absenteeism and increased health care utilization were not included in the total cost. Subsequent research has found these expenses to be substantial.[8] Given that all indirect costs of insomnia were not accounted for, it is fair to consider Stoller's[7] estimate as an equivalent or conservative estimate of overall costs.

Center for Sleep Medicine, Weill Cornell Medical College, 425 East 61st Street, 5th Floor, New York, NY 10065, USA
* Corresponding author.
E-mail address: sar9072@med.cornell.edu

Sleep Med Clin 12 (2017) 39–46
http://dx.doi.org/10.1016/j.jsmc.2016.10.011
1556-407X/17/© 2016 Elsevier Inc. All rights reserved.

Assuming that insomnia-related expenses are steady, Stoller's[7] figures can be adjusted to an annual cost of $150.36 to $174.89 billion when adjusted for inflation to 2016 US dollars (inflation calculated using online calculator: bls.ghttp://www.bls.gov/data/inflation_calculator.htmov). This is 0.95% of the predicted US gross domestic product for 2016, based on the predicted figure of $18,494 billion (http://www.statista.com/statistics/216985/forecast-of-us-gross-domestic-product/).

Other calculations of the financial costs of insomnia have been done. Daley and colleagues[6] estimated the total direct and indirect costs of insomnia in Quebec to be equivalent to 1% of the province's gross domestic product. In this study, the three greatest costs associated with insomnia were lost productivity, absenteeism, and use of alcohol as a sleep aid. Together, these three indirect costs comprised 96% of the total cost of insomnia in the population over 1 year. This reinforces the importance of including indirect costs in assessing the true price of insomnia to society. A 2011 study estimated the annual cost of decreased productivity caused by insomnia in the United States to be $63.2 billion.[9] Insomnia-related accidents and errors in the workplace in the United States were estimated to have an annual cost of $31.1 billion.[10] Anyone either suffering from or seeing patients suffering from insomnia can understand how easily reduced focus caused by lack of sleep can translate into reduced productivity and increased workplace errors.

Pollack and colleagues[11] compared the health care utilization and productivity costs between patients with a diagnosis of insomnia and/or a prescription for a sleep medication with patients with neither, and found that costs were 24% greater for the insomnia and/or sleep medication group when controlling for comorbidities. Prescription of a sleep medication served as a proxy for an actual insomnia diagnosis in this study because of the frequent association of insomnia with other conditions for which a visit may be billed. The difference in cost within the insomnia group between those being prescribed medications and those not was not reported; therefore, this study did not determine whether being prescribed a sleep medication was associated with any change in cost. However, another study that looked at health care utilization costs of people newly diagnosed with insomnia found that, among the insomnia group, patients who were prescribed sleep medication actually had a higher increase in cost over the course of 1 year when compared with those who were not prescribed medication.[12] Whether patients used any other treatments is not known. The expenses associated with insomnia are a catch 22. Untreated insomnia results in the high direct and indirect costs mentioned previously. However, if insomnia is treated with prescription medication, to the extent to which patients need to continue pharmacotherapy to receive lasting benefit, the cost of medication becomes an ongoing expenditure. Insomnia tends to be a persistent condition, which can significantly contribute to its price tag. A 3-year survey of people reporting insomnia at baseline found 74% of respondents to have insomnia after 1 year and 46% still had insomnia after 3 years.[13] Of the 54% of respondents who had remission, 27% had a relapse by the time of the 3-year follow-up. Another longitudinal survey found that, of the people who had insomnia at baseline, more than half of them reported having insomnia 10 years later.[14]

GOALS OF TREATMENT

Although insomnia is characterized by poor sleep quality and/or inadequate time spent sleeping because of difficulty falling asleep or remaining asleep within the desired sleep period, it is often, in a broader sense, a state of psychophysiologic hyperarousal that persists during daytime and nighttime.[15] People suffering from insomnia also experience impaired daytime functioning and often fatigue.[16] Often, the impaired sleep at night becomes the primary focus of efforts by the sufferer to correct. This often leads to behaviors that inadvertently perpetuate insomnia, such as devoting excessive time, effort, and thought to trying to attain more sleep.[17]

The main goals of treating insomnia are to improve sleep quality and daytime function.[18] In many studies of insomnia treatment with patients reporting subjective improvement in sleep quality and an increase in subjective sleep time, a significant increase in objectively measured sleep time is not usually seen.[19] Still, the benefits of improved subjective sleep have been associated with improvement in other objectively tested variables. Belief that one had good quality sleep, regardless of actual sleep quality, was associated with better performance on cognitive function tests the following day.[20]

The secondary goals of treatment are to lessen the risk of somatic and psychiatric comorbidities and injuries and accidents associated with insomnia. A third goal of insomnia treatment is to lessen the associated financial losses to the individual and society.

LIMITATIONS OF SEDATIVE-HYPNOTIC USE

The predominant treatment of insomnia is sedative-hypnotics.[21] Although the number of outpatient visits to physicians with a primary complaint of insomnia increased by 13% from 1999 to 2010, the number of prescriptions for sleep medications increased by 293% over the same time period.[22] This indicates a disproportionate increase in hypnotic use in insomnia sufferers. Part of this increase may be caused by the release of blockbuster drugs, such as eszopiclone (Lunesta), ramelteon (Rozerem), and zolpidem controlled release (Ambien CR), and the availability of generic zolpidem during this time period in the United States. However, it is worth noting that drastic increase in prescription sleep aid use may reflect an increase in the use of prescription sleep aids for occasional sleeplessness in addition to treating persistent insomnia.[23] However, anyone who watched television in the United States around the time eszopiclone, ramelteon, and zolpidem controlled release were released can likely remember the advertisements, which probably had an effect on prescribing trends.

In terms of the treatment efficacy of medication for difficulty sleeping, a meta-analysis on pharmacologic treatment of chronic insomnia determined that benzodiazepines and nonbenzodiazepines were effective treatments. However, they were both found to have significantly higher adverse events when compared with placebo. There continues to be a lack of evidence that sleep medication use improves daytime function or health-related quality of life.[24,25] Of note, only 18 of the 105 studies analyzed had a duration greater than or equal to 30 days and only three studies were 12 weeks or longer.[26] Therefore, little is known about tolerance and the long-term effects of hypnotics.

Given the high persistence and relapse rate of insomnia, longer studies are ideal in assessing the effectiveness of any intervention. The actual use of sleep medications in people with chronic insomnia can last for years. One small survey of patients who had been treated for insomnia at a multidisciplinary sleep center found that 53% of the respondents continued to use sleep medications for the 3 to 5 years that had lapsed since their initial treatment.[27] A Japanese study of psychiatric outpatients with comorbid insomnia who were regular benzodiazepine receptor agonist users found that 30.5% of their sample used these medications for 1 to 5 years and 46.6% used them for greater than 5 years.[28] Many patients continue to take sleep medications for many years even when the drug has not improved their sleep.

Among a group of patients who had moderate to severe insomnia for an average of almost 10 years, 60.4% were regular users of sleep medications and 13.9% used sleep medications occasionally.[29] All who were on prescription or nonprescription sleep aids were determined to have pharmacotherapeutic failure.[29]

Multiple health risks and increased mortality have been associated with sleep medication use.[24] People taking sedatives are at increased risk for adverse cognitive and psychomotor events and daytime fatigue.[30] An increased risk of developing psychiatric disorders has been linked with sleep medication use,[31] which is problematic because there is a high association of psychiatric comorbidity with insomnia. Insomnia is often comorbid with sleep-disordered breathing and the common symptoms of awakenings in the night and nonrestorative sleep make it easy for sleep-disordered breathing to be misinterpreted as insomnia. Among a group of patients with chronic, drug resistant insomnia, polysomnography (PSG) found that 77.6% had obstructive sleep apnea and 22.4% had upper airway resistance syndrome.[29] Use of sedating medications with uncontrolled sleep-disordered breathing can worsen its severity. Use of sleep medication has also been associated with increased risk for infections and cancer.[24,32]

COGNITIVE BEHAVIORAL THERAPY FOR INSOMNIA

Cognitive behavioral therapy for insomnia (CBT-I) is an intervention that helps the patient improve their sleep by teaching them to change dysfunctional thought patterns and behaviors, which are contributing to their poor sleep. The components of CBT-I are stimulus control, sleep-restriction therapy, cognitive therapy for dysfunctional thoughts, sleep hygiene, and relaxation techniques.[33]

The National Institutes of Health, American Academy of Sleep Medicine, and the American College of Physicians all recommend CBT-I as first-line treatment of insomnia.[1–3] Multiple meta-analyses have found CBT-I to be an effective treatment of insomnia.[19,34] A meta-analysis has also found that CBT-I is effective in treating insomnia that is comorbid with psychiatric and medical conditions.[35] Although the clinical phase of the intervention typically lasts no more than several weeks, improvement in sleep time has been seen to continue to improve for up to 1 year.[19] The treatment effects of CBT-I have been found to be sustained for up to 3 years.[36]

A study of the effect of CBT-I for comorbid insomnia and posttraumatic stress disorder showed that CBT-I, when compared with a waitlist control, yielded improvements in sleep time by sleep diary and PSG. The CBT-I group also had a decrease in disruptive nocturnal behaviors and an improvement in interpersonal functioning. Of note, all treatment benefits were maintained at 6-month follow-up. Improvements were also seen in posttraumatic stress disorder symptoms and nightmares; however, these variables improved equally in the control group.[37] There is also evidence that the risk for medical comorbidities associated with insomnia can be reduced. A randomized controlled trial on older adults with chronic insomnia and elevated risk for diabetes and cardiovascular disease showed improvement in sleep and biomarker levels associated with co-morbid disease risk with CBT-I.[38]

There is little risk associated with CBT-I. There is usually a period of acute sleep deprivation associated with the sleep-restriction therapy during which the patient may be at increased risk for accident or errors.[39] This sleep deprivation is contraindicated in bipolar disorder with mania and may not be appropriate in people with severe illness.

COST EFFECTIVENESS OF INSOMNIA TREATMENT

CBT-I is an intervention that alleviates suffering (over the long-term, but often creates short-term discomfort), increases safety, diminishes a risk factor for chronic disease, has minimal potential for harm, and requires nothing more than the time of a skilled professional and the determination of the patient. Discussion of the cost effectiveness of treating insomnia, however, adds to the support for CBT-I. Three studies[40–42] have shown evidence that CBT-I is cost effective solely on the savings in health care utilization costs. Lost productivity may be the greatest indirect cost associated with insomnia.[6] To illustrate the productivity savings that CBT-I treatment would yield would potentially make a stronger case for payers to allocate more resources toward making CBT-I accessible. A study of an Internet-delivered CBT-I program estimated at costing $245 per person yielded a net cost savings of $512 per person over 6 months because of increased productivity and decreased absenteeism.[43]

Comparing the cost effectiveness of behavioral versus pharmacologic interventions for insomnia is complicated because of the number of indirect costs that are associated with both. Pharmacologic and behavioral treatments for insomnia have been found to be cost-effective with analysis of direct costs and utilization of health care, but inclusion of the cost of adverse effects of sleep medications is lacking.[44] When formulating a true

cost-effectiveness analysis of treatment options for insomnia, the variables that must be considered go far beyond improvement of sleep and daytime function. Measuring the impact on indirect costs in relation to specific interventions further supports the use of CBT-I. McCrae and coworkers[42] conducted a small experiment comparing subsequent health care utilization costs between people completing a brief CBT-I series and people who did not complete treatment and found that the health care utilization expenses were lower in the group that completed the treatment. For insomnia with comorbid depression there is evidence that including CBT-I plus standard treatment is more cost effective than standard treatment alone.[45]

Only one study, thus far, has compared the cost-effectiveness of CBT-I versus sedative-hypnotic use for insomnia treatment with consideration of indirect costs.[46] Tannenbaum and colleagues[46] compared the cost effectiveness of CBT-I versus sedative hypnotic use in Medicare patients. When including the expenses associated with falls for insomnia treated with CBT-I, insomnia treated with sedative-hypnotics, and untreated insomnia, they found that sedative-hypnotic treatment is 1.669 times more costly than CBT-I and no treatment is 1.741 times more costly than CBT-I.

RE-EVALUATION OF DIRECT COSTS OF INSOMNIA TREATMENT

The practice of placing a monetary value on all health care interventions has unfortunately created the drive to minimize the reliance on what may be perceived as a high utilization of clinician hours. This certainly adds to the explanation of why sedative-hypnotics are so highly used versus CBT-I. Because of the common presumption that the direct cost of CBT-I is more expensive than pharmacotherapy, it is worthwhile to re-examine this in terms of chronicity. A very conservative hypothetical scenario is presented.

It is difficult to describe the cost of CBT-I sessions in the United States because of variations in payer reimbursement. The 2016 Medicare reimbursement for psychotherapy sessions is $60.03 for a 30-minute session and $119.39 for a 60-minute session. Based on a 60-minute initial session and five 30-minute follow-up sessions, the average Medicare cost for in-person CBT-I is $419.54 (**Table 1**).

The direct expense of medication use is variable, although it is thought to be low, because the most common agents used are available as generics. Generic zolpidem is available at a low cost, with a 30-day supply costing from $6.90 (with use of an Internet-available coupon) to $159.00 at major

Table 1 Insomnia treatment estimated direct costs	
Pharmacologic	**3 y**
Generic zolpidem, 10 mg at $6.90 per 30-d supply	36.5 prescriptions = $251.85
Level 3 initial visit at $77.75	× 1 = $77.75
Level 2 follow-up visit at $25.80	× 2 = $51.60
Total	$381.20
CBT-I	**3 y**
60-min psychotherapy session at $119.39	× 1 = $119.39
30-min psychotherapy session at $60.03	× 5 = $300.15
Total	$419.54

Adapted from http://www.goodrx.com/ambien. Accessed August 7, 2016; and http://gi.org/wp-content/uploads/2016/01/Medicare-2016-RVU-breakdown-Nov-20152.pdf. Accessed August 7, 2016.

chain retailers.[47] The newer medication suvorexant, which is not available in the generic form, costs $291.87 to $376.00 for a 30-day supply of 20-mg tablets at major chain retailers.[48]

Based on the lowest prescription cost for generic zolpidem, 10-mg tablets, 3 years of nightly usage would add up to $251.85. The addition of minimal monitoring office visits (one level 3 initial visit and two level 2 follow-up visits) based on the 2016 Medicare reimbursement schedule[49] adds $129.35 to the 3-year direct expense cost for a total of $381.20 (see **Table 1**). A 3-year period was used because that is the longest amount of time that CBT-I treatment effects have been found to be sustained. The effects of CBT-I for periods longer than 3 years have not been reported. Were nightly zolpidem use to continue for 5 years with an additional two level 2 follow-up visits, the combined costs would be $600.70. Therefore, based on our rough cost estimate, CBT-I is likely to be more cost effective over time than hypnotic medication for the treatment of insomnia. However, pharmacotherapy is likely to have less direct treatment costs for acute insomnia (as long as maladaptive behaviors do not occur causing the insomnia to become chronic).

BARRIERS TO COGNITIVE BEHAVIORAL THERAPY FOR INSOMNIA AND EFFORTS TO INCREASE ACCESS

Although CBT-I is the gold standard[1–3] for treatment of primary and comorbid insomnia, there is

a need to increase its availability to patients. The two major barriers to more widespread use of CBT-I are the lack of CBT-I practitioners and that many physicians are not aware of its efficacy.[50] Despite the expectations of many patients and referring providers, not all sleep clinics offer CBT-I. For example, of all the sleep programs within the Veterans Affairs system, only 54% of these programs offer CBT-I.[51]

In the interest of increasing access and reducing cost, many groups have developed simplified or abbreviated versions of CBT-I, training more master's level practitioners including nurse practitioners and physician assistants,[52] and/or using technology, such as Interned-based programs.

A randomized controlled trial of Internet-based CBT-I intervention showed that the improvements were sustained for 3 years, and the intervention group used less sleep medications than the control group.[53] A meta-analysis on 15 studies of CBT-I found that it is effective in improving total sleep time, sleep efficiency, insomnia severity, and depression severity when compared with control subjects, and all but total sleep time were maintained at up to 48 weeks posttreatment.[54]

Community-based workshops have also been demonstrated to be effective and cost effective.[12,41] A small study on sleep-restriction therapy alone on patients with an objective total sleep time of less than 6 hours by PSG found improvements in subjective insomnia severity and subjective total sleep time at 3 months.[39] However, this study did not include a PSG measurement at the 3-month mark.

A stepped care model of behavioral insomnia treatment has been proposed as a way to quickly increase access to cost-effective, evidence-based care.[55] Most patients would be triaged to self-administered CBT-I as the first step, which can be made readily available for anyone who needs it, and sessions with trained providers and behavioral specialists would be arranged for those who self-administered care is not suitable or has not yielded adequate improvement.[55] Stepped care models have been tested in other psychiatric disorders. A meta-analysis has found that stepped care is equal to care as usual for depression and superior to care as usual for anxiety.[56] Payers should cover the cost of access to evidence-based self-administered CBT-I. However, it is also important that they do not turn coverage of online CBT-I into a barrier for clinician-administered treatment.

SUMMARY

The recognition of insomnia as a separate comorbid condition rather than a secondary condition of mood and anxiety disorders and other health problems points to the need for a durable treatment rather than temporary symptomatic relief. Insomnia medications are most suitable for alleviation of transient sleep disturbances in people who otherwise have a low degree of dysfunctional sleep-related thoughts and behaviors.

Based on current data available, CBT-I is more effective, safer, and more cost-effective than pharmacotherapy or nontreatment of insomnia. Despite this, and recommendations from multiple national and international institutions for CBT-I as first-line therapy, nontreatment and pharmacotherapy continue to be the predominant treatment approach for insomnia sufferers. The main reasons for this are lack of awareness of CBT-I and lack of treatment providers. A more comprehensive cost-effectiveness analysis on insomnia treatment can be expected to demonstrate that CBT-I is less expensive than pharmacologic treatment. This is because of a reduction in indirect and long-term costs of insomnia.

Several therapy sessions of CBT-I are probably not more expensive than pharmacotherapy (based on our rough calculations). However, self-administered, group, and stepped care models of CBT-I are being developed and evaluated as a means to make this intervention have a lower direct cost, and more critically, available to meet the needs of the population. A large initial investment would expedite the availability of evidence-based programs. The stakeholders, aside from the sufferers themselves, who stand to reap the most financial benefit from improved treatment of insomnia are employers and health insurance companies. Growing evidence of the superiority of CBT-I over nontreatment and pharmacotherapy with regard to recovery of the financial losses associated with indirect costs of lost productivity, absenteeism, and increased health care utilization because of comorbidities and injuries can help influence key stakeholders.

REFERENCES

1. National Institutes of Health. National Institutes of Health State of the Science Conference statement on manifestations and management of chronic insomnia in adults, June 13-15, 2005. Sleep 2005; 28(9):1049–57.
2. Schutte-Rodin S, Broch L, Buysse D, et al. Clinical guideline for the evaluation and management of chronic insomnia in adults. J Clin Sleep Med 2008; 4(5):487–504.
3. Qaseem A, Kansagara D, Forciea MA, et al, Clinical Guidelines Committee of the American College of Physicians. Management of chronic insomnia disorder in adults: a clinical practice guideline from the American College of Physicians. Ann Intern Med 2016;165(2):125–33.
4. Chung KF, Yeung WF, Ho FY, et al. Cross-cultural and comparative epidemiology of insomnia: the Diagnostic and Statistical Manual (DSM), International Classification of Diseases (ICD) and International Classification of Sleep Disorders (ICSD). Sleep Med 2015;16(4):477–82.
5. Leger D, Bayon V. Societal costs of insomnia. Sleep Med Rev 2010;14(6):379–89.
6. Daley M, Morin CM, LeBlanc M, et al. The economic burden of insomnia: direct and indirect costs for individuals with insomnia syndrome, insomnia symptoms, and good sleepers. Sleep 2009;32(1): 55–64.
7. Stoller MK. Economic effects of insomnia. Clin Ther 1994;16(5):873–97 [discussion: 854].
8. Ozminkowski RJ, Wang S, Walsh JK. The direct and indirect costs of untreated insomnia in adults in the United States. Sleep 2007;30(3):263–73.
9. Kessler RC, Berglund PA, Coulouvrat C, et al. Insomnia and the performance of US workers: results from the America Insomnia Survey. Sleep 2011;34(9):1161–71.
10. Shahly V, Berglund PA, Coulouvrat C, et al. The associations of insomnia with costly workplace accidents and errors: results from the America Insomnia Survey. Arch Gen Psychiatry 2012;69(10):1054–63.
11. Pollack M, Seal B, Joish VN, et al. Insomnia-related comorbidities and economic costs among a commercially insured population in the United States. Curr Med Res Opin 2009;25(8):1901–11.
12. Anderson LH, Whitebird RR, Schultz J, et al. Healthcare utilization and costs in persons with insomnia in a managed care population. Am J Manag Care 2014;20(5):e157–65.
13. Morin CM, Belanger L, LeBlanc M, et al. The natural history of insomnia: a population-based 3-year longitudinal study. Arch Intern Med 2009;169(5):447–53.
14. Janson C, Lindberg E, Gislason T, et al. Insomnia in men: a 10-year prospective population based study. Sleep 2001;24(4):425–30.
15. Basta M, Chrousos GP, Vela-Bueno A, et al. Chronic insomnia and stress system. Sleep Med Clin 2007; 2(2):279–91.
16. Riedel BW, Lichstein KL. Insomnia and daytime functioning. Sleep Med Rev 2000;4(3):277–98.
17. Spielman AJ. Assessment of insomnia. Clin Psychol Rev 1986;6(1):11–25.
18. Edinger JD, Buysse DJ, Deriy L, et al. Quality measures for the care of patients with insomnia. J Clin Sleep Med 2015;11(3):311–34.
19. Okajima I, Komada Y, Inoue Y. A meta-analysis on the treatment effectiveness of cognitive behavioral therapy for primary insomnia. Sleep Biol Rhythms 2011;9(1):24–34.

20. Draganich C, Erdal K. Placebo sleep affects cognitive functioning. J Exp Psychol Learn Mem Cogn 2014;40(3):857–64.
21. Ma Y, Dong M, Mita C, et al. Publication analysis on insomnia: how much has been done in the past two decades? Sleep Med 2015;16(7):820–6.
22. Ford ES, Wheaton AG, Cunningham TJ, et al. Trends in outpatient visits for insomnia, sleep apnea, and prescriptions for sleep medications among US adults: findings from the National Ambulatory Medical Care survey 1999-2010. Sleep 2014;37(8):1283–93.
23. Moloney ME, Konrad TR, Zimmer CR. The medicalization of sleeplessness: a public health concern. Am J Public Health 2011;101(8):1429–33.
24. Kripke DF. Hypnotic drug risks of mortality, infection, depression, and cancer: but lack of benefit. F1000Res 2016;5:918.
25. DiBonaventura M, Richard L, Kumar M, et al. The association between insomnia and insomnia treatment side effects on health status, work productivity, and healthcare resource use. PLoS One 2015;10(10): e0137117.
26. Buscemi N, Vandermeer B, Friesen C, et al. The efficacy and safety of drug treatments for chronic insomnia in adults: a meta-analysis of RCTs. J Gen Intern Med 2007;22(9):1335–50.
27. Rosenthal LD, Dolan DC, Taylor DJ, et al. Long-term follow-up of patients with insomnia. Proc (Bayl Univ Med Cent) 2008;21(3):264–5.
28. Murakoshi A, Takaesu Y, Komada Y, et al. Prevalence and associated factors of hypnotics dependence among Japanese outpatients with psychiatric disorders. Psychiatry Res 2015;230(3):958–63.
29. Krakow B, Ulibarri VA, McIver ND. Pharmacotherapeutic failure in a large cohort of patients with insomnia presenting to a sleep medicine center and laboratory: subjective pretest predictions and objective diagnoses. Mayo Clin Proc 2014;89(12): 1608–20.
30. Glass J, Lanctot KL, Herrmann N, et al. Sedative hypnotics in older people with insomnia: meta-analysis of risks and benefits. BMJ 2005;331(7526):1169.
31. Chung KH, Li CY, Kuo SY, et al. Risk of psychiatric disorders in patients with chronic insomnia and sedative-hypnotic prescription: a nationwide population-based follow-up study. J Clin Sleep Med 2015;11(5):543–51.
32. Kripke DF, Langer RD, Kline LE. Hypnotics' association with mortality or cancer: a matched cohort study. BMJ open 2012;2(1):e000850.
33. Ebben MR, Narizhnaya M. Cognitive and behavioral treatment options for insomnia. Mt Sinai J Med 2012; 79(4):512–23.
34. Smith MT, Perlis ML, Park A, et al. Comparative meta-analysis of pharmacotherapy and behavior therapy for persistent insomnia. Am J Psychiatry 2002;159(1):5–11.
35. Geiger-Brown JM, Rogers VE, Liu W, et al. Cognitive behavioral therapy in persons with comorbid insomnia: a meta-analysis. Sleep Med Rev 2015; 23:54–67.
36. Backhaus J, Hohagen F, Voderholzer U, et al. Long-term effectiveness of a short-term cognitive-behavioral group treatment for primary insomnia. Eur Arch Psychiatry Clin Neurosci 2001;251(1):35–41.
37. Talbot LS, Maguen S, Metzler TJ, et al. Cognitive behavioral therapy for insomnia in posttraumatic stress disorder: a randomized controlled trial. Sleep 2014;37(2):327–41.
38. Carroll JE, Seeman TE, Olmstead R, et al. Improved sleep quality in older adults with insomnia reduces biomarkers of disease risk: pilot results from a randomized controlled comparative efficacy trial. Psychoneuroendocrinology 2015;55: 184–92.
39. Kyle SD, Miller CB, Rogers Z, et al. Sleep restriction therapy for insomnia is associated with reduced objective total sleep time, increased daytime somnolence, and objectively impaired vigilance: implications for the clinical management of insomnia disorder. Sleep 2014;37(2):229–37.
40. Morgan K, Dixon S, Mathers N, et al. Psychological treatment for insomnia in the regulation of long-term hypnotic drug use. Health Technol Assess 2004;8(8):iii–iv, 1–68.
41. Bonin EM, Beecham J, Swift N, et al. Psycho-educational CBT-Insomnia workshops in the community. A cost-effectiveness analysis alongside a randomised controlled trial. Behav Res Ther 2014;55:40–7.
42. McCrae CS, Bramoweth AD, Williams J, et al. Impact of brief cognitive behavioral treatment for insomnia on health care utilization and costs. J Clin Sleep Med 2014;10(2):127–35.
43. Thiart H, Ebert DD, Lehr D, et al. Internet-based cognitive behavioral therapy for insomnia: a health economic evaluation. Sleep 2016;39(10):1769–78.
44. Wickwire EM, Shaya FT, Scharf SM. Health economics of insomnia treatments: the return on investment for a good night's sleep. Sleep Med Rev 2015; 30:72–82.
45. Watanabe N, Furukawa TA, Shimodera S, et al. Cost-effectiveness of cognitive behavioral therapy for insomnia comorbid with depression: analysis of a randomized controlled trial. Psychiatry Clin Neurosci 2015;69(6):335–43.
46. Tannenbaum C, Diaby V, Singh D, et al. Sedative-hypnotic medicines and falls in community-dwelling older adults: a cost-effectiveness (decision-tree) analysis from a US Medicare perspective. Drugs Aging 2015;32(4):305–14.
47. Available at: http://www.goodrx.com/ambien. Accessed August 7, 2016.
48. Available at: http://www.goodrx.com/belsomra?drugname=belsomra. Accessed August 7, 2016.

49. Available at: http://gi.org/wp-content/uploads/2016/01/Medicare-2016-RVU-breakdown-Nov-20152.pdf. Accessed August 7, 2016.

50. Conroy DA, Ebben MR. Referral practices for cognitive behavioral therapy for insomnia: a survey study. Behav Neurol 2015;2015:819402.

51. Sarmiento K, Rossettie J, Stepnowsky C, et al. The state of Veterans Affairs sleep medicine programs: 2012 inventory results. Sleep Breath 2016;20(1):379–82.

52. Fields BG, Schutte-Rodin S, Perlis ML, et al. Master's-level practitioners as cognitive behavioral therapy for insomnia providers: an underutilized resource. J Clin Sleep Med 2013;9(10):1093–6.

53. Blom K, Jernelöv S, Rück C, et al. Three-year follow-up of insomnia and hypnotics after controlled internet treatment for insomnia. Sleep 2016;39(6):1267–74.

54. Seyffert M, Lagisetty P, Landgraf J, et al. Internet-delivered cognitive behavioral therapy to treat insomnia: a systematic review and meta-analysis. PLoS One 2016;11(2):e0149139.

55. Espie CA. "Stepped care": a health technology solution for delivering cognitive behavioral therapy as a first line insomnia treatment. Sleep 2009;32(12):1549–58.

56. Ho FY, Yeung WF, Ng TH, et al. The efficacy and cost-effectiveness of stepped care prevention and treatment for depressive and/or anxiety disorders: a systematic review and meta-analysis. Sci Rep 2016;6:29281.

Hypersomnia
Evaluation, Treatment, and Social and Economic Aspects

Prabhjyot Saini, MSPH[a],*, David B. Rye, MD, PhD[b]

KEYWORDS

- Idiopathic hypersomnia • Sleep drunkenness • Narcolepsy • Hypersomnolence disorder
- Excessive daytime sleepiness • Quality of life • Economic costs • Psychosocial factors

KEY POINTS

- The literative classification of hypersomnolence disorders renders it difficult to ensure equivalence between disease terms when studies are separated in time. This evolution in taxonomies reflects growing understanding of this complex, and possibly heterogeneous, disorder.
- Current treatments for hypersomnia are targeted at symptomatic management of excessive daytime sleepiness rather than curtailing the duration of habitual sleep, or combating the closely related sleep inertia and sleep drunkenness.
- Although there are multiple treatments approved by the Food and Drug Administration for narcolepsy, there are none for the other recognized hypersomnias, and off-label use of these medications is inadequate to alleviate symptoms in many patients.
- Patients with idiopathic hypersomnia struggle with a cornucopia of symptoms, from an inability to wake up promptly, working memory and attention issues, compromised alertness when driving, and being in a constant "brain fog" that affects their daily roles and functioning.

INTRODUCTION

As defined by the International Classification of Sleep Disorders, third edition (ICSD-3), hypersomnolence or excessive daytime sleepiness is "the inability to stay awake and alert during the major waking episodes of the day, resulting in periods of irrepressible need for sleep or unintended lapses into drowsiness or sleep." Hypersomnolence may be associated with or presumptively due to, an underlying, secondary cause, or it may occur as a symptom sui generis (**Table 1**). Although ancillary symptoms vary, core features of sleepiness and/or prolonged sleep times are present across these diagnoses.

The classification of hypersomnolence disorders has been iterative and continues to evolve. Idiopathic hypersomnia (IH) was referred to as "intrinsic sleep disorder" in the first revision of the ICSD.[1] In the ensuing years, distinct IH phenotypes of "classic," "narcolepticlike," and "mixed" were proposed,[2] and later differentiated into

Disclosure Statement: Nothing to disclose (P. Saini). D.B. Rye has served as an advisory board member and unpaid consultant for Jazz Pharmaceuticals, as well as a consultant or advisory board member for Balance Therapeutics, UCB Pharma, Xenoport, and Flamel Technologies. He is a coinventor on US Patent Application 20110028418 that describes the use of GABA-A receptor antagonists for the treatment of excessive sleepiness and sleep disorders associated with excessive sleepiness.
This work was partially funded by NIH (R01-NS089719), and the Mind Science Foundation.
a Department of Neurology, Emory University School of Medicine, 12 Executive Park Drive Northeast, Room 426, Atlanta, GA 30329, USA; b Department of Neurology and Program in Sleep, Emory University School of Medicine, 12 Executive Park Drive Northeast, Room 427, Atlanta, GA 30329, USA
* Corresponding author.
E-mail address: Prabhjyot.saini@emory.edu

1556-407X/17/© 2016 Elsevier Inc. All rights reserved.

Table 1
Central disorders of hypersomnolence (International Classification of Sleep Disorders, third edition)

Primary	Associated with Another Condition
Narcolepsy type 1	Medical disorder
Narcolepsy type 2	Medication or substance
Idiopathic hypersomnia	Psychiatric disorder
Kleine-Levin syndrome	Insufficient sleep

"complete" and "incomplete" forms.[3,4] The ICSD-2 identified 2 forms of IH based on habitual sleep length of 6 to 10 versus more than 10 hours.[5] Great difficulty terminating sleep in the morning or after naps, known as sleep drunkenness, was noted to be common in both forms, but was included only in diagnostic criteria for the long sleep type. Because sleep testing and epidemiologic features did not support a 10-hour cutoff,[6] the ICSD-3 abandoned this subdivision, but added objectively measured long sleep times as a diagnostic criterion.

The Diagnostic and Statistical Manual of Mental Disorders (DSM) also recognizes a syndrome akin to IH, the newly named "hypersomnolence disorder" (HD). The DSM-5 places a greater emphasis on utility to the busy clinician, relying more on symptom-based criteria; in this instance, how hypersomnia causes distress or impacts daytime function, as opposed to objective testing, so diagnostic criteria differ somewhat between IH and HD.

The evolution and variety of nosologies present a challenge to the clinician, researcher, and writer attempting to succinctly and accurately summarize an extensive literature. The changing distinctions render it difficult, for example, to ensure equivalence between disease terms when studies are separated in time. However, this evolution also reflects growing understanding of this complex, and possibly heterogeneous, disorder. This article focuses on IH, its epidemiology, clinical evaluation, treatment, and social and economic aspects.

EPIDEMIOLOGY OF IDIOPATHIC HYPERSOMNIA

Estimating IH prevalence is difficult because of the requirement for objective sleep measurement and absence of a biomarker. Prevalence estimates extrapolated from diverse sleep centers are confounded by reporting and referral biases.

Among patients referred for excessive daytime sleepiness (EDS), the prevalence of IH varies from 10.3% to 28.5%.[7–11] In the general population, IH prevalence has been estimated at 0.002% to 0.010%.[2,12–14] However, in a population sample of 15,929 adults, 1.6% reported excessive quantity of sleep (ie, >9 hours per 24), and 0.5% met DSM criteria for hypersomnia.[15]

The mean age of onset is 21.9 years,[16–22] although diagnosis is often quite delayed.[2,12–14,22–25] There is a female predominance.[2,25,26] Approximately 29.4% of patients report a family history,[8,21,22,24,25] suggesting a significant genetic component. Heritability estimates from twin studies are unavailable.

The core feature of IH is EDS, alone or with prolonged, unrefreshing sleep. Sleep drunkenness, that is, extraordinary difficulty awakening, is frequently present[27] and may be more prominent than EDS itself.[15,28] Cognitive difficulties are common and include an inability to focus continuously for more than 1 hour, frequent memory lapses, forgotten appointments and tasks, and lost personal items.[27] In addition, manifestations of autonomic dysfunction, such as Raynaudlike syndrome, migraine, orthostatic syncope,[2,28,29] cold extremities, feeling of faintness, temperature dysregulation, palpitations, and digestive problems, are sometimes present.[27]

Such symptoms may be seen in a variety of disorders, however, so that differentiation as attributable to IH is rarely straightforward. Therefore, comprehensive evaluation by sleep medicine clinicians is preferred.

DIFFERENTIAL DIAGNOSIS OF IDIOPATHIC HYPERSOMNIA

Evaluation of patients who present with EDS should begin with a careful history and examination to assess for potential medical causes. EDS affects 16% to 50% of patients with Parkinson disease,[30–32] up to 28% of patients with multiple systems atrophy,[32,33] and 50% to 80% of patients with myotonic dystrophy.[34–36]

The differentiation between hypersomnolence associated with psychiatric disease and IH can be difficult. One common symptom of major depression, especially with atypical features (ie, mood reactivity, leaden paralysis, carbohydrate cravings with weight gain, and interpersonal rejection sensitivity) is a major sleep period of 10 hours or more. Yet, given the psychosocial burden and diagnostic delay in IH, some patients with IH may subsequently develop depression.[26,27] Our preference in these cases is to ensure that both depressive symptoms and hypersomnolence are addressed.

EDS due to other sleep disorders must be ruled out, particularly delayed sleep phase syndrome (DSPS), obstructive sleep apnea (OSA), and insufficient sleep syndrome. Similar to patients with IH, patients with DSPS may present with sleep inertia/sleep drunkenness, and EDS, each of which appears due to curtailed sleep times.[3,37] OSA commonly results in EDS, which resolves in most cases with treatment of OSA.[38] Insufficient sleep syndrome results in EDS due to sleep time restriction and is associated with afternoon and evening EDS, impaired concentration, and decreased energy.[3,39]

In the absence of other disorders, the differential diagnosis of EDS centers on IH and 2 narcolepsy disorders (type 1 [NT1] and type 2 [NT2]). The characteristics of sleepiness can differ among these 3 disorders, especially between IH and NT1. Specifically, daytime naps in patients with NT1 are generally short and refreshing, whereas patients with IH are more likely to have daytime naps exceeding 1 hour,[24] longer unwanted naps, and more difficulty waking up from naps.[40]

The classic symptom tetrad for NT1 includes EDS and features of rapid eye movement (REM)-sleep dissociation including cataplexy, sleep paralysis, and hypnagogic or hypnopompic hallucinations. Cataplexy, that is, sudden loss of muscle tone in response to emotion, typically laughter, is specific for NT1.[41] Cataplexy ranges from partial, mild face, and neck weakness to complete weakness in the limbs and trunk resulting in falls.[41] However, cataplexy is confounded by mimics, including basilar migraine, syncope, and conversion disorder.[41–44] Furthermore, onset of cataplexy may follow the onset of EDS by weeks, months, years, or even decades.[45–47]

The remaining features of REM-sleep dissociation (ie, sleep paralysis and hallucinations) are nonspecific and insensitive (**Table 2**). Sleep paralysis occurs more commonly in minorities than in Caucasians, can occur in 7.6% of the general population, 28.3% of students, and 31.9% of a psychiatric patient population,[48] compared with 35% and 69% of patients with NT2 and NT1, respectively. Hallucinations are present in 77% of patients with NT1 and 42% of patients with NT2. Most patients with IH do not have sleep paralysis,[2,17,21,24–27,49–51] or hypnogogic hallucinations,[17,21,24–27,49,50,52] but their presence does not exclude an IH diagnosis. Differentiation of NT2 from IH cannot convincingly be made on clinical symptomatology alone.[40]

DIAGNOSTIC TESTING

The overlapping clinical features of the Central Disorders of Hypersomnia (CDH) necessitate objective testing with the nocturnal polysomnogram (PSG) followed by the multiple sleep latency test (MSLT). The PSG allows identification of disorders believed to cause sleepiness (eg, OSA), ensures sufficient sleep time before MSLT (ie, >360–420 minutes), and can identify features suggestive of narcolepsy, including REM sleep behavior disorder and a short nocturnal REM latency (<15 minutes).[53] The MSLT involves a series of 4 or 5 nap opportunities, during which the mean latency to sleep and the number of naps containing REM sleep are quantified.

According to ICSD-3, 2 diagnostic criteria should be met to confirm a clinical diagnosis of IH:

1. The MSLT shows fewer than 2 sleep-onset REM periods (including the REM latency from the preceding PSG if less than or equal to 15 minutes).
2. At least 1 of the following:
   a. A mean sleep latency of less than or equal to 8 minutes on MSLT.
   b. Total 24-hour sleep time is greater than or equal to 660 minutes on 24-hour PSG or by wrist actigraphy averaged over 7 days.

The MSLT has long been the gold standard for the diagnosis of narcolepsy, but like many diagnostic modalities, it has its flaws. The MSLT has been best validated in NT1.[54] It has false positives for both NT1 and IH[55] and test-retest reliability outside of the context of NT1 appears poor.[56,57] False negatives are also a substantial problem, and may be as high as 71% for those with IH with long sleep.[49] The MSLT requires discontinuation of psychoactive medications,[53] which can be clinically challenging. The ICSD-3 criterion allowing alternate diagnosis by sleep time longer than 660 minutes offers a partial solution to these issues, but additional validation studies are needed.

The new ICSD-3 criteria therefore allow for alternate second and third pathways to a diagnosis in requiring objective documentation of more than 11 hours of total sleep in a 24-hour period either by PSG or actigraphy. Unfortunately, further specific recommendations on how to modify the traditional PSG/MSLT protocol to capture these 11 hours are not available. Alternatively, an average derived from at least 7 days of conventional actigraphy can be used. Whether these 3 different means to an IH diagnosis yield a homogeneous population has not been established. The reliability and validity of these new criteria are also unknown.

TREATMENT OF IDIOPATHIC HYPERSOMNIA

Treatments for hypersomnia are generally targeted at EDS, rather than at sleep duration or sleep

Table 2
Clinical features of the narcolepsies and idiopathic hypersomnia

Feature	Narcolepsy Type 1	Narcolepsy Type 2	Idiopathic Hypersomnia
Excessive daytime sleepiness	Present	Present	Present
Cataplexy	Generally present (cataplexy plus characteristic MSLT features, or hypocretin deficiency, are necessary for diagnosis)	Absent (by definition)	Absent (by definition)
Sleep paralysis	Present in 69%	Present in 35%	Present in 21%[22]
Sleep hallucinations	Present in 77%	Present in 42%	Present in 20%[22]
Tetrad of all 4 of the above symptoms	Present in 42% (rarely presents together)	Absent	Absent
Fragmented nocturnal sleep	Significantly lower sleep efficiency than narcolepsy without cataplexy	May be common	Atypical
REM sleep behavior disorder	Present in 45%–61%; significantly more PSG-measured REM sleep without atonia than in IH	Significantly more PSG-measured REM sleep without atonia than in IH	Not studied
Sleep drunkenness	Rare, but occasionally reported	May be common	Present in almost 50%[22]
Long nocturnal sleep time	Present in 18% of patients with narcolepsy with or without cataplexy	Present in 18% of patients with narcolepsy with or without cataplexy	Present in 75%[6]
Effect and duration of naps	Refreshing, short		Unrefreshing and long, often exceeding an hour

Abbreviations: IH, idiopathic hypersomnia; MSLT, multiple sleep latency test; PSG, polysomnography; REM, rapid eye movement.

Adapted from Khan Z, Trotti LM. Central disorders of hypersomnolence: focus on the narcolepsies and idiopathic hypersomnia. Chest 2015;148(1):264; with permission.

drunkenness. Although there are multiple treatments approved by the Food and Drug Administration (FDA) for narcolepsy, there are none for IH, so treatment generally defaults to off-label use of medications approved for narcolepsy. The pharmacologic options include wakefulness-promoting agents (modafinil and armodafinil), traditional psychostimulants (amphetamines, methylphenidate, and their derivatives), and several emerging therapies for treatment-refractory cases (sodium oxybate, clarithromycin, and flumazenil).

Modafinil

Modafinil is FDA-approved for EDS in narcolepsy (type 1 or 2), shift-work sleep disorder, and when EDS persists after treating sleep apnea. In addition to use in IH, it is also used off-label for sleepiness in Parkinson disease,[58] multiple sclerosis,[59] and myotonic dystrophy.[60]

To date, modafinil has been the most studied treatment for IH.[18,24,25,61–65] Clinical series have demonstrated that modafinil decreases naps,[63] and as many as 72% of patients with IH report complete response (after accounting for dropouts due to factors such as cost).[25] The American Academy of Sleep Medicine's most recent recommendation is that modafinil may be effective for IH.[66] Subsequently, 2 recent randomized controlled trials (RCTs) have confirmed the efficacy of modafinil in patients with IH, decreasing subjective sleepiness, improving driving safety, reducing the number of crashes,[67] and increasing sleep latency on the maintenance of wakefulness test (MWT). Cost information is listed in **Table 3**.[61,64]

Mechanism of action
The primary mechanism of action is thought to be inhibition of dopamine reuptake via the dopamine transporter,[68] although other mechanisms may contribute.

Standard dosage
Dosing ranges between 100 and 400 mg, as a single or divided dose, titrated from 100 mg once a day. For patients with evening sleepiness, split-dose regimens are more effective than once-daily dosing.[69–72]

Side effects
Modafinil has limited dependency and abuse potential, and promotes wakefulness with less psychomotor agitation than conventional psychostimulants.[63] In RCTs for non-IH indications, the most common adverse reactions (≥5%) were headache, nausea, nervousness, rhinitis, diarrhea, back pain, anxiety, insomnia, dizziness, and dyspepsia.[73] Severe rash, including Stevens-Johnson Syndrome, has been reported in postmarketing experience.[73]

Children and women
Modafinil is not FDA approved for individuals younger than 18 years because of reports of serious side effects,[74] although clinical series have demonstrated safe use in children and adolescents.[75] Modafinil is pregnancy class C and should be avoided or used with caution in pregnant women. In addition, it decreases hormonal contraceptive effectiveness up to even 1 month after discontinuing the drug.[73]

Armodafinil

Armodafinil is the R-enantiomer of racemic modafinil and is FDA approved for the same indications. The 2 enantiomers have similar pharmacologic properties, but substantially different pharmacokinetic profiles, as a result of the differing rates at which the enantiomers are metabolized.[76] To date, there are no trials, clinical reviews or literature studying armodafinil as treatment for IH. Cost information is listed in **Table 4**.

Mechanism of action
See modafinil.

Standard dosage
Dosing for armodafinil is 150 to 250 mg every morning. Armodafinil results in higher drug concentrations later after dosing and an increased steady-state concentration compared with modafinil.[77]

Side effects
In RCTs for non-IH indications, the most common adverse reactions (≥5%) were headache, nausea, dizziness, and insomnia.[78]

Children and women
Armodafinil is not approved and has not been studied in pediatric patients for any indication. Similar to modafinil, armodafinil is a pregnancy class C drug, so should be avoided or used with caution in pregnant women, and decreases

Table 3 Prices based on NADAC for modafinil as of July 6, 2016	
Drug	**NADAC per 30 Units (USD)**
Modafinil 100-mg tablet	89.86
Modafinil 200-mg tablet	103.58

Abbreviation: NADAC, national average drug acquisition cost.
Data from NADAC weekly reference data from November 2013 to current week. Centers for Medicare & Medicaid Services. (2016). National Average Drug Acquisition Cost. Available at: https://data.medicaid.gov/Drug-Prices/NADAC-as-of-2016-07-06/k2t8-c68j.

Table 4 Prices based on NADAC for armodafinil (Nuvigil) as of July 6, 2016	
Drug	**NADAC per 30 Units (USD)**
Nuvigil 50-mg tablet	200.89
Nuvigil 150-mg tablet	588.11
Nuvigil 200-mg tablet	583.66
Nuvigil 250-mg tablet	587.04

Abbreviation: NADAC, national average drug acquisition cost.
Data from NADAC weekly reference data from November 2013 to current week. Centers for Medicare & Medicaid Services. (2016). National Average Drug Acquisition Cost. Available at: https://data.medicaid.gov/Drug-Prices/NADAC-as-of-2016-07-06/k2t8-c68j.

plasma levels of hormonal contraceptives even up to 1 month after discontinuation.[78]

Traditional Psychostimulants

Several sympathomimetic stimulants (eg, methylphenidate, amphetamine) are FDA approved for the treatment of sleepiness in narcolepsy.[79] There is a paucity of literature supporting the efficacy of amphetamines in IH, but they are often considered second- or third-line therapies.[66]

Before the availability of modafinil, methylphenidate was first-line treatment for IH. In a retrospective chart review, 61 (72%) of 85 patients with IH were prescribed methylphenidate, 40 (51%) of 78 as monotherapy at the last visit. Of those on monotherapy, 38 (95%) reported a positive response, higher than those on modafinil monotherapy (88%). Cost information is listed in **Table 5**.

Mechanism of action

Promotion of wakefulness is through presynaptic enhancement of dopamine release and prevention of reuptake through binding to dopamine and norepinephrine transporters.[80]

Standard dosage

Dosing varies by type of amphetamine and preparation, which include immediate release, extended release, and transdermal formulations.

Side effects

Tachycardia, hypertension, palpitations, and sweating are common.[81] Anorexia, weight loss, seizures, and anxiety can occur. Unlike modafinil, amphetamines can cause vasoconstriction and cardiac stimulation from increased peripheral noradrenaline. At high doses, amphetamines inhibit monoamine oxidase, further increasing synaptic dopamine and leading to cytotoxicity or psychosis.[82,83]

Children and women

Some stimulants are approved for pediatric narcolepsy treatment. Stimulants are classified as pregnancy class C drugs. Adequate studies in pregnant women have not been conducted and they should be used during pregnancy only if the potential benefit justifies the potential risk.

Sodium Oxybate

Sodium oxybate (SXB), the sodium salt of gamma-hydroxybutyrate, is the only drug approved by the FDA for both cataplexy and EDS in narcolepsy.[84–86] In narcolepsy RCTs, it reduced cataplexy, sleepiness, naps, and nighttime awakenings.[87] It increases slow-wave sleep and decreases the frequency of hypnogogic hallucinations and sleep paralysis.[86]

Unlike modafinil and psychostimulants, it is not considered first or second line for IH treatment, but may be considered in individual, treatment-refractory cases. In the one retrospective SXB study in 46 patients with IH,[88] 15% chose not to fill the prescription because of side-effect concerns. Compared with patients with NT1, patients with IH took a lower daily dose of SXB (mean final dose of 4.3 g) and more frequently took only a single dose. Overall, 65% reported a good/very good response and 47% of patients continued SXB. Epworth sleepiness scale scores improved by 3.5 points (clinically significant), and 71% reported waking more easily. Cost information is listed in **Table 6**.

Mechanism of action

The mechanism of action of SXB has not yet been elucidated. SXB is an endogenous cerebral inhibitory neurotransmitter, which activates its own receptors and modulates gamma-aminobutyric acid (GABA)-B receptors.[88,89] Therapeutic efficacy may be mediated by the increase in slow-wave sleep.

Table 5
Prices based on NADAC for methylphenidate as of July 6, 2016

Drug	NADAC per 30 Units, USD
Methylphenidate 5-mg tablet	13.39
Methylphenidate 10-mg tablet	17.53
Methylphenidate 20-mg tablet	25.24

Abbreviation: NADAC, national average drug acquisition cost.
Data from NADAC weekly reference data from November 2013 to current week. Centers for Medicare & Medicaid Services. (2016). National Average Drug Acquisition Cost. Available at: https://data.medicaid.gov/Drug-Prices/NADAC-as-of-2016-07-06/k2t8-c68j.

Table 6
Prices based on NADAC for sodium oxybate (Xyrem) as of July 6, 2016

Drug	Cost per Unit, USD
Xyrem, 1-y cost	143,604[93]
Xyrem, 500 mg/mL	19.40[93,94]

Abbreviation: NADAC, national average drug acquisition cost.

Standard dosage

SXB dosing for narcolepsy ranges from 4.5 to 9.0 g nightly, divided into 2 doses of no more than 4.5 g each. Starting dose is 2 doses of 2.25 g, separated by 2.5 to 4.0 hours. Patients should use an alarm to wake for the second dose, although for patients with IH, this may be problematic.[27,88] SXB prescription requires registration and education through an FDA Risk Evaluation and Mitigation Strategy (REMS) program.

Side effects

Most common adverse reactions ($\geq$5%) were nausea, dizziness, vomiting, somnolence, enuresis, and tremor.[90] Postmarketing experience suggests additional rare, seemingly dose-related, acute anxiety or depression inclusive of suicidal ideation.[91,92]

Children and women

SXB is not approved for use in children. There are no adequate and well-controlled studies in pregnant women.

Clarithromycin

The finding of a presumptive small peptide in cerebrospinal fluid (CSF) of subjects with hypersomnolence that enhances GABA-A receptor function in vitro[95] has led to the use of negative allosteric modulators or antagonists of the GABA-A receptor, including clarithromycin, for treatment of otherwise-refractory IH. Clarithromycin is not FDA approved for the treatment of any CDH.

In a retrospective review of 53 patients, 64% reported improvement in EDS and 38% elected to continue clarithromycin therapy.[96] In an RCT, clarithromycin resulted in improvements in subjective measures of sleepiness, functional status, and health-related quality of life.[97] As with 1 of the 2 modafinil RCTs, these 2 studies included patients with IH and those with other CDH. Cost information is listed in **Table 7**.

Mechanism of action

Clarithromycin's mechanism for relieving sleepiness is currently unknown, but might reflect its action as a negative allosteric modulator of GABA-A receptors. Alternatively, clarithromycin's effects may be mediated by anti-inflammatory properties or alteration of gut flora composition.[97]

Standard dosage

Dosage for clarithromycin begins as 500 mg taken orally with breakfast and lunch, with possible increase as high as 1000 mg twice daily, depending on therapeutic response and side effects. In published reports, patients typically added clarithromycin to their existing medication regimen.[96,97]

Table 7 Prices based on NADAC for clarithromycin as of July 6, 2016	
Drug	NADAC per 30 Units, USD
Clarithromycin 250-mg tablet	62.59
Clarithromycin 500-mg tablet	26.60

Abbreviation: NADAC, national average drug acquisition cost.

Data from NADAC weekly reference data from November 2013 to current week. Centers for Medicare & Medicaid Services. (2016). National Average Drug Acquisition Cost. Available at: https://data.medicaid.gov/Drug-Prices/NADAC-as-of-2016-07-06/k2t8-c68j.

Side effects

Clarithromycin is associated with central nervous system excitation, such as insomnia, mania, delirium, and psychosis.[98] Other side effects reported in patients with CDH include dysgeusia/dysosmia, gastrointestinal distress, nausea, and headache.[96,97]

Children and women

Clarithromycin has not been studied in children with CDH. There is a twofold increase in miscarriages in women exposed to clarithromycin during early pregnancy.[99,100]

Flumazenil

Flumazenil is a GABA-A receptor antagonist that competitively inhibits activity at the benzodiazepine site on the GABA/benzodiazepine receptor complex. It is FDA approved for the reversal of benzodiazepine sedation, either in general anesthesia or in the case of benzodiazepine overdose.[101] As with clarithromycin, flumazenil is hypothesized to have benefit in IH through its effects at GABA-A receptors, but published support for this treatment is presently limited. A single-blind, placebo-controlled, fixed-order challenge with intravenous injections of placebo, and low (0.35–0.5 mg) and high (1.5–2.0 mg) flumazenil doses demonstrated that flumazenil improved psychomotor vigilance (decreased attention lapses and increased reaction speed) and subjective alertness.[95]

Future Therapies

Pitolisant

Alternative therapies in development that speak to biological findings are becoming accessible in Europe. Cerebrospinal fluid histamine levels are reduced[102,103] or unchanged in IH,[17] and also reduced in narcolepsy with or without hypocretin deficiency, suggesting that low histamine levels may be a mediator of somnolence of central origin. Pitolisant is an inverse agonist of the Histamine H3 autoreceptor that increases histamine release in the hypothalamus and cortex. Pitolisant has been shown to be effective in patients with IH and symptomatic central hypersomnia and EDS refractory to stimulants.[19] Pitolisant holds promise as an alternative treatment option as the European Commission granted a marketing authorization for NT1 and NT2 valid throughout the European Union for Wakix on March 31, 2016.[104]

Transcranial direct current stimulation

Another potential approach is transcranial direct current stimulation. Transcranial direct current stimulation encompasses the induction of a relatively weak constant current flow through the cerebral cortex via scalp electrodes. Dependent on stimulation polarity, this results in a modulation of cortical excitability and spontaneous neural activity.[105] A recent pilot study demonstrated objective improvement in reaction times and improving attentional domain. This nonpharmacological approach can be a possible intervention to address the significant symptoms that are not addressed by current therapeutics.

SOCIAL AND ECONOMIC ASPECTS OF IDIOPATHIC HYPERSOMNIA

The effects of hypersomnia are not limited to health, but seep deeply into the social aspects of life. Because hypersomnia is a chronic illness without a cure, its burdens become a permanent part of a patient's life.

Before diagnosis, individuals with hypersomnia are often stigmatized as lazy, inattentive, or unmotivated.[3] The average age of onset is 21.9 and the average age of diagnosis ranges from 15 to 58.[18,19,22,24,25,88] No published studies have specifically focused on characterizing the factors that contribute to this delay.

Most patients with IH never feel fully awake during the daytime. Their alertness is modulated by external conditions (eg, sun, indoor lighting) in the same way as healthy controls, but they often report feeling more sedated than healthy controls in dark environments. Patients with IH prefer standing to sitting, walking while learning or speaking, and report multitasking more often than controls; that is, patients with IH rely on multimodal arousal strategies to sustain alertness.[27]

Almost half of patients with IH report difficulties waking up[22] and many do not hear alarm clocks. This sleep drunkenness can constitute a very important problem that interferes with the demands of school start times and day-shift employment. Patients with sleep drunkenness may use multiple alarm clocks or place alarms in hard to reach or obstructed places, or may require other interventions. For example, loud voices or other auditory stimulation alone or together with somatic stimulation (ie, multimodal stimuli methods) may be required to facilitate waking up.[27,49] Such arousal methods can make affected individuals dependent on others, strain close interpersonal relationships with supporters, and detract from a sense of independence.[27]

Decrements in daytime alertness, difficulty waking in the morning, and cognitive symptoms challenge patients' ability to excel at school, to work and generate income, to participate in recreational activities, and to achieve socially optimal outcomes in their personal and professional lives.[106–109] These same factors may restrict the range of available occupations, as prolonged sitting and soporific work environments can be challenging for patients with IH. As a result, patients with IH may require longer to attain educational and professional goals.[27] One quarter of patients with IH report being forced to relocate or having been dismissed because of their symptoms.[110]

Sleepiness also heightens the risk for road accidents. Adequate alertness is a key prerequisite to safe driving, and sleepiness has a strong causal role in road accidents.[67] Patients with IH report more driving accidents and near misses within the prior 5 years than do controls, and accident occurrence is associated with higher subjective sleepiness measures.[67,106]

Given all of these factors, it is perhaps not surprising that quality of life is decreased in patients with IH. Short Form-36 scores for NT2 and IH are similar in most domains.[26] Even patients with IH receiving medicinal treatment exhibit lower scores than national normative data on nearly all domains.[106]

The effects of IH can be challenging for both patients and their supporters. Most patients with IH (65%) report receiving adequate support from family, friends, or coworkers. Unfortunately, 13% of patients with IH report having divorced or broken up with a partner because of their symptoms.[106]

In addition to the interpersonal and intrapersonal difficulties, obtaining treatment can be a financial challenge. Under each drug described previously, the retail pharmacy price is given for 30 pills.

Coverage for off-label usage of medications varies by insurance provider. Many patients with IH need to try several medications/dosages or use multidrug combinations for symptomatic control,[24,25] which can add to the overall cost of treatment. Moreover, the refractory nature of IH in a subset of patients leaves them financially vulnerable to spikes in health care spending (eg, pursuing new treatment, additional visits). The cost of failed IH therapies has not been formally studied, but clinical experience and patient support group meetings give the impression that the cost is problematic and high.

IH can be a very disabling condition with negative consequences on the physical, mental, and social well-being of some affected individuals. Patients are largely left on their own to alleviate the compound effects of this disorder, as treatment may not be optimal.

WOMEN AND PREGNANCY

There is a general lack of adequate, well-controlled human studies of medications during pregnancy. Two retrospective studies of patients with NT1 or NT2, a minority of whom were treated through pregnancy, did not find significant differences in complication rates between treated and untreated patients,[111,112] but certainty about risk is difficult to achieve without large numbers of medication-exposed pregnancies. As a result, doctors may find it difficult to advise patients with IH who are planning pregnancy. Although one approach may be to advise women to discontinue treatment because of potential teratogenicity, the implications of being untreated for the duration of pregnancy (eg, inability to drive, inability to maintain employment) can be quite dramatic in some patients and must also factor into decision making.

TREATMENT RESPONSE

Regular assessment after treatment initiation is important, to allow dose adjustment or adding/switching medications when necessary. Patients with IH are more likely to be resistant to wake-promoting medications[19] and to try a greater number of stimulants for a shorter amount of time than narcoleptic patients.[18,20,88]

Assessment should focus on symptoms and goals of the patient, using tools that are sensitive to change. Objective measures, such as the MWT, the Sustained Attention to Response Task,[113] and the Psychomotor Vigilance Test,[114,115] may be useful for quantitatively evaluating clinical outcomes[97] but do not necessarily correlate with symptom reports or subjective measures.

CHALLENGES IN THE DEVELOPMENT

To improve drug development to target IH, it is important to recognize the barriers targeting the disorder. First, there has been historical confusion of IH as a distinct diagnostic entity, often described as multiple subgroups of varying symptomatic presentations[2,4,15] and identified in published classification manuals with ever-changing criteria of these symptoms.[1,5,6] There is no pathognomic sign or symptom that is diagnostic of IH.

Second, IH does not have clearly defined, sensitive and specific criteria that can be used in clinical and research settings, and its identification remains as a diagnosis of exclusion of other sleep disorders, principally NT1. The MSLT was developed and validated as an aid in the diagnosis of narcolepsy,[54] and since then it has been shown to possess significant flaws of accuracy and precision,[55–57] as described previously.

Third, there is no identifiable etiology of IH. Recent experimental and clinical findings have suggested a bioactive, peptidelike component in the CSF of patients with primary hypersomnia that potentiates GABA-A receptor activity that is attenuated in the presence of the benzodiazepine antagonist flumazenil.[95]

Fourth, with a lack of an etiology, the development of animal models that can be used as proof of principle or therapeutic development is not possible nor is the ability to recapitulate various symptoms of IH. Particularly critical for future therapeutic development are proof-of-principle studies that can use animal models to demonstrate mitigation/modulation of symptoms through genetic, pharmacologic, or noninvasive means.

Fifth, perhaps the paramount obstacle is the relative low prevalence of the disorder, which limits the number of companies willing to invest in new therapeutic development for a disorder with a small market. The low prevalence of IH renders it a rare disorder, and even under the FDA's Orphan Drug Designation program, there has been only 1 drug that has recently garnered orphan drug status for the indication of IH and is currently in phase 2 clinical trials for the treatment of IH and NT2 (NCT02512588).

Despite these barriers, the clinical implications have left patients with few resources to manage their symptoms while continuing to maintain their roles in their personal and professional lives.

Since the publication of a putative substance that enhances the GABA-A receptor in subjects with disorders of central hypersomnolence, patients have used social media (eg, Facebook) to initiate regional and national support groups around the world. Shortly thereafter, the Hypersomnia Foundation was incorporated. The Hypersomnia Foundation strives to improve the lives of people with hypersomnia by advocating on their behalf, providing support, educating the public and health care professionals, raising awareness, and funding research into effective treatments, better diagnostic tools, and, ultimately, a cure for these debilitating conditions.[116] This patient-centered collaborative action plan has enabled patients to take initiative to bring awareness to the medical community about IH, the impact of IH on daily life, and the difficulties faced in the medical system when seeking care. The Hypersomnia Foundation holds an annual meeting connecting patients, families, professionals, and all stakeholders together to update.

SUMMARY

Given all these barriers and circumstances, a fluctuating disease definition, insensitive and nonspecific diagnostic criteria, treatments and guidelines borrowed from narcolepsy, which have little overlap, IH remains a diagnosis of exclusion with a limited number of RCTs and no approved drugs. The field and patients are sorely in need of improved diagnostics and treatment modalities ideally driven by a greater knowledge of its underlying pathophysiology.

Drug development programs should have a firm scientific foundation and understanding the natural history of the disease is a critical element in this foundation. In rare disorders, the small number of patients affected and clinical experience dispersed among a small number of clinical referral centers, the natural history of rare diseases is often poorly described. It is critical to know, for example, which disease manifestations are likely to develop and when, and which are likely to persist. It is critical to identify disease signs that predict the development of the most important disease manifestations. Also, there is a substantial phenotypic variability that must be accounted for.

Knowledge about the disease's natural history can inform important aspects of disease that are important for drug development and for filling the knowledge gaps that remain. For example, defining the target disease population, including the full range of the disease manifestation and any subtypes, developing outcome measures that are sensitive and specific to changes in the manifestations of the disease with and without treatment, develop

genotypic-phenotypic correlates and possible biomarkers that can serve as surrogate endpoints.

The clinician should have familiarity with the mechanisms of action, dosing regimens, and side effects of IH treatments. Rendering a definitive diagnosis affects the choice of treatment, inclusive of cost, and is relevant for informing patients of their prognosis and potential need for accommodations in their personal and professional lives.

ACKNOWLEDGMENTS

The authors gratefully acknowledge Lynn Marie Trotti, MD, MSc, for providing helpful feedback on this article.

REFERENCES

1. Thorpy MJ. International classification of sleep disorders: diagnostic and coding manual. Rochester (MN): American Sleep Disorders Association; 1990.
2. Bassetti C, Aldrich MS. Idiopathic hypersomnia. A series of 42 patients. Brain 1997;120(Pt 8):1423–35.
3. Billiard M, Sonka K. Idiopathic hypersomnia. Sleep Med Rev 2015;29:23–33.
4. Billiard M, Merle C, Carlander B, et al. Idiopathic hypersomnia. Psychiatry Clin Neurosci 1998; 52(2):125–9.
5. American Academy of Sleep Medicine. International classification of sleep disorders: diagnostic and coding manual. 2nd edition. Westchester (IL): American Academy of Sleep Medicine; 2005.
6. American Academy of Sleep Medicine. International classification of sleep disorders. 3rd edition. Darien (IL): American Academy of Sleep Medicine; 2014.
7. Boon P, Pevernagie D, Schrans D. Hypersomnolence and narcolepsy; a pragmatic diagnostic neurophysiological approach. Acta Neurol Belg 2002;102(1):11–8.
8. Roth B. Idiopathic hypersomnia: a study of 187 personally observed cases. Int J Neurol 1981; 15(1–2):108–18.
9. van Den Hoed J, Kraemer H, Guilleminault C, et al. Disorders of excessive daytime somnolence: polygraphic and clinical data for 100 patients. Sleep 1981;4(1):23–37.
10. Kaveh Moghadam K, Pizza F, Vandi S. Utility of 24-hour continuous polygraphic recording in the differential diagnosis of hypersomnias of central origin. Sleep 2011;34:A212.
11. Kim D, Yoon S, Joo E, et al. Clinical and polysomnographic characteristics of patients with daytime sleepiness. Sleep 2012;35:A272.

12. Billiard M, Dauvilliers Y. Idiopathic hypersomnia. Sleep Med Rev 2001;5(5):351–60.

13. Harris SF, Monderer RS, Thorpy M. Hypersomnias of central origin. Neurol Clin 2012;30(4):1027–44.

14. Masri TJ, Gonzales CG, Kushida CA. Idiopathic hypersomnia. Sleep Med Clin 2012;7(2):283–9.

15. Roth B. Narcolepsy and hypersomnia: review and classification of 642 personally observed cases. Schweiz Arch Neurol Neurochir Psychiatr 1976; 119(1):31–41.

16. Bruck D, Parkes JD. A comparison of idiopathic hypersomnia and narcolepsy-cataplexy using self report measures and sleep diary data. J Neurol Neurosurg Psychiatry 1996;60(5):575–8.

17. Dauvilliers Y, Delallee N, Jaussent I, et al. Normal cerebrospinal fluid histamine and tele-methylhistamine levels in hypersomnia conditions. Sleep 2012;35(10):1359–66.

18. Lavault S, Dauvilliers Y, Drouot X, et al. Benefit and risk of modafinil in idiopathic hypersomnia vs. narcolepsy with cataplexy. Sleep Med 2011;12(6):550–6.

19. Leu-Semenescu S, Nittur N, Golmard JL, et al. Effects of pitolisant, a histamine H3 inverse agonist, in drug-resistant idiopathic and symptomatic hypersomnia: a chart review. Sleep Med 2014;15(6):681–7.

20. Nittur N, Konofal E, Dauvilliers Y, et al. Mazindol in narcolepsy and idiopathic and symptomatic hypersomnia refractory to stimulants: a long-term chart review. Sleep Med 2013;14(1):30–6.

21. Vaňková J, Nevšímalová S, Šonka K, et al. Increased REM density in narcolepsy-cataplexy and the polysymptomatic form of idiopathic hypersomnia. Sleep 2001;24(6):707–11.

22. Sowa NA. Idiopathic hypersomnia and hypersomnolence disorder: a systematic review of the literature. Psychosomatics 2016;57(2):152–64.

23. Aldrich MS. The clinical spectrum of narcolepsy and idiopathic hypersomnia. Neurology 1996; 46(2):393–401.

24. Anderson KN, Pilsworth S, Sharples LD, et al. Idiopathic hypersomnia: a study of 77 cases. Sleep 2007;30(10):1274–81.

25. Ali M, Auger RR, Slocumb NL, et al. Idiopathic hypersomnia: clinical features and response to treatment. J Clin Sleep Med 2009;5(6):562–8.

26. Dauvilliers Y, Paquereau J, Bastuji H, et al. Psychological health in central hypersomnias: the French Harmony study. J Neurol Neurosurg Psychiatry 2009;80(6):636–41.

27. Vernet C, Leu-Semenescu S, Buzare MA, et al. Subjective symptoms in idiopathic hypersomnia: beyond excessive sleepiness. J Sleep Res 2010; 19(4):525–34.

28. Roth B, Nevsimalova S, Rechtschaffen A. Hypersomnia with "sleep drunkenness". Arch Gen Psychiatry 1972;26(5):456–62.

29. Matsunaga H. Clinical study on idiopathic CNS hypersomnolence. Jpn J Psychiatry Neurol 1987; 41(4):637–44.

30. Arnulf I. Excessive daytime sleepiness in parkinsonism. Sleep Med Rev 2005;9(3):185–200.

31. Arnulf I, Konofal E, Merino-Andreu M, et al. Parkinson's disease and sleepiness: an integral part of PD. Neurology 2002;58(7):1019–24.

32. Moreno-Lopez C, Santamaria J, Salamero M, et al. Excessive daytime sleepiness in multiple system atrophy (SLEEMSA study). Arch Neurol 2011; 68(2):223–30.

33. Shimohata T, Nakayama H, Tomita M, et al. Daytime sleepiness in Japanese patients with multiple system atrophy: prevalence and determinants. BMC Neurol 2012;12:130.

34. Hilton-Jones D. Myotonic dystrophy–forgotten aspects of an often neglected condition. Curr Opin Neurol 1997;10(5):399–401.

35. Quera Salva MA, Blumen M, Jacquette A, et al. Sleep disorders in childhood-onset myotonic dystrophy type 1. Neuromuscul Disord 2006;16(9–10):564–70.

36. Romigi A, Albanese M, Liguori C, et al. Sleep-wake cycle and daytime sleepiness in the myotonic dystrophies. J Neurodegener Dis 2013;2013:692026.

37. Nevšímalová S, Blažejová K, Illnerová H, et al. A contribution to pathophysiology of idiopathic hypersomnia. Suppl Clin Neurophysiol 2000;53:366–70.

38. Gasa M, Tamisier R, Launois SH, et al. Residual sleepiness in sleep apnea patients treated by continuous positive airway pressure. J Sleep Res 2013;22(4):389–97.

39. Roehrs T, Zorick F, Sicklesteel J, et al. Excessive daytime sleepiness associated with insufficient sleep. Sleep 1983;6(4):319–25.

40. Sonka K, Susta M, Billiard M. Narcolepsy with and without cataplexy, idiopathic hypersomnia with and without long sleep time: a cluster analysis. Sleep Med 2015;16(2):225–31.

41. Scammell TE. Narcolepsy. N Engl J Med 2015; 373(27):2654–62.

42. Pizza F, Vandi S, Poli F, et al. Narcolepsy with cataplexy mimicry: the strange case of two sisters. J Clin Sleep Med 2013;9(6):611–2.

43. Krahn LE. Reevaluating spells initially identified as cataplexy. Sleep Med 2005;6(6):537–42.

44. Shankar R, Jalihal V, Walker M, et al. Pseudocataplexy and transient functional paralysis: a spectrum of psychogenic motor disorder. J Neuropsychiatry Clin Neurosci 2010;22(4):445–50.

45. Sours JA. Narcolepsy and other disturbances in the sleep-waking rhythm: a study of 115 cases with review of the literature. J Nerv Ment Dis 1963;137:525–42.

46. Luca G, Haba-Rubio J, Dauvilliers Y, et al. Clinical, polysomnographic and genome-wide association analyses of narcolepsy with cataplexy: a European Narcolepsy Network study. J Sleep Res 2013; 22(5):482–95.

47. Rye DB, Dihenia B, Weissman JD, et al. Presentation of narcolepsy after 40. Neurology 1998;50(2): 459–65.

48. Sharpless BA, Barber JP. Lifetime prevalence rates of sleep paralysis: a systematic review. Sleep Med Rev 2011;15(5):311–5.

49. Vernet C, Arnulf I. Idiopathic hypersomnia with and without long sleep time: a controlled series of 75 patients. Sleep 2009;32:753–9.

50. Sasai T, Inoue Y, Komada Y, et al. Comparison of clinical characteristics among narcolepsy with and without cataplexy and idiopathic hypersomnia without long sleep time, focusing on HLA-DRB1*1501/DQB1*0602 finding. Sleep Med 2009; 10(9):961–6.

51. Hong S, Kim T, Joo S, et al. Comparisons of clinical and polysomnographic findings between narcolepsy without cataplexy and idiopathic hypersomnia. Sleep Med 2013;14:e153.

52. Honda M, Honda Y. Clinical characteristics of nocturnal sleep and concomitant symptoms in hypersomnias of central origin; analysis on self-completed questionnaire. Sleep 2011;34:A211.

53. Littner MR, Kushida C, Wise M, et al. Practice parameters for clinical use of the multiple sleep latency test and the maintenance of wakefulness test. Sleep 2005;28(1):113–21.

54. Folkerts M, Rosenthal L, Roehrs T, et al. The reliability of the diagnostic features in patients with narcolepsy. Biol Psychiatry 1996;40(3):208–14.

55. Baumann CR, Mignot E, Lammers GJ, et al. Challenges in diagnosing narcolepsy without cataplexy: a consensus statement. Sleep 2014;37(6):1035–42.

56. Trotti LM, Staab BA, Rye DB. Test-retest reliability of the multiple sleep latency test in narcolepsy without cataplexy and idiopathic hypersomnia. J Clin Sleep Med 2013;9(8):789–95.

57. Mignot E, Lin L, Finn L, et al. Correlates of sleep-onset REM periods during the multiple sleep latency test in community adults. Brain 2006; 129(6):1609–23.

58. Trotti LM, Bliwise DL. Treatment of the sleep disorders associated with Parkinson's disease. Neurotherapeutics 2014;11(1):68–77.

59. Kraft GH, Bowen J. Modafinil for fatigue in MS: a randomized placebo-controlled double-blind study. Neurology 2005;65(12):1995–7 [author reply: 1995–7].

60. Orlikowski D, Chevret S, Quera-Salva MA, et al. Modafinil for the treatment of hypersomnia associated with myotonic muscular dystrophy in adults: a multicenter, prospective, randomized, double-blind, placebo-controlled, 4-week trial. Clin Ther 2009;31(8):1765–73.

61. Mayer G, Benes H, Young P, et al. Modafinil in the treatment of idiopathic hypersomnia without long sleep time–a randomized, double-blind, placebo-controlled study. J Sleep Res 2015;24(1):74–81.

62. Janackova S, Motte J, Bakchine S, et al. Idiopathic hypersomnia: a report of three adolescent-onset cases in a two-generation family. J Child Neurol 2011;26(4):522–5.

63. Bastuji H, Jouvet M. Successful treatment of idiopathic hypersomnia and narcolepsy with modafinil. Prog Neuropsychopharmacol Biol Psychiatry 1988; 12(5):695–700.

64. Philip P, Chaufton C, Taillard J, et al. Modafinil improves real driving performance in patients with hypersomnia: a randomized double-blind placebo-controlled crossover clinical trial. Sleep 2014;37(3):483–7.

65. Yaman M, Karakaya F, Aydin T, et al. Evaluation of the effect of modafinil on cognitive functions in patients with idiopathic hypersomnia with P300. Med Sci Monit 2015;21:1850–5.

66. Morgenthaler TI, Kapur VK, Brown T, et al. Practice parameters for the treatment of narcolepsy and other hypersomnias of central origin: an American Academy of Sleep Medicine report. Sleep 2007; 30(12):1705–11.

67. Pizza F, Jaussent I, Lopez R, et al. Car crashes and central disorders of hypersomnolence: a French study. PLoS One 2015;10(6):e0129386.

68. Wisor J. Modafinil as a catecholaminergic agent: empirical evidence and unanswered questions. Front Neurol 2013;4:139.

69. Broughton RJ, Fleming JA, George CF, et al. Randomized, double-blind, placebo-controlled crossover trial of modafinil in the treatment of excessive daytime sleepiness in narcolepsy. Neurology 1997;49(2):444–51.

70. Schwartz JR, Feldman NT, Bogan RK. Dose effects of modafinil in sustaining wakefulness in narcolepsy patients with residual evening sleepiness. J Neuropsychiatry Clin Neurosci 2005;17(3):405–12.

71. Schwartz JR, Feldman NT, Bogan RK, et al. Dosing regimen effects of modafinil for improving daytime wakefulness in patients with narcolepsy. Clin Neuropharmacol 2003;26(5):252–7.

72. Randomized trial of modafinil for the treatment of pathological somnolence in narcolepsy. US Modafinil in Narcolepsy Multicenter Study Group. Ann Neurol 1998;43(1):88–97.

73. Cephalon Inc. Provigil: highlights of prescribing information. 2007. Available at: https://www.accessdata.fda.gov/drugsatfda_docs/label/2015/020717s037s038lbl.pdf.

74. Wise MS, Arand DL, Auger RR, et al. Treatment of narcolepsy and other hypersomnias of central

origin: an American Academy of Sleep Medicine review. Sleep 2007;30(12):1712–27.

75. Lecendreux M, Bruni O, Franco P, et al. Clinical experience suggests that modafinil is an effective and safe treatment for paediatric narcolepsy. J Sleep Res 2012;21(4):481–3.

76. Darwish M, Kirby M, Hellriegel ET, et al. Pharmaco-kinetic profile of armodafinil in healthy subjects: pooled analysis of data from three randomized studies. Clin Drug Investig 2009;29(2):87–100.

77. Bogan RK. Armodafinil in the treatment of excessive sleepiness. Expert Opin Pharmacother 2010; 11(6):993–1002.

78. Cephalon Inc. Nuvigil: highlights of prescribing information. 2007. Available at: https://www.accessdata.fda.gov/drugsatfda_docs/label/2015/021875s021lbledt.pdf.

79. Mitler MM, Hajdukovic R, Erman M, et al. Narcolepsy. J Clin Neurophysiol 1990;7(1):93–118.

80. Seiden LS, Sabol KE, Ricaurte GA. Amphetamine: effects on catecholamine systems and behavior. Annu Rev Pharmacol Toxicol 1993;33:639–77.

81. Stiefel G, Besag FM. Cardiovascular effects of methylphenidate, amphetamines and atomoxetine in the treatment of attention-deficit hyperactivity disorder. Drug Saf 2010;33(10):821–42.

82. Leviel V. Dopamine release mediated by the dopamine transporter, facts and consequences. J Neurochem 2011;118(4):475–89.

83. Mignot EJM. A practical guide to the therapy of narcolepsy and hypersomnia syndromes. Neurotherapeutics 2012;9(4):739–52.

84. Barateau L, Lopez R, Dauvilliers Y. Treatment options for narcolepsy. CNS Drugs 2016;30(5):369–79.

85. Khan Z, Trotti LM. Central disorders of hypersomnolence: focus on the narcolepsies and idiopathic hypersomnia. Chest 2015;148(1):262–73.

86. Boscolo-Berto R, Viel G, Montagnese S, et al. Narcolepsy and effectiveness of gamma-hydroxybutyrate (GHB): a systematic review and meta-analysis of randomized controlled trials. Sleep Med Rev 2012;16(5):431–43.

87. A randomized, double blind, placebo-controlled multicenter trial comparing the effects of three doses of orally administered sodium oxybate with placebo for the treatment of narcolepsy. Sleep 2002;25(1):42–9.

88. Leu-Semenescu S, Louis P, Arnulf I. Benefits and risk of sodium oxybate in idiopathic hypersomnia versus narcolepsy type 1: a chart review. Sleep Med 2016;17:38–44.

89. Alshaikh MK, Tricco AC, Tashkandi M, et al. Sodium oxybate for narcolepsy with cataplexy: systematic review and meta-analysis. J Clin Sleep Med 2012; 8(4):451–8.

90. Jazz Pharmaceuticals. Xyrem: highlights of prescribing information. 2002. Available at: https://www.accessdata.fda.gov/drugsatfda_docs/label/2012/021196s013lbl.pdf.

91. Ortega-Albás JJ, López-Bernabé R, García AL. Suicidal ideation secondary to sodium oxybate. J Neuropsychiatry Clin Neurosci 2010;22(3). 352r. e26–352.e26.

92. Rossetti AO, Heinzer RC, Tafti M, et al. Rapid occurrence of depression following addition of sodium oxybate to modafinil. Sleep Med 2010;11(5): 500–1.

93. Helfand C. Xyrem—Jazz pharmaceuticals. 2014. Available at: http://www.fiercepharma.com/special-report/xyrem-jazz-pharmaceuticals. Accessed August 16, 2016.

94. Langreth R. Drug prices defy gravity, doubling for dozens of products. 2014. Available at: http://www.bloomberg.com/news/articles/2014-04-30/drug-prices-defy-gravity-doubling-for-dozens-of-pro-ducts; http://www.bloomberg.com/graphics/info graphics/drug-prices-soar-for-top-selling-brands. html#xyrem. Accessed August 15, 2016.

95. Rye DB, Bliwise DL, Parker K, et al. Modulation of vigilance in the primary hypersomnias by endogenous enhancement of GABAA receptors. Sci Transl Med 2012;4(161):161ra151.

96. Trotti LM, Saini P, Freeman AA, et al. Improvement in daytime sleepiness with clarithromycin in patients with GABA-related hypersomnia: clinical experience. J Psychopharmacol 2014;28(7):697–702.

97. Trotti LM, Saini P, Bliwise DL, et al. Clarithromycin in gamma-aminobutyric acid-related hypersomnolence: a randomized, crossover trial. Ann Neurol 2015;78(3):454–65.

98. Bandettini Di Poggio M, Anfosso S, Audenino D, et al. Clarithromycin-induced neurotoxicity in adults. J Clin Neurosci 2011;18(3):313–8.

99. Einarson A, Phillips E, Mawji F, et al. A prospective controlled multicentre study of clarithromycin in pregnancy. Am J Perinatol 1998;15(9):523–5.

100. Andersen JT, Petersen M, Jimenez-Solem E, et al. Clarithromycin in early pregnancy and the risk of miscarriage and malformation: a register based nationwide cohort study. PLoS One 2013;8(1): e53327.

101. Roche Laboratories Inc. Romazicon: package information. 2007. Available at: https://www.accessdata.fda.gov/drugsatfda_docs/label/2007/020073s016lbl.pdf.

102. Kanbayashi T, Kodama T, Kondo H, et al. CSF histamine contents in narcolepsy, idiopathic hypersomnia and obstructive sleep apnea syndrome. Sleep 2009;32(2):181–7.

103. Bassetti CL, Baumann CR, Dauvilliers Y, et al. Cerebrospinal fluid histamine levels are decreased in patients with narcolepsy and excessive daytime sleepiness of other origin. J Sleep Res 2010;19(4): 620–3.

104. European Medicines Agency. Wakix: summary for the public. 2016. Available at: http://www.ema.europa.eu/docs/en_GB/document_library/EPAR_-_Summary_for_the_public/human/002616/WC500204748.pdf.

105. Nitsche MA, Boggio PS, Fregni F, et al. Treatment of depression with transcranial direct current stimulation (tDCS): a review. Exp Neurol 2009;219(1):14–9.

106. Ozaki A, Inoue Y, Hayashida K, et al. Quality of life in patients with narcolepsy with cataplexy, narcolepsy without cataplexy, and idiopathic hypersomnia without long sleep time: comparison between patients on psychostimulants, drug-naïve patients and the general Japanese population. Sleep Med 2012;13(2):200–6.

107. Jennum P, Ibsen R, Avlund K, et al. Health, social and economic consequences of hypersomnia: a controlled national study from a national registry evaluating the societal effect on patients and their partners. Eur J Health Econ 2014;15(3):303–11.

108. Jennum P, Kjellberg J. The socio-economical burden of hypersomnia. Acta Neurol Scand 2010;121(4):265–70.

109. Jennum P, Knudsen S, Kjellberg J. The economic consequences of narcolepsy. J Clin Sleep Med 2009;5(3):240–5.

110. Ozaki A, Inoue Y, Hayashida K. Quality of life in patients with narcolepsy with cataplexy, narcolepsy without cataplexy, and idiopathic hypersomnia without long sleep time. Sleep Biol Rhythms 2011;9(4):311.

111. Romigi A, Liguori C, Izzi F, et al. Oral L-carnitine as treatment for narcolepsy without cataplexy during pregnancy: a case report. J Neurol Sci 2015;348(1–2):282–3.

112. Thorpy M, Zhao CG, Dauvilliers Y. Management of narcolepsy during pregnancy. Sleep Med 2013;14(4):367–76.

113. Fronczek R, Middelkoop HA, van Dijk JG, et al. Focusing on vigilance instead of sleepiness in the assessment of narcolepsy: high sensitivity of the Sustained Attention to Response Task (SART). Sleep 2006;29(2):187–91.

114. Dinges DF, Powell JW. Microcomputer analyses of performance on a portable, simple visual RT task during sustained operations. Behav Res Meth Instrum Comput 1985;17(6):652–5.

115. Basner M, Dinges DF. Maximizing sensitivity of the psychomotor vigilance test (PVT) to sleep loss. Sleep 2011;34(5):581–91.

116. Hypersomnia Foundation. 2015. Available at: http://www.hypersomniafoundation.org/. Accessed October 08, 2016.

Reducing the Clinical and Socioeconomic Burden of Narcolepsy by Earlier Diagnosis and Effective Treatment

CrossMark

Michael Thorpy, MD*, Anne Marie Morse, MD

KEYWORDS

- Burden - Narcolepsy - Socioeconomic - Sleepiness - Cataplexy - Psychosocial - Comorbidities
- Diagnosis

KEY POINTS

- Narcolepsy is a rare condition that carries a significant burden.
- The burden of narcolepsy is the result of clinical difficulties and disability directly related to the disorder and the socioeconomic liability.
- Time to appropriate diagnosis and treatment is generally prolonged and contributes to the burden.
- Effective treatment results in long-term benefits by improving clinical outcomes, potentially enabling improved education, increased employment opportunity, and improved work productivity and quality of life.
- Improved awareness about the diagnosis and tailored therapies improve clinical and socioeconomic outcomes by reducing time to effective treatment.

CLINICAL BURDEN

Age of Onset

The burden of narcolepsy varies with the age of onset. Although narcolepsy can begin at any age from infancy to the 80s or older, there is generally a bimodal distribution of symptom onset with an initial main peak at 15 years old and a lesser second peak at approximately 35 years old.[1,2] An analysis of 1000 patients with narcolepsy of all ages showed a median onset at 16 years and a median age of diagnosis of 33 years,[3] consistent with the known epidemiology and also suggesting the additional challenge of delay in diagnosis.

When narcolepsy begins in childhood, not only are the symptoms more difficult to recognize but the disorder is often misdiagnosed. In addition, even when appropriately identified, many of the medications prescribed for the treatment of narcolepsy are not approved for use in the pediatric population. Therefore, treatment is often delayed and less effective, commonly resulting in compromised learning and impaired education, as well as the development of psychosocial difficulties.[4] Similarly, consequences seen in the working age group (18–65 years old) can include impairment that may lead to loss of employment with frequent job changes, and, in the elderly (>65 years old), retirement may be earlier than desired and postretirement activities may be curtailed and adversely affected because of symptoms.

Symptom Evolution and Effects

The 5 main symptoms of narcolepsy are sleepiness, cataplexy, hypnagogic hallucinations, sleep paralysis, and disturbed nocturnal sleep.

Sleep-Wake Disorders Center, Montefiore Medical Center, and Albert Einstein College of Medicine, Bronx, NY, USA
* Corresponding author. Sleep-Wake Disorders Center, Montefiore Medical Center, 111 East 210th Street, Bronx, NY 10467.
E-mail address: michael.thorpy@einstein.yu.edu

Sleep Med Clin 12 (2017) 61–71
http://dx.doi.org/10.1016/j.jsmc.2016.10.001
1556-407X/17/© 2017 Elsevier Inc. All rights reserved.

Cataplexy, the pathognomonic symptom of narcolepsy, is the abrupt loss of muscle tone provoked by a strong emotion. Cataplexy in adults is mainly precipitated by positive emotions such as laughter, elation, or happiness, although it can be precipitated by negative emotions such as anger. When obvious, such as when a person laughs and falls to the ground, cataplexy often leads to a rapid diagnosis of narcolepsy. However, most patients do not have falls associated with cataplexy; instead, they have more subtle symptoms such as facial, head, or limb weakness, which may be more difficult to diagnose. Cataplexy can be misdiagnosed as a drop attack, seizure, or a psychogenic symptom.

In children, the triggers and symptoms of cataplexy can differ from adults; precipitating factors can include exhaustion, tiredness, and stress, and symptoms can be described as the child having puppetlike movements.[5] However, symptoms usually evolve into the more typical form of cataplexy as the child ages.[6] Patients describe knee buckling that may lead to falls, but sometimes cataplexy may be only an abnormal sensation felt in the muscles with emotion. Other features of cataplexy may be facial weakness, with the inability to smile or drooping of the eyelids or head, and facial twitching or grimacing. In addition, objects may be dropped from the hands, or stumbling or incoordination can cause falls.

Sleepiness is not only the most common feature of narcolepsy but also generally the most disabling. In children, the initial presentation of abnormal sleepiness can be increased total sleep during the 24-hour day.[6] The sleepiness of narcolepsy is an unrelenting persistent symptom that can have fluctuations in severity but is always present. Typically, it is most evident when the patient is sedentary or inactive, such as when watching television, reading, sitting quietly, or when a passenger in a car. However, patients can also experience a momentary sleep, in which they can continue wakeful activities, such as driving, but memory formation may be impaired, thereby leading to automatic behavior episodes, behaviors for which the patient has no memory. The patient is capable of acting appropriately, but has no recall for the activity.

Vivid dreams at sleep onset are a common feature and often occur before falling asleep, leading to hypnagogic hallucinations, which are usually visual but can be auditory. Dreams on awakening (hypnopompic dreams) also occur, but are less specific to narcolepsy. Frequent dreams, nightmares, and lucid dreams are common.[7,8] Delusional dreams, in which the patient after awakening believes the activity really occurred, are more common than hypnopompic dreams in narcolepsy.[9]

Patients with narcolepsy have disturbed nocturnal sleep, which is characterized by sleep fragmentation, increased lighter sleep, and reduced deep sleep.[10] There are frequent fragmented, brief, nightly awakenings with difficulty returning to sleep and overall poor sleep quality. The sleep disturbance may be a major concern of the patient and often requires specific treatment.

In addition, patients with narcolepsy have abnormalities of rapid eye movement (REM) sleep and REM sleep motor regulation.[11] For example, sleep paralysis is a partial manifestation of REM sleep leading to an inability to move for seconds or minutes and can occur in the transition from sleep to wakefulness or from wakefulness to sleep, often in association with dreams or hallucinations. However, sleep paralysis occurs frequently in healthy individuals and so may not raise a suspicion of narcolepsy. In contrast, REM sleep behavior, which is dream-driven activity that occurs while asleep,[10] is a pathologic feature that can manifest as a part of disrupted REM sleep and can also be a cause of bodily injury to the patient and potentially the bed partner.

Cognitive Deficits

Patients with narcolepsy frequently complain of memory difficulties, trouble with attention, and deterioration of executive function. Memory problems are among the most frequent complaints in patients with narcolepsy. Complaints include forgetfulness and problems in following conversations.[12] However, it is possible that the disturbed sleep patterns in narcolepsy, rather than daytime sleepiness, are responsible for impaired memory.[13] Attention is affected on tasks that require an extended period of time or that require the ability to focus, or divided attention. In simple tasks narcoleptic patients seem to be able to compensate for arousal fluctuations by increases in alertness for short periods of time. More demanding tasks require the need to use effort to keep high arousal levels but this leads to speed-accuracy trade-offs, with patients performing less accurately or more slowly.

Executive function impairments are caused by attentional and cognitive resources that have to be allocated to the continuous maintenance of alertness, with the result that tasks are not performed quickly or accurately. Decision making is also affected in narcoleptics with a tendency toward risky choices possibly caused by changes in reward processing associated with reduced hypocretin levels.[14–17]

In the light of these self-report data, it is surprising that memory assessment by standardized tests has not consistently revealed significant impairments.[13] For instance, earlier studies did not identify significant group differences on either immediate or delayed recall for verbal and visual memory between narcoleptic patients and healthy control subjects.[18,19] Other studies suggest a modality-specific effect, with more pronounced problems for verbal compared with visual memory.[20]

Delay in Diagnosis

Narcolepsy is typically associated with a delay in diagnosis of approximately 8 to 15 years, and may be more delayed in female patients.[21,22] The delay seems to be related to numerous causes, such as mildness of initial symptoms, gradual onset, lack of recognition of the condition by the patient or clinician, and mistaken diagnosis because of alternative disorders of sleepiness such as sleep deprivation or obstructive sleep apnea (OSA). The high comorbidity burden in patients with narcolepsy with some disorders that have symptom overlap with narcolepsy also contribute to the lack of recognition. The delayed diagnosis leads to delayed treatment, which increases the burden of the disease with detrimental effects on health care resource use, employment, and quality of life.[21]

Although approximately 70% of the US general public know about the diagnosis of narcolepsy, rarely can all 5 symptoms be identified.[23] Narcolepsy ranks lowest in awareness compared with all other chronic diseases requiring long-term treatment. In 2012, only 7% of primary care physicians in the United States could identify all 5 main narcolepsy symptoms.[23] However, reduced knowledge among medical professionals is not limited to primary care physicians. The 2014 AWAKEN (The Awareness and Knowledge of Narcolepsy) study showed similar deficiencies among sleep specialists; only 63% identified excessive daytime sleepiness (EDS) and cataplexy as 2 primary narcolepsy symptoms and less than one-quarter could identify all 5 symptoms of narcolepsy.[23]

Identification and characterization of symptoms can be challenging for both physicians and patients. For instance, cataplexy can be difficult for physicians to recognize as well as challenging for patients to describe. Therefore, it should be explored on more than 1 occasion because many patients fail to recall the symptom when first asked, and the symptom has great variability. The ancillary symptoms, when present, of sleep paralysis, hypnagogic hallucinations, automatic behavior, and frequent and vivid dreaming can all help establish the clinical diagnosis.

In order to improve time to diagnosis, questions about frequency of sleepiness, sleepiness while sedentary, dreaming during naps, and the age of onset of sleepiness help in identifying patients with narcolepsy. In addition, the diagnosis is less likely to be missed by clinicians if narcolepsy is included in the differential diagnosis of the complaint of sleepiness. Especially because other comorbid sleep disorders are commonly seen in narcolepsy, clinicians have to consider that more than 1 sleep disorder may be present.[24]

Diagnostic Criteria

In the International Classification of Sleep Disorders, Third Edition (ICSD-3), there are 2 forms of idiopathic narcolepsy: type 1 and type 2. Type 1 is consistent with hypocretin reduction or loss and requires the presence of cataplexy or reduced cerebrospinal fluid levels of orexin/hypocretin.[25]

Type 2 does not have cataplexy or hypocretin reduction, but polysomnogram (PSG) findings are essential. The Diagnostic and Statistical Manual of Mental Disorders, Fifth Edition, does not require objective polysomnographic criteria, whereas the ICSD-3 requires both a PSG and multiple sleep latency test (MSLT). Type 2 narcolepsy is more difficult to diagnose because the pathognomonic symptom of cataplexy is not present and false-negative objective testing can occur. A detailed clinical history with accurate knowledge of alternative diagnoses is essential to rule out other possible causes of chronic sleepiness.[26]

The MSLT with a short mean sleep latency (≤8 minutes) and 2 or more sleep onset REM periods (SOREMPs) is the most important diagnostic measure, and prior sleep deprivation, shift work, or circadian disorders should be excluded by actigraphy or sleep logs. On nocturnal polysomnography, a short REM sleep latency (≤15 minutes) can aid in the diagnosis of narcolepsy without cataplexy, although sensitivity is low. Hypocretin levels can be helpful, because levels are low to intermediate in 10% to 30% of patients with narcolepsy without cataplexy, but access to hypocretin analysis is limited.[27]

Misdiagnosis

It is common for patients with narcolepsy to first be misdiagnosed with a variety of mental and neurologic conditions.[28] Frequently children are misdiagnosed as having attention deficit/hyperactivity disorder (ADHD).[29,30] The variable level of activity and alertness is common to both disorders. In addition, the treatment of ADHD can mask the symptoms of narcolepsy, leading to a more prolonged delay in diagnosis and inappropriate treatment. Children may also be misdiagnosed with epilepsy and treated with anticonvulsant therapy[31] because of the paroxysmal nature of some of the symptoms of narcolepsy, most specifically the episodes of cataplexy and automatic behavior.

Psychiatric disorders, especially depression, are also common misdiagnoses in patients with narcolepsy.[32] For instance, Carter and colleagues[33] found that 60% of the 252 patients with narcolepsy interviewed were initially diagnosed with other conditions, such as depression and insomnia, despite visits with multiple health care providers. This finding is likely related to the high degree of neuropsychiatric comorbidity that can be present in these patients.

Sleep disturbance and resulting daytime fatigue cause some patients to be misdiagnosed with a primary form of insomnia. Alternatively, weight gain, which is common at the onset of narcolepsy, can lead to a misdiagnosis of OSA if the patient also develops sleep disordered breathing (SDB). Narcolepsy and OSA can occur together because OSA is very common and many patients with narcolepsy have SDB as well. However, the misdiagnosis of sleep apnea as being the primary cause of the sleepiness can cause a delay in the diagnosis of narcolepsy and in initiation of appropriate treatment.

Comorbidities

Patients with narcolepsy have a significant risk for comorbid medical conditions. Potential comorbidities include eating disorders; obesity; hypercholesterolemia; gastrointestinal disorders; diabetes; psychiatric conditions, including schizophrenia and depression; fibromyalgia; neurologic symptoms, including migraine headaches and cognitive dysfunction; other autoimmune disorders; and impairment of psychosocial function.[34] Among adults with narcolepsy, there is a greater prevalence of medical and psychiatric comorbidities,[29] as well as a statistically significant 1.5-fold excess mortality ($P<.001$) relative to a non-narcolepsy population, for reasons that are unclear.[29]

Psychiatric comorbidity, commonly anxiety and depression, is reported up to 4 times more often in patients with narcolepsy. Note that these patients can be at risk for suicidality and the use of sedative neuropsychiatric medications in combination with medication for the treatment of narcolepsy can increase this risk.[35]

There is a growing body of evidence showing that both children and adults with narcolepsy are more likely to be overweight or obese. One explanation may be that there is increased body mass index (BMI) and leptin levels indicating altered energy homeostasis, particularly in hypocretin-deficient patients with narcolepsy.[36] In addition, compared with idiopathic hypersomnia, patients with narcolepsy also have a greater waist circumference, increased waist/hip ratio, increase of diastolic blood pressure, and high cholesterol and triglyceride values independent of BMI.[37]

OSA, insomnia, and other sleep disorders can be present in patients with narcolepsy and contribute to the EDS. These other disorders may be overlooked during the focus on management strategies for narcolepsy. This possibility is especially important because pharmaceutical intervention for treatment of narcolepsy can exacerbate or precipitate other sleep disorders, such as OSA, periodic limb movements, restless legs syndrome (RLS), and REM behavioral disorder (RBD).[38,39]

Incorrect, Delayed, and Ineffective Treatment

It is important that the treating physicians have complete familiarity with the mechanism of action, dosing regimens, and rationale for specific use of medication used to treat narcolepsy[40] in order to improve the comfort, compliance, and safety of patients. Methylphenidate and amphetamines predate the use of modafinil/armodafinil, and, although they are less costly than the newer drugs, they are associated with a potential for abuse, as well as side effects that include growth suppression in children and cardiovascular disease in adults.[41,42] However, despite the risk for abuse, in clinical practice, patients with narcolepsy rarely abuse drugs for narcolepsy or develop addictions.[16,17] These stimulants are considered second-line (methylphenidate) or third-line (amphetamines) therapy for narcolepsy and should be considered after failure of treatment with sodium oxybate and/or modafinil/armodafinil.

Antidepressants are frequently used for treatment of cataplexy, despite few data being available regarding efficacy and lack of US Food and Drug Administration (FDA) approval for this indication. Clinically, case reports suggest that they can be effective, with long-acting serotonin-norepinephrine reuptake inhibitors being favored.[43-45] In addition, use of these medications may be limited by side effects that include insomnia, mental stimulation, and reduced sexual function, as well as precipitation of RBD and RLS.[46,47]

It is common for patients to be given a diagnosis of depression or ADHD as the primary cause of the symptoms, as opposed to narcolepsy. The challenge here is that the therapy for depression or

ADHD may mask the symptoms of narcolepsy and lead to delayed and ineffective therapy.

An additional layer of difficulty leading to delayed, ineffective, or incorrect management is health insurance companies that are not knowledgeable about current therapy for narcolepsy. In this circumstance, physicians may be forced to use lesser therapy options because of a company's belief that stimulants are first-line therapy, particularly because these medications are cheaper than newer, more effective medications. Additional limitations that may be encountered with some newer medications, such as sodium oxybate, are that they may not only require a prior authorization for dispensing (thereby delaying treatment) but they may also require the expertise of a clinician who has extensive experience in their administration in order to achieve maximal benefit for the patient.

SOCIOECONOMIC BURDEN

Patients with narcolepsy have significantly higher rates of health-related contact and medication use, and a higher socioeconomic cost. Narcolepsy is associated with impaired function, a lower quality of life, and reductions in employment and work productivity that result in indirect costs that further increase the economic burden.[48–50] Interpersonal relationships and psychological well-being are impaired in narcoleptic patients.[51] The sleepiness and impaired function also likely contribute to the higher risk of vehicular and work-related accidents among adults with narcolepsy.[52,53]

Educational Compromise

Adjusting to narcolepsy as a student can adversely affect education, particularly because the narcolepsy diagnosis is often delayed. Before diagnosis, a student's grades and relationship and trust with teachers and administrators may have deteriorated because of several factors, including symptoms that interfere with the child's ability to keep pace with peers or the misperception of sleepiness as laziness, ADHD,[54] and oppositional behavior or disruptive conduct disorder that may lead to disciplinary action. School staff may not be knowledgeable about narcolepsy and not know how to help the diagnosed student. Educating school administrators and teachers greatly improves these students' ability to manage their conditions and succeed in school.[55]

Employment and Productivity, and Retirement Challenges

Patients with narcolepsy have lower employment rates, and those in employment have a lower income level than control individuals.[56] There is an increase in absenteeism (the percentage of time people miss work because of health problems), as well as presenteeism (the percentage of time people's work productivity is affected by health problems).[57] Irresistible sleepiness is typically associated with work absences.[22] Narcolepsy is the cause of unemployment for many patients. For instance, in patients with sleep attacks, there is a significant correlation between early retirement and higher indirect costs compared with patients without these attacks.[49]

Many patients with narcolepsy need to go on full disability compensation.[49] This burden results in an impact on patients, their families, partners, and caregivers, and there are substantial economic effects on the health care system caused by the direct medical costs.[48–50,56]

Health Care Use and Costs, Direct and Indirect

People with narcolepsy have higher annual rates of inpatient admissions; emergency department visits, with or without admission; hospital outpatient visits; other outpatient services; and physician visits than control populations.[50] There is an increase in traditional health care professional visits, neurologist visits, and psychiatrist visits.[57]

The rate of total annual drug prescriptions was doubled in narcolepsy versus controls, including a 337% and 72% higher usage rate of narcolepsy drugs and non-narcolepsy drugs, respectively (both $P<.0001$). Mean yearly costs are significantly higher in narcolepsy compared with controls for medical services ($8346 vs $4147; $P<.0001$) and drugs ($3356 vs $1114; $P<.0001$). Narcolepsy is associated with substantial personal and economic burdens, as indicated by significantly higher rates of health care use and medical costs.[50]

Effects on health care costs can be identified up to 11 years before the first diagnosis and become more pronounced as the disease advances. Narcolepsy causes socioeconomic consequences, not only for patients but also for their partners, which occur years before disease diagnosis, confirming a diagnostic delay.[56]

This high socioeconomic burden is comparable with other chronic neurologic diseases, and the indirect health care costs are considerably higher than the direct costs.[49]

Psychosocial Consequences and Quality of Life

There is reduced quality of life in patients with narcolepsy.[57] Issues regarding interpersonal relationships and psychological well-being are also well documented, with problem areas including sexual dysfunction, depression, low levels of self-esteem, anxiety, social and emotional withdrawal, poor psychosocial adjustment, and irritability.[51] Depressive symptoms are strongly associated with lower quality-of-life scores.[22]

REDUCING THE BURDEN OF NARCOLEPSY
Early, Rapid, and Accurate Diagnosis

In addition to clinicians' lack of symptom recognition, which can be improved through educational initiatives to expand symptom awareness, a barrier to diagnosis is the lack of readily available and accurate biomarkers and diagnostic tests for narcolepsy, especially in the absence of cataplexy. The diagnostic challenges of narcolepsy in the absence of cataplexy are well recognized. The ICSD-3 distinguishes between 2 types of narcolepsy, and these criteria endorse a greater reliance on biomarkers and electrophysiologic testing than symptom recognition. Limitations occur in making a clinical diagnosis of cataplexy, which is largely a patient-reported symptom that is rarely witnessed by clinicians and is subject to mistaken recognition, lack of awareness, or denial of symptoms by the patient.

In the absence of cataplexy, and with negative MSLT findings diagnostic for type 2 narcolepsy, the presence of severe EDS usually leads to a diagnosis of idiopathic hypersomnia if other causes of EDS are excluded and the MSLT shows an MSL less than or equal to 8 minutes.[25] Idiopathic hypersomnia can be as disabling as narcolepsy and can evolve into type 1 or type 2 narcolepsy. This possibility was also suggested by a case history that documented an initial diagnosis of idiopathic hypersomnia. Electrophysiologic features and diagnostic symptoms characteristic of type 2 narcolepsy occurred, and ultimately there was the development of cataplexy and reduced cerebrospinal fluid hypocretin levels indicating narcolepsy type 1.[58]

The implication of this case is that narcolepsy may represent a continuum, and, as discussed by the investigators, type 2 narcolepsy may represent an intermediate stage. Such a concept has also been suggested by postmortem data from a patient with narcolepsy without cataplexy showing only a 33% loss of hypocretin neurons, in contrast with greater than 90% loss in type 1.[59]

Although cataplexy is the pathognomonic symptom for narcolepsy, it is present in only up to 70% of patients with narcolepsy, and many patients have EDS as their main symptom. EDS may be more debilitating and also can be caused by several sleep disorders, including chronic sleep deprivation and OSA.[25] It is important that clinicians recognize the presence of the ancillary symptoms of narcolepsy, such as hypnagogic hallucinations, automatic behavior, excessive and unusual dreaming, and sleep paralysis that can help establish a presumptive clinical diagnosis that can lead to ordering of appropriate confirmatory diagnostic tests.

Barriers that may unduly delay treatment, such as an absolute requirement for positive diagnostic biomarkers, should be avoided by health care companies, who should accept the most appropriate clinical criteria that can enable a timely diagnosis. Such criteria may include the presence of narcolepsy-associated symptoms, including cataplexy, sometimes allowing treatment to begin before definitive positive testing can be obtained. The strongest rationale for objective testing is the absence of cataplexy in the presence of other narcolepsy-related symptoms, and the PSG and MSLT in this situation should be recognized without restrictions, such as prior authorization by health care companies. Appropriate use of polysomnographic tests may provide additional objective support of a narcolepsy diagnosis in the presence of cataplexy, reducing the chance of a false-positive result if relying exclusively on patient-reported presence of cataplexy.

Although sleep studies are useful in the pediatric population, their specificity and sensitivity in children and adolescents has not been confirmed, suggesting that symptomatic presentation may be a useful diagnostic indicator, and that reliance on sleep studies should be individualized depending on the clinical situation.

Negative objective tests for narcolepsy should never be considered conclusive in the presence of clinical features of narcolepsy, especially because there are limitations of the MSLT.[4,60–64] Confounding factors, such as the use of some medications and the presence of other medical and psychiatric disorders, such as anxiety, can affect test results. Although patients with narcolepsy may display negative objective findings, the consequences of symptoms are nevertheless disabling, and patients presenting with symptoms and other characteristics consistent with narcolepsy should be initiated on therapy and the testing repeated at a later date as recommended by the ICSD-3.[25]

Timely, Effective, and Comprehensive Treatment

In the United States, several medications are approved by the FDA for management of narcolepsy, and there are additional drugs that may be effective for some symptoms but are not currently

FDA approved. Modafinil and armodafinil are FDA approved only for EDS. Methylphenidate and amphetamines, approved for narcolepsy although they only have benefit for EDS, predate the use of modafinil/armodafinil. Although they are less costly than the newer drugs, they are considered second-line (methylphenidate) or third-line (amphetamines) therapy.

Modafinil and armodafinil may be considered first-line therapy, although neither of these drugs is effective as monotherapy for symptoms other than EDS. Their efficacy may be enhanced with concomitant use of sodium oxybate,[65] which is approved for both EDS and cataplexy in adults with narcolepsy.[66]

Sodium oxybate is the only medication approved by the FDA in the United States for the treatment of both EDS and cataplexy associated with narcolepsy, for which it is considered first-line therapy.[67] It is also the only medication recommended in the American Academy of Sleep Medicine and European Federation of Neurological Societies guidelines for all the symptoms of narcolepsy.[67,68] Sodium oxybate usually requires titration, and although rapid initial benefit typically occurs, it may take up to 7 months to see maximum benefit.[69] Therefore, the sooner the patient is started on the medication and the better the clinical supervision the more rapid the maximal beneficial response.

Other treatments can include antidepressants, such as selective serotonin reuptake inhibitors, serotonin-norepinephrine reuptake inhibitors, and tricyclic antidepressants, for the treatment of cataplexy, sleep paralysis, and hypnagogic hallucinations.[67] However, these drugs are not FDA approved for the treatment of narcolepsy and there is less evidence for their efficacy than for first-line or FDA-approved drugs for narcolepsy.[67]

There is no single management strategy for initiating treatment. Therefore, treatment decisions have to be customized based on clinician-patient discussions regarding the symptoms, needs, and goals of individual patients.

Management of Adverse Medication Effects

Almost all patients use prescription medications to treat their narcolepsy. For many, these drugs drastically improve their symptoms; however, the side effects can be significant. Many patients have had to give up a beneficial drug because of intolerable side effects or because of the development of tolerance.

Modafinil and armodafinil use may cause allergic reactions and severe rashes, notably in children, although these are rare occurrences, and can reduce the efficacy of oral contraceptives.[70,71] Sodium oxybate can cause nausea and abnormal neuropsychiatric effects and its use may be limited because of potential interactions with alcohol, sedative hypnotics, and other central nervous system depressants.[66]

As mentioned earlier, methylphenidate and amphetamines are associated with a potential for tolerance, abuse, and side effects that include growth suppression in children and cardiovascular disease in adults.[41,42]

In addition, nondrug therapies such as scheduled naps, diet modifications, and exercise play an important role in helping patients with narcolepsy manage their condition, but they do not eliminate the symptoms.[51]

School/Work Accommodations

Educating school administrators and teachers greatly improves students' ability to manage their conditions and succeed in school. Children with narcolepsy are eligible for 504 classifications. This designation entitles the child, through the board of education, to school-based accommodations to allow the child the same opportunity as other children to excel in school. Accommodations should be tailored to meet each individual's needs. Possible accommodations include scheduled nap breaks, designated nap location, recording devices such as a smart pen, shared notes from teacher or classmates, extended time on tests and homework assignments, breaks during tests, and excused absenteeism.[55]

For work, a reasonable accommodation is a change or adjustment to a job or a workplace that allows people with narcolepsy to apply for jobs or to perform the essential work duties. These patients should be protected by the Americans with Disabilities Act to help achieve accommodations necessary for a safe and effective work environment. Examples of reasonable accommodations may include changing an employee's work schedule; assigning nonessential functions of the job to other employees; providing the employee with special equipment, devices, or software; restructuring the employee's job; providing the employee with additional training; and providing the employee with paid or unpaid leave needed because of the disability.

Psychosocial Management

The difficulty of gaining a correct and early diagnosis and the detrimental psychosocial impact of delayed diagnosis and effective treatment of narcolepsy has formed a consistent barrier to understanding the basis of problems in narcolepsy.

Box 1
Summary of narcolepsy burden and reduction strategies

Narcolepsy burden:

- Narcolepsy is a lifelong, incurable, disabling neurologic disorder that typically begins in childhood and is not rare in patients presenting with excessive sleepiness
- Diagnosis is delayed 8 to 15 years because of limitations in accuracy and availability of diagnostic biomarkers
- Symptoms develop over time, and initial diagnostic tests may be falsely negative despite severe and specific clinical symptoms and signs
- Narcolepsy produces impaired psychosocial development, education, and employment, and can result in permanent disability
- There is a high burden of illness associated with comorbidities, increased mortality, and high health care resource use and associated costs
- Narcolepsy is a spectrum and narcolepsy without cataplexy can be as debilitating as that with cataplexy

To reduce the burden of narcolepsy:

General:

- Public and clinician education about the clinical features of narcolepsy is essential to improve early diagnosis
- Diagnostic electrophysiologic tests should be performed whenever the disorder is suspected, and awareness of the limitations of the tests is essential in avoiding a falsely negative diagnosis
- Medication treatment should be initiated early, especially when cataplexy is present, primarily because of safety concerns but also to improve quality of life
- Multiple concurrent medications should be considered and may be required using a therapeutic approach that needs to be individualized
- Older narcolepsy medications, such as methylphenidate and amphetamines, should be regarded as second-line or third-line treatment options because of their potential for abuse and severe adverse effects
- Structure days to maintain entrainment of the circadian sleep-wake rhythm and limit length of naps to avoid disrupting nighttime sleep
- Screening for development of comorbid medical and psychiatric illness
- Psychosocial support is necessary for most patients with narcolepsy

School-aged population:

- Physician involvement with school teachers and faculty to improve understanding of narcolepsy
- Education accommodations (eg, 504 classification)
- Scheduled and strategic naps to improve school day performance in a designated nap area
- Recording devices such as a smart pen and shared notes from teacher or classmates
- Extended time on tests and homework assignments and breaks during tests
- Excused absenteeism

Working population:

- Workplace accommodations, such as changing the employee's work schedule
- Assigning nonessential functions of the job to other employees
- Providing the employee with special equipment, devices, or software
- Restructuring the employee's job
- Providing the employee with additional training
- Providing the employee with paid or unpaid leave needed because of the disability

Patients with narcolepsy experience difficulties with posttreatment medication regimens and there is a need for pretreatment and posttreatment psychoeducation and support. Considerable psychosocial challenges can arise for patients with narcolepsy, and addressing these challenges should form part of treatment, because, if left unattended, they may interfere with longer-term psychosocial functioning and outcome.[72]

Once effective treatment has begun, continuous psychosocial management is essential.[72] Patients with narcolepsy adjust following successful treatment as the patient discards perceptions of illness and behaviors associated with being sick and learns to become well. Recognition of the burden of normality has important clinical implications for maximizing the posttreatment care and outcome of patients with narcolepsy.[72]

Measures should be taken to increase public and clinician awareness of this disease. Appropriate treatment must be provided in order to increase quality of life and to assist patients continuing with a functional working life[49] (**Box 1**).

SUMMARY

As summarized in **Box 1**, although narcolepsy has a low prevalence, it is a debilitating disease with a substantial clinical and socioeconomic burden resulting from its early onset, severe symptoms, delay in diagnosis, lack of cure, and a need for lifelong therapy. This need for lifelong therapy, in particular, requires the establishment of health care policies that shorten the time to finding an effective treatment plan. Appropriate treatment results in long-term benefits from both patient and societal perspectives by improving clinical outcomes, potentially enabling improved education and increased employment and work productivity, and quality of life.

REFERENCES

1. Okun ML, Lin L, Pelin Z, et al. Clinical aspects of narcolepsy-cataplexy across ethnic groups. Sleep 2002;25(1):27–35.
2. Dauvilliers Y, Montplaisir J, Molinari N, et al. Age at onset of narcolepsy in two large populations of patients in France and Quebec. Neurology 2001; 57(11):2029–33.
3. Thorpy MJ, Cronin S, Temple H. Age of onset and time to diagnosis of narcolepsy [abstract S20.002]. Neurology 1999;52(Suppl 2):A110.
4. Aran A, Einen M, Lin L, et al. Clinical and therapeutic aspects of childhood narcolepsy-cataplexy: a retrospective study of 51 children. Sleep 2010;33(11): 1457–64.
5. Anic-Labat S, Guilleminault C, Kraemer HC, et al. Validation of a cataplexy questionnaire in 983 sleep-disorders patients. Sleep 1999;22(1):77–87.
6. Pizza F, Franceschini C, Peltola H, et al. Clinical and polysomnographic course of childhood narcolepsy with cataplexy. Brain 2013;136(Pt 12):3787–95.
7. Schredl M. Dreams in patients with sleep disorders. Sleep Med Rev 2009;13(3):215–21.
8. Mazzetti M, Bellucci C, Mattarozzi K, et al. REM-dreams recall in patients with narcolepsy-cataplexy. Brain Res Bull 2010;81(1):133–40.
9. Wamsley E, Donjacour CE, Scammell TE, et al. Delusional confusion of dreaming and reality in narcolepsy. Sleep 2014;37(2):419–22.
10. Roth T, Dauvilliers Y, Mignot E, et al. Disrupted nighttime sleep in narcolepsy. J Clin Sleep Med 2013; 9(9):955–65.
11. Dauvilliers Y, Rompré S, Gagnon J-F, et al. REM sleep characteristics in narcolepsy and REM sleep behavior disorder. Sleep 2007;30(7):844–9.
12. Ganado W. The narcolepsy syndrome. Neurology 1958;8(6):487–96.
13. Bellebaum C, Daum I. Memory and cognition in narcolepsy. In: Meeta G, Thorpy MJ, Pandi-Perumal SR, editors. Narcolepsy: a clinical guide. Switzerland: Springer International Publishing; 2016. p. 233–43.
14. Delazer M, Hogl B, Zamarian L, et al. Executive functions, information sampling, and decision making in narcolepsy with cataplexy. Neuropsychology 2011;25(4):477–87.
15. Bayard S, Abril B, Yu H, et al. Decision making in narcolepsy with cataplexy. Sleep 2011;34(1):99–104.
16. Bayard S, Langenier MC, Dauvilliers Y. Effect of psychostimulants on impulsivity and risk taking in narcolepsy with cataplexy. Sleep 2013;36(9):1335–40.
17. Bayard S, Dauvilliers YA. Reward-based behaviors and emotional processing in human with narcolepsy-cataplexy. Front Behav Neurosci 2013;7:50.
18. Rogers AE, Rosenberg RS. Tests of memory in narcoleptics. Sleep 1990;13(1):42–52.
19. Aguirre M, Broughton R, Stuss D. Does memory impairment exist in narcolepsy-cataplexy? J Clin Exp Neuropsychol 1985;7(1):14–24.
20. Naumann A, Bellebaum C, Daum I. Cognitive deficits in narcolepsy. J Sleep Res 2006;15(3):329–38.
21. Thorpy MJ, Krieger AC. Delayed diagnosis of narcolepsy: characterization and impact. Sleep Med 2014;15(5):502–7.
22. Ingravallo F, Gnucci V, Pizza F, et al. The burden of narcolepsy with cataplexy: how disease history and clinical features influence socio-economic outcomes. Sleep Med 2012;13(10):1293–300.
23. Rosenberg R, Kim AY. The AWAKEN survey: knowledge of narcolepsy among physicians and the general population. Postgrad Med 2014;126(1):78–86.
24. Daniels E, King MA, Smith IE, et al. Health-related quality of life in narcolepsy. J Sleep Res 2001;10(1):75–81.

25. American Academy of Sleep Medicine. International classification of sleep disorders. 3rd edition. Darien (IL): American Academy of Sleep Medicine; 2014.

26. Baumann CR, Mignot E, Lammers GJ, et al. Challenges in diagnosing narcolepsy without cataplexy: a consensus statement. Sleep 2014;37(6):1035–42.

27. Mignot E, Lammers GJ, Ripley B, et al. The role of cerebrospinal fluid hypocretin measurement in the diagnosis of narcolepsy and other hypersomnias. Arch Neurol 2002;59(10):1553–62.

28. Kryger MH, Walid R, Manfreda J. Diagnoses received by narcolepsy patients in the year prior to diagnosis by a sleep specialist. Sleep 2002;25(1):36–41.

29. Ohayon MM. Narcolepsy is complicated by high medical and psychiatric comorbidities: a comparison with the general population. Sleep Med 2013; 14(6):488–92.

30. Modestino EJ, Winchester J. A retrospective survey of childhood ADHD symptomatology among adult narcoleptics. J Atten Disord 2013;17(7):574–82.

31. Macleod S, Ferrie C, Zuberi SM. Symptoms of narcolepsy in children misinterpreted as epilepsy. Epileptic Disord 2005;7(1):13–7.

32. Morrish E, King MA, Smith IE, et al. Factors associated with a delay in the diagnosis of narcolepsy. Sleep Med 2004;5(1):37–41.

33. Carter LP, Acebo C, Kim A. Patients' journeys to a narcolepsy diagnosis: a physician survey and retrospective chart review. Postgrad Med 2014;126(3): 216–24.

34. Panossian LA, Avidan AY. Narcolepsy and other comorbid medical illnesses. In: Meeta G, Thorpy MJ, Pandi-Perumal SR, editors. Narcolepsy: a clinical guide. Switzerland: Springer International Publishing; 2016. p. 147–59.

35. Wang YG, Swick TJ, Carter LP, et al. Safety overview of postmarketing and clinical experience of sodium oxybate (Xyrem): abuse, misuse, dependence, and diversion. J Clin Sleep Med 2009;5(4):365–71.

36. Nishino S, Ripley B, Overeem S, et al. Low cerebrospinal fluid hypocretin (Orexin) and altered energy homeostasis in human narcolepsy. Ann Neurol 2001;50(3):381–8.

37. Poli F, Plazzi G, Di Dalmazi G, et al. Body mass index-independent metabolic alterations in narcolepsy with cataplexy. Sleep 2009;32(11):1491–7.

38. Abril B, Carlander B, Touchon J, et al. Restless legs syndrome in narcolepsy: a side effect of sodium oxybate? Sleep Med 2007;8(2):181–3.

39. Thorpy MJ, Dauvilliers Y. Clinical and practical considerations in the pharmacologic management of narcolepsy. Sleep Med 2015;16(1):9–18.

40. Mignot EJ. A practical guide to the therapy of narcolepsy and hypersomnia syndromes. Neurotherapeutics 2012;9(4):739–52.

41. Auger RR, Goodman SH, Silber MH, et al. Risks of high-dose stimulants in the treatment of disorders of excessive somnolence: a case-control study. Sleep 2005;28(6):667–72.

42. Vitiello B. Understanding the risk of using medications for attention deficit hyperactivity disorder with respect to physical growth and cardiovascular function. Child Adolesc Psychiatr Clin N Am 2008;17(2): 459–74, xi.

43. Frey J, Darbonne C. Fluoxetine suppresses human cataplexy: a pilot study. Neurology 1994;44(4): 707–9.

44. Izzi F, Placidi F, Marciani MG, et al. Effective treatment of narcolepsy-cataplexy with duloxetine: a report of three cases. Sleep Med 2009;10(1):153–4.

45. Moller LR, Ostergaard JR. Treatment with venlafaxine in six cases of children with narcolepsy and with cataplexy and hypnagogic hallucinations. J child Adolesc Psychopharmacol 2009;19(2):197–201.

46. Ju YE, Larson-Prior L, Duntley S. Changing demographics in REM sleep behavior disorder: possible effect of autoimmunity and antidepressants. Sleep Med 2011;12(3):278–83.

47. Drug-induced restless legs syndrome. Prescrire Int 2010;19(108):164–5.

48. Dodel R, Peter H, Spottke A, et al. Health-related quality of life in patients with narcolepsy. Sleep Med 2007;8(7–8):733–41.

49. Dodel R, Peter H, Walbert T, et al. The socioeconomic impact of narcolepsy. Sleep 2004;27(6):1123–8.

50. Black J, Reaven NL, Funk SE, et al. The Burden of Narcolepsy Disease (BOND) study: health-care utilization and cost findings. Sleep Med 2014;15(5): 522–9.

51. Buttoo K, Pandi-Perumal SR, Guilleminault C. Narcolepsy and mental illness. In: Meeta G, Thorpy Michael J, Pandi-Perumal SR, editors. Narcolepsy: a clinical guide. Switzerland: Springer International Publishing; 2016. p. 277–84.

52. Philip P, Sagaspe P, Lagarde E, et al. Sleep disorders and accidental risk in a large group of regular registered highway drivers. Sleep Med 2010; 11(10):973–9.

53. Smolensky MH, Di Milia L, Ohayon MM, et al. Sleep disorders, medical conditions, and road accident risk. Accid Anal Prev 2011;43(2):533–48.

54. Dahl RE, Pelham WE, Wierson M. The role of sleep disturbances in attention deficit disorder symptoms: a case study. J Pediatr Psychol 1991;16(2):229–39.

55. Flygare J. Succeeding in school and in the workplace with narcolepsy. In: Meeta G, Thorpy MJ, Pandi-Perumal SR, editors. Narcolepsy: a clinical guide. Switzerland: Springer International Publishing; 2016. p. 395–406.

56. Jennum P, Ibsen R, Petersen ER, et al. Health, social, and economic consequences of narcolepsy: a controlled national study evaluating the societal effect on patients and their partners. Sleep Med 2012;13(8):1086–93.

57. Flores NM, Villa KF, Black J, et al. The humanistic and economic burden of narcolepsy. J Clin Sleep Med 2016;12(3):401–7.

58. Pizza F, Vandi S, Liguori R, et al. Primary progressive narcolepsy type 1: the other side of the coin. Neurology 2014;83(23):2189–90.

59. Thannickal TC, Nienhuis R, Siegel JM. Localized loss of hypocretin (orexin) cells in narcolepsy without cataplexy. Sleep 2009;32(8):993–8.

60. Stores G, Montgomery P, Wiggs L. The psychosocial problems of children with narcolepsy and those with excessive daytime sleepiness of uncertain origin. Pediatrics 2006;118(4):e1116–23.

61. Dorris L, Zuberi SM, Scott N, et al. Psychosocial and intellectual functioning in childhood narcolepsy. Dev Neurorehabil 2008;11(3):187–94.

62. Peraita-Adrados R, Garcia-Penas JJ, Ruiz-Falco L, et al. Clinical, polysomnographic and laboratory characteristics of narcolepsy-cataplexy in a sample of children and adolescents. Sleep Med 2011;12(1):24–7.

63. Nevsimalova S. The diagnosis and treatment of pediatric narcolepsy. Curr Neurol Neurosci Rep 2014;14(8):469.

64. Inocente CO, Lavault S, Lecendreux M, et al. Impact of obesity in children with narcolepsy. CNS Neurosci Ther 2013;19(7):521–8.

65. Black J, Houghton WC. Sodium oxybate improves excessive daytime sleepiness in narcolepsy. Sleep 2006;29(7):939–46.

66. Xyrem [package insert]. Palo Alto CJP, Inc; 2014.

67. Morgenthaler TI, Kapur VK, Brown T, et al. Practice parameters for the treatment of narcolepsy and other hypersomnias of central origin. Sleep 2007;30(12):1705–11.

68. Billiard M, Bassetti C, Dauvilliers Y, et al. EFNS guidelines on management of narcolepsy. Eur J Neurol 2006;13(10):1035–48.

69. Bogan RK, Roth T, Schwartz J, et al. Time to response with sodium oxybate for the treatment of excessive daytime sleepiness and cataplexy in patients with narcolepsy. J Clin Sleep Med 2015;11(4):427–32.

70. Nuvigil [packet insert]. Frazer PC, Inc; 2010.

71. Provigil [packet insert]. Frazer PC, Inc; 2010.

72. Wilson SJ, Frazer DW, Lawrence JA, et al. Psychosocial adjustment following relief of chronic narcolepsy. Sleep Med 2007;8(3):252–9.

Neurologic Diseases and Sleep

Daniel A. Barone, MD[a],*, Sudansu Chokroverty, MD[b]

KEYWORDS

- Stroke • Migraine • Chronic pain • Epilepsy • Neurodegenerative disease • Dementia
- Socioeconomic

KEY POINTS

- Sleep disorders are often comorbid with neurologic illness, either of which may negatively impact socioeconomic status.
- Reductions in workplace attendance and productivity, public safety, and personal well-being may occur with either set of conditions, more so when combined.
- The socioeconomic burden of sleep disorders and neurologic illness can be identified, but the real cost of these conditions lies far beyond the financial realm.

INTRODUCTION

Sleep disorders are commonly associated with various comorbid conditions, including general medical, psychiatric, and neurologic disorders,[1] all of which may impact socioeconomic status negatively. Additionally, sustained sleep deprivation results in reduced workplace productivity, public safety,[2] and personal well-being,[3] as well as performance deficits, poor vigilance, excessive daytime sleepiness, depressed mood, and impairments in concentration and memory.[4,5] This review focuses on the relationship that sleep has on the socioeconomic impact of common neurologic illnesses including stroke, migraines and chronic pain, epilepsy, restless legs syndrome (RLS), and neurodegenerative diseases and dementia. Other conditions existing within the neurologic and sleep realms, particularly narcolepsy, will be discussed elsewhere in this issue of *Sleep Medicine Clinics*.

SOCIOECONOMIC IMPACT OF VARIOUS SLEEP DISORDERS

Sleep disorders affect approximately 35% to 40% of the US adult population annually, and are a significant cause of morbidity and mortality. However, there is an underappreciation and undertreatment of these conditions, and the socioeconomic implications may be immense, particularly with regard to obstructive sleep apnea (OSA), insomnia, and sleep deprivation.

Obstructive Sleep Apnea

The socioeconomic burden of OSA is significant, given its high prevalence and its association with increased cardiovascular disease morbidity and mortality.[6] The costliest and the sickest upper one-third of patients with OSA consume 65% to 82% of all medical costs, and untreated OSA may double the medical expenses mainly because of cardiovascular disease.[7] One study, using data from the Danish National Patient Registry (1998–2006), found that snoring, OSA, and obesity hypoventilation syndrome were associated with significantly higher rates of health-related contact, medication use, and unemployment, and accounted for increased socioeconomic costs. It was found that these socioeconomic effects increased proportionally with the severity of OSA, and the consequences were present up to 8 years before diagnosis. It was concluded that despite

[a] Center for Sleep Medicine, Weill Cornell Medical College, 425 East 61st, 5th Floor, New York, NY 10065, USA;
[b] JFK Neuroscience Institute/Seton Hall University, 65 James Street, Edison, NJ 08818, USA
* Corresponding author.
E-mail address: dab9192@med.cornell.edu

Sleep Med Clin 12 (2017) 73–85
http://dx.doi.org/10.1016/j.jsmc.2016.10.007
1556-407X/17/© 2016 Elsevier Inc. All rights reserved.

sleep.theclinics.com

treatment with continuous positive airway pressure (CPAP), which does reduce mortality, earlier disease detection could have a greater impact on socioeconomic factors.[8] Furthermore, in an analysis of 82,178 elderly veterans diagnosed with OSA, there was a higher incidence of health care use compared with those without OSA, and veterans with a new diagnosis of OSA had an higher rate of health care use in the year of diagnosis compared with patients with chronic OSA and patients without OSA.[9]

Insomnia

As with OSA, several studies have shown that insomnia affects the workforce. Absenteeism in those with insomnia is a major problem, and the economic impact may be severe. One study demonstrated that, compared with good sleepers, severe insomniacs reported more medical problems, had more physician office visits, were hospitalized twice as often, and used more medication. Furthermore, the severe insomniacs in this study had a higher rate of absenteeism (missing work twice as often as good sleepers), as well as decreased concentration and difficulty performing duties.[10] The impact of insomnia on workers affects their daytime functioning, and many studies have found a higher rate of work accidents in insomniacs.[11]

Sleep Deprivation

Sleep deprivation is associated with a range of metabolic abnormalities,[12] especially regarding glucose metabolism[13]; sleep-deprived patients have increased blood glucose and decreased insulin, contributing to insulin resistance, type 2 diabetes mellitus,[14] obesity,[15] and hypertension,[16] all of which may increase the risk of stroke.[16] Even 1 night of reduced sleep has been reported to increase food intake and to reduce energy expenditure in healthy subjects,[17] and studies using functional MRI have demonstrated acute sleep deprivation enhances hedonic stimulus processing, which may increase the drive to consume food.[18] Thus, an increase in hedonic food consumption combined with a reduction in energy expenditure may contribute to the development of obesity.[16] It has also been demonstrated that sleep deprivation is associated with a moderately increased risk of acute myocardial infarction[19] and other vascular events.[20] Although problems falling asleep or daytime sleepiness affect 35% to 40% of the population,[6] and sleep deprivation may significantly impact socioeconomic status, compared with healthy individuals, individuals suffering from sleep deprivation are less productive, have an increased health care use, and an increased likelihood of accidents. Nearly 20% of all serious car crash injuries are associated with driver sleepiness, independent of alcohol effects.[21] Chronic sleep deprivation, like other sleep disorders, places a significant burden on the health care system through increased use; patients in the highest quartile of the Epworth Sleepiness Scale are associated with an 11% increase in health care use.[22]

NEUROLOGIC DISORDERS, SLEEP DYSFUNCTION, AND SOCIOECONOMIC IMPACT

In this section, we address the bidirectional relationship between sleep and common neurologic illnesses, and how this relationship may increase socioeconomic burden.

Stroke

The worldwide impact of stroke is considerable, and it is estimated that there are 4.5 million deaths per year from stroke and more than 9 million stroke survivors. To this point, approximately 1 in 4 men and nearly 1 in 5 women aged 45 years can expect to have a stroke if they live to 85 years of age. The overall incidence rate of stroke is roughly 2 to 25 per thousand, and the risk of recurrence is 15% to 40% over 5 years; the total prevalence rate is approximately 5 per thousand. After a stroke, 65% of survivors are functionally independent at 1 year, with stroke comprising the major cause of disability.[23] Approximately one-fourth of strokes occur in people less than 65 years of age, which may have tremendous consequences in the socioeconomic realm. In the United States, cost of stroke has been estimated at greater than $65 billion. Direct costs, including that of physicians and other health professionals, acute and long-term care, and medications and other medical supplies, account for 67% of total costs, and the remaining 33% is due to indirect costs, which includes lost productivity.[24,25] A metaanalysis of 70 studies reported data on return to work after a stroke with ranges from 0% to 100%. Additional social consequences reported in this analysis included negative impact on family relationships (5%–54%), deterioration in sexual life (5%–76%), economic difficulties (24%–33%), and deterioration in leisure activities (15%–79%).[26] Although the literature linking stroke with sleep abnormalities has been focused mostly on sleep deprivation/insomnia and OSA (which is reviewed elsewhere in this article), sleep-related movement disorders such as RLS and periodic leg movements in sleep may also increase the risk of hypertension and cardiovascular disease,[27] potentially leading to increased morbidity that could eventually result in cerebrovascular events.[5]

Large-scale epidemiologic studies have established associations between OSA and cardiovascular disease.[28–31] The pathophysiology might be based on the alterations on the modulation of the autonomic nervous system during apneic events,[32] in that activation of the sympathetic nervous system occurs in association with respiratory events and predisposes to the development of cardiovascular disease and stroke,[33–36] although endocrine pathways may also be implicated.[37] Additionally, it is well-known that obesity is strongly linked with OSA, which has in turn been identified as an independent risk factor for stroke and all-cause mortality.[38] For example, a study of more than 6000 participants demonstrated that those with OSA had a 2-fold increase in odds ratio for having hypertension,[30] and the odds ratio for developing ischemic heart disease and cerebrovascular disease was increased by 3-fold and 4-fold, respectively, compared with the control population.[28–31]

Although there exist robust data linking OSA with stroke, the link between insomnia and stroke is more controversial. For example, 1 German study failed to demonstrate that the presence of insomnia led to increased incident stroke outcome in either sex. This study had a mean follow-up of 14 years, and 917 strokes (710 nonfatal strokes and 207 fatal strokes) were observed. Among men, the hazard ratio for the association between short ($\leq$5 hours) daily sleep duration and stroke was 1.44 (95% confidence interval [CI], 1.01–2.06). Among women, the quantity of sleep was also not related to any stroke outcome based on multivariate analysis.[39] However, a metaanalysis was performed including 122,501 subjects with 6332 cardiovascular events followed over 3 to 20 years and demonstrated that insomnia resulted in an increased risk of developing or dying from cardiovascular disease (relative risk, 1.45; 95% CI, 1.29–1.62; $P < .00001$).[40] In another study using information from a random sample of 1 million people during a 10-year follow-up, 1049 stroke events were identified, and in those with insomnia, there was a reported increased incidence of stroke (8.01 vs 3.69 per 1000 person-years; $P<.001$).[41]

Migraines and Chronic Pain

Migraines

Migraines are a form of chronic headaches that are moderate to severe in intensity, usually affecting one-half of the head, with a pulsating nature, and lasting from 2 to 72 hours. Associated symptoms may include nausea, vomiting, and sensitivity to light, sound, or smell. The pain is generally made worse by physical activity, and up to one-third of sufferers report an aura.[42] Approximately 18% of women and 6% of men suffer from migraine (an estimated 23.6 million Americans).[43] Migraine prevalence varies with age (highest in 35- to 45-year-olds), household income (highest in the lowest income group, which earned less than $10,000 annually), and race (higher in whites than in blacks).[44–49] Migraine may have major implications on the workforce; in a large telephone survey, it was reported loss of work time owing to migraine was 5.7 days per year per person affected.[50] This estimate takes no account of reduced effectiveness in those at work despite being in a migraine attack, otherwise known as presenteeism, nor does it include losses attributable to headache disorders other than migraine. Thus, it has been estimated that migraine, and other headache disorders, continuously reduce workforce capacity by greater than 1%.[51] However, despite the commonality and known burden of migraine, many sufferers remain underdiagnosed and undertreated, and suffer with substantial disability.[52–55]

Sleep has long been recognized to both provoke and relieve headaches,[5] and epidemiologic research has demonstrated an association between sleep disorders with more frequent and severe headaches.[56] The interactions between headache and sleep can be summarized as either sleep disturbances as the cause of headache (eg, sleep deprivation aggravating migraine, or OSA causing morning headaches), headache syndromes as the cause of sleep disturbances (eg, hypnic headaches), or sleep disturbances and headache existing in the same patient with similar causes (eg, tension-type headache and insomnia induced by depression).[5]

Most headaches related to sleep deprivation are usually diffuse or poorly localized, and do not have distinguishing features.[5] Dull, frontal-aching headaches may result in both normal subjects and in those who suffer from an underlying headache disorder in the context of sleep deprivation,[57] and there is an established relationship between sleep complaints, sleep disruption, and short nocturnal sleep duration[58,59] and migraines. Problems with initiating sleep or with maintaining a healthy sleep pattern may be factors migraine precipitation,[60,61] and short sleepers exhibit more migraine attacks than long sleepers and are also more likely to experience morning attacks at awakening.[62] Sleep has also been shown to provide migraine relief.[62] Similarly, sleep deprivation may be a precipitating factor for tension-type headaches,[63] but, given the fact that anxiety and depression are usually comorbid features, it is difficult to fully explain which is the main culprit.[5]

Regarding specific sleep disorders, the presence of a headache upon awakening is a nonspecific symptom in sleep-related respiratory disorders (eg, OSA, sleep-related alveolar hypoventilation, chronic obstructive pulmonary disorder), simple snoring,[64] and in other primary sleep disorders such as insomnia or periodic leg movements in sleep.[65] A retrospective study comprising 82 patients with headache and OSA showed that successful treatment with CPAP reduced headaches in up to 80% of patients, supporting OSA as a cause for the morning headaches,[66] and suggesting that the pathogenesis of headaches in patients with OSA is more likely related to hypoxia/hypercapnia rather than to a disturbance in sleep physiology.[5] In chronic headaches, the association between sleep deprivation and headache is stronger and more common than in episodic ones,[62,67] and a shorter sleep duration may predict severity in patients suffering from chronic headache.[68] Finally, data have shown that there exist genes that increase the risk of RLS, and a recent study demonstrated an association of the MEIS1 genetic variant with the comorbidity of RLS and migraine in patients, possibly secondary to an imbalance in iron homeostasis and the dopaminergic system may represent a link between RLS and migraines.[69]

The socioeconomic impact of migraines has been associated with disability and decreased functional status and consequent indirect costs to employers.[70–72] It has been found that those suffering with migraine required 3.8 bed rest days for men and 5.6 days for women each year, resulting in a total of 112 million bedridden days. Migraine costs American employers about $13 billion per year secondary to missed days of work and impaired work function. Annual direct medical costs for migraine care were about $1 billion, with approximately $100 spent on each diagnosed patient. Thus, the economic burden of migraine falls mostly on patients and their employers in the form of bedridden days and lost productivity.[73]

Chronic pain

As with headaches and headache syndromes, there exists a complex relationship between chronic pain and sleep, in that pain can disrupt sleep and poor sleep can exaggerate pain intensity. Sleep disturbances are often seen in the context of chronic pain, and includes changes in sleep continuity and sleep architecture, as well as increased sleepiness during the daytime.[5] It is well-known that pain disturbs sleep, and a reciprocal relationship has been proposed[74]; sleep deprivation has been hypothesized to produce hyperalgesic changes, and may interfere with analgesic treatments involving the opioid and serotoninergic systems.[5] There have been reports suggesting that disturbance of sleep continuity, not simply sleep restriction, impairs endogenous pain-inhibitory function and increases spontaneous pain,[75] and that, in healthy individuals, sleep deprivation, particularly of REM sleep, may induce hyperalgesia[76] and spontaneous pain.[77]

The report of sleep disturbance in those with chronic pain is a common finding, occurring in two-thirds of patients. In 1 study, chronic pain patients (n = 221) were recruited from a secondary care outpatient clinic, aged between 20 and 84 years (mean, 52). The majority were found to be "poor sleepers" (86%) with increased pain severity, depressive symptoms, and attention to pain. It was concluded that sleep disturbance may contribute to clinical pain severity indirectly through changes in mood and attention.[78] Other studies show that at least 50% (≤70%–88%) of patients suffering with chronic pain complain of significant sleep disturbance.[79–83] In a study analyzing 1090 chronic pain patients referred to the Pain Clinic of the Karlovac General Hospital, Karlovac, Croatia, it was found that those with musculoskeletal pain accounted for the highest percentage (n = 316; 29%), followed by those with neuropathic pain (n = 253; 23.20%), and those with low back pain (n = 225; 20.60%). Moderate to severe sleep impairment was present in patients over 65 years of age (P = .007), and in patients with musculoskeletal pain, neuropathic pain, and back pain (P = .001).[84]

Insomnia and chronic pain are major health problems worldwide, and are linked independently to significant reductions in quality of life,[85–87] psychiatric morbidity,[88,89] medical morbidity,[90] disability,[91,92] and estimated to cost the US economy well over $70 billion annually.[93–95] When they occur together, lost productivity is likely magnified.[96] The socioeconomic costs of chronic pain make it one of the costliest conditions,[97] and underscores the critical importance of identifying strategies to prevent these disorders and their consequences.[98]

Epilepsy

Epilepsy affects more than 50 million individuals worldwide, and there is strong evidence characterizing the relationship between sleep chronobiology and seizure disorders[5,99] Because sleep deprivation results in an increase in interepileptic discharges in those with epilepsy,[100] sleep deprivation has become an established method to elicit epileptiform activity in electroencephalography,[5] but exactly how sleep deprivation activates epileptic regions remains unclear.[5] Various sleep disorders may coexist with epilepsy, including OSA, RLS, narcolepsy, and insomnia,[101] and these disorders may contribute to sleep deprivation, which may worsen seizure frequency.[5] One investigation revealed that sleep disturbances were twice as common (38.6%) in 486 adult patients with focal epilepsy as compared with 492 nonepileptic controls (18%).[102]

The burden of epilepsy may be due to the physical hazards resulting from the unpredictability of seizures, social exclusion as a result of negative toward people with epilepsy, and the stigma of having epilepsy. Furthermore, there are associated psychological consequences, with increased levels of anxiety, depression, and poor self-esteem compared with people without epilepsy.[103] One prospective survey of 400 patients with epilepsy found that 62% reported at least 1 seizure precipitant[104]; of them, sleep deprivation was the second most common precipitant overall (stress was first), and reported by 18% of patients. Another survey of 71 subjects concluded that seizure occurrence was related significantly to lack of sleep, and higher stress and anxiety levels.[105] How sleep deprivation may increase the risk of epileptic seizures is not well-known, although the culprit may be a reduction of intracortical inhibition.[106] However, in another study of 84 patients with medically refractory focal epilepsy who underwent inpatient electroencephalography–polysomnographic monitoring, participants were assigned to either sleep deprivation every other night or to normal sleep, and seizures per day did not differ between the 2 groups.[107]

OSA is present in approximately 40% to 70% of epileptic patients, which may be a result of several factors, including a sedentary lifestyle and/or the effects of antiepileptic medications.[108] Antiepileptic medications may contribute to or worsen OSA given their effects on respiratory centers, their reduction on the threshold for awakening, and their effect of weight gain.[109] Additionally, it was demonstrated that epileptic patients greater than 50 years of age who concomitantly suffered with OSA had poorer control of seizures as compared with epileptic patients without OSA,[110] highlighting the relationship between epilepsy and OSA, in which the sleep fragmentation and sleep deprivation caused by OSA may facilitate the occurrence of seizures.[5] Treatment with CPAP improves daytime somnolence and quality of life, and results in better control of epileptic seizures,[111] as demonstrated by a pilot trial

conducted in 35 adults with refractory epilepsy and concurrent OSA, which revealed a 50% reduction in seizures in approximately 28% of the patients using CPAP therapy compared with those using sham therapy.[112] This and other reports have led to the thought that approximately one-third of patients with the combination of epilepsy and OSA will experience a beneficial effect on their seizures if OSA is treated.[5]

It is known that sleep deprivation decreases the odds of seizure remission. For example, in 1 cohort study, it was demonstrated that, for each hour of increased sleep on the preceding night, the relative odds of a seizure the following day decreased (odds ratio, 0.91; 95% CI, 0.82–0.99).[105] Similarly, there is evidence from small cohort studies that several risk factors may reduce significantly the likelihood of terminal remission, including the presence of symptomatic epilepsy, focal seizures or syndromes, slow waves on an electroencephalograph, greater seizure frequency, high stress or anxiety, and lack of sleep.[113] The findings of another study demonstrated that poor sleep quality, excessive daytime sleepiness, and insomnia were significantly associated with epilepsy (odds ratio, 3.52 [95% CI, 2.45–5.05]; 2.10 [95% CI, 1.41–3.12]; and 5.91 [95% CI, 3.43–10.16], respectively).[114] A report on 270 consecutive adult patients with epilepsy demonstrated that fatigue was more severe in epilepsy patients than in healthy controls without epilepsy, especially when seizures were not controlled. Concordantly, sleep-related impairments and depression aggravated fatigue in epilepsy patients.[115] In people with epilepsy, it was found that inadequate sleep hygiene is related independently to reduced quality of life, but indirectly related to anxiety and depressive symptoms through sleep quality.[116]

Epilepsy has important socioeconomic costs to a population, as 1 study assessing the burden of illness at the community level demonstrated. Patients assessed were those with established epilepsy (n = 1628), who were identified through the National Epilepsy Survey, and patients with newly diagnosed epilepsy (n = 602), from the National General Practice Study of Epilepsy. Per patient, initial direct costs of $917 per patient per year were found, which decreased after 8 years of follow-up to $254. The cost to the UK of newly diagnosed epilepsy in the first year was $27 million, and the total annual cost of established epilepsy was estimated at $2.895 billion; 69% of this total cost was secondary to indirect costs (unemployment and excess mortality).[117] Another study based on Arizona Medicaid claims, which included subjects who were aged 65 years or older, provided an estimated epilepsy incidence and prevalence for this population at 7.9 and 19.3 per 1000 person-years, respectively. This patient population had higher epilepsy incidence and prevalence compared with the general US population. It was concluded that these differences may be at least in part attributable to their low socioeconomic status.[118]

Restless Legs Syndrome

RLS is a common and often underestimated neurologic, sensory motor, and movement disorder, with a prevalence ranging from approximately 2.5% to 10% in Western industrialized countries. It was found in 1 metaanalysis that RLS is associated with reductions in quality of life similar to those seen in patients with other chronic conditions, and can result in a substantial economic burden.[12] RLS may affect quality and duration of sleep, which can impair next-day performance in such areas as activities of daily living (ie, work, household chores), cognitive functioning (ie, concentration, forgetfulness, mental tiredness, alertness), emotional functioning (ie, irritability, depressed mood), physical functioning (ie, physical tiredness, active leisure activities), energy, daytime sleepiness, and social functioning (ie, relationships, social activities/situations).[13] A more detailed discussion regarding the socioeconomic impact of RLS can be found elsewhere in this issue of *Sleep Medicine Clinics*.

Neurodegeneration and Dementia

There exists much data linking the relationship between disrupted sleep, cognitive performance, and neurodegenerative disease.[5] The fact that sleep–wake disruption is one of the earliest reported symptoms of many neurodegenerative disorders provides insight into the underlying pathophysiology of these disorders, because sleep–wake abnormalities are sometimes accompanied by neurodegenerative or neurotransmitter changes. In addition to being a symptom of the underlying neurodegenerative condition, there is also emerging evidence that sleep disturbance itself may contribute to the development and facilitate the progression of neurodegeneration. As such, the sleep–wake cycle may be an ideal target for further study for potential interventions, not only to lessen the burden of these diseases, but also to slow their progression. The most important entities include circadian disruption associated with Alzheimer's disease (AD), rapid eye movement behavior disorder, and sleep fragmentation associated with Parkinson's disease (PD).[119]

Neurocognitive domains such as executive attention and other higher cognitive functions are especially vulnerable to sleep loss,[120] and it is known that sleep is needed for memory consolidation,[121] with sleep deprivation being linked to memory and learning deficits.[122]

Sleep fragmentation owing to conditions such as OSA and RLS similarly results in neurocognitive performance decrements akin to those noted in studies regarding sleep restriction.[4] Sleep disturbances and sleep disorders may disrupt neuronal pathways, as exemplified by the fact that sleep deprivation studies in normal subjects demonstrate that sleep loss can cause impairment in attention and working memory. Furthermore, untreated sleep disturbances and sleep disorders such as OSA can also result in cognitive impairment. Thus, poor sleep and sleep disorders may present a significant risk factor for the development of dementia.[123] For example, a retrospective longitudinal study of 604 Taiwanese patients with sleep related movement disorder, who were shown to have a 3.952 times (95% CI, 1.124–4.767) higher risk of developing all-cause dementia compared with individuals without, and which increased progressively over time.[124]

Although sleep disturbances are common in older adults, little is known about the sleep of cognitively intact older adults and its relationship to subsequent cognitive impairment. A prospective cohort study was performed encompassing 4 US sites, 1245 women (mean age, 82.6 years) without dementia from the Study of Osteoporotic Fractures. These participants completed actigraphy at the baseline visit and comprehensive cognitive assessment at follow-up. A total of 473 women (38%) developed cognitive impairment during an average follow-up of 4.9 years (0.6), 290 (23.3%) developed MCI, and 183 (14.7%) developed dementia. It was found that women in the lowest quartile of average sleep efficiency (<74%) had a 1.5-fold higher odds of developing MCI or dementia compared with women in the highest quartile of sleep efficiency. Additionally, longer sleep latency was associated with increased odds of developing cognitive impairment, as was greater variability in sleep efficiency and total sleep time.[125] Finally, epidemiologic research has demonstrated that sleep and circadian traits correlate with cognitive performance even among those without neurologic illness.[126]

Alzheimer's disease

AD[127] is a debilitating and increasingly common neurodegenerative disorder resulting in progressive loss of memory, cognition, language skills, and personality traits.[128] It is characterized by progressive accumulation of extracellular "plaques" composed of the amyloid-β protein and intraneuronal "tangles" comprising hyperphos-phorylated forms of tau, which is a microtubule-associated protein.[128] Currently, there are more than 35 million people worldwide afflicted with AD,[129] including 5.3 million in the United States.[130]

Pathologic and imaging studies in patients with AD have shown brain abnormalities in areas regulating sleep,[131] and circadian abnormalities feature prominently in this neurodegenerative disorder.[132] The relationship between AD and sleep loss may be bidirectional[5]; for example, a study in animals demonstrated that during slow wave sleep, the brain "glymphatic" system cleared β-amyloid from the central nervous system.[133] Another study demonstrated that brain β-amyloid plaque formation in mice coincides with disordered sleep, and that clearance of the plaques restored normal sleep patterns.[134] Investigations in humans have yielded conflicting results.[5] In several longitudinal studies, subjects with sleep disturbance had a greater risk of cognitive decline[135] or AD[136] compared with those without sleep disturbance. Others have reported that prolonged sleep duration[137] and the presence of excessive daytime sleepiness[138] were associated with a higher risk of cognitive decline, but negative studies have been reported as well.[139] A recent study revealed that amyloid protein in the brain may interfere with sleep quality and long-term memory formation.[140] Another study demonstrated that variation in the circadian organization of rest–activity patterns as measured via actigraphy may predict the subsequent risk of dementia or mild cognitive impairment.[141] Additionally, sleep-disordered breathing may confer an increased risk of developing cognitive impairment in older women, particularly those with the apolipoprotein E4 allele.[142]

There are considerable financial, social, and emotional costs associated with caring for AD patients, both at home and institutionally. The care needed by AD patients, which is often through family and friends, ranges from help with managing finances in the early stages, to activities such as bathing, dressing, and feeding in the later disease stages.[143] Those caring for community-based patients spend approximately 60 hours per week in their supportive role.[144] Additionally, the time committed to caring for the patient can lead to the reduction or even complete cessation of payment for caregivers working hours[145]; and the extra but unavoidable out-of-pocket expenses, including housing alterations and transportation, also strain caregivers.[146] The excessive strain of providing such care can result in caregivers themselves requiring treatment from the health care system.[146] The AD patient may be placed in a long-term care facility when the burden on caregivers is too great, which contributes to the enormous total economic cost of AD. The provision of care to large numbers of elderly patients with AD accounts for 3.5% of total in-patient National Health Service expenditure in England.[146]

Parkinson's disease

PD is a chronic, progressive, degenerative, neurologic condition characterized by slowness of movement, rigidity, tremor, and postural disturbances[147]; the incidence ratio in European-derived populations is approximately 20 new cases per 100,000 people per year and the prevalence is 160 per 100,000 with no differences between sexes or countries.[119,148]

Studies in PD, using both imaging and pathology, have shown abnormalities in areas of the brain known to regulate sleep and circadian rhythms,[149] and complaints such as daily hypersomnolence, insomnia, periodic leg movements in sleep, rapid eye movement behavior disorder, and sleep-disturbed breathing are common in those with PD.[150] Two prospective studies have analyzed the unclear relationship that PD patients have regarding their sleep; do atypical or altered sleep habits exist before their clinical diagnosis, or do these sleep habits constitute a risk factor for PD[5]? In one, which was a large cohort of nurses on shift work, it was found that shift working was associated with a lower risk of PD, and that a long average duration of sleep was associated with an increased risk.[151] In the other, which included a large cohort of older Americans, longer daytime napping, and not nighttime sleep duration, was associated with future risk of PD[152]; this confirmed the results of a prior analysis, which noted that excessive daytime sleepiness may be associated with an increased risk of PD.[153] Furthermore, those with AD who reported more daytime napping had an increase in parkinsonian motor signs, which suggests that this subgroup of patients may have an increased propensity for sleepiness, resembling PD.[5,154]

In the United States, the economic burden of PD has been estimated to be at least $14.4 billion per year, or $22,800 per person on average. Whereas the economic burden of only disease-related medical expenses (not accounting for reduced employment, etc) for people with PD is approximately $8.1 billion total, or $12,800 per person, the economic burden of nonmedical costs is an additional $6.3 billion, or $10,000 per person. Approximately 9% of all residents aged 75 to 84 live nursing homes, but 15% of those with PD do so, and nursing home care accounted for more than $5 billion of PD-related medical costs.[155]

A retrospective 3-month German clinic-based analysis reported on the direct costs of 40 PD outpatients, which broke down to be 45% for medications, 39% for inpatient treatment, and 8% for other medical aids and appliances, 5% for outpatient visits, and 4% for physiotherapy. These costs were positively correlated with disease severity,[156] which has been corroborated by 2 other US-based studies.[157,158]

SUMMARY

Although both sleep disorders and neurologic illness are common and burdensome in their own right, when combined they can have tremendous negative impact at an individual level as well as societally. The socioeconomic burden of sleep disorders and neurologic illness can be identified,[159] but the real cost of these conditions lies far beyond the financial realm. There is an urgent need for comprehensive care and support systems to help with the burden of disease. Further research in improving patient outcomes in those who suffer with these conditions will help patients and their families, and society in general.

REFERENCES

1. Chokroverty S. Diagnosis and treatment of sleep disorders caused by co-morbid disease. Neurology 2000;54(5 Suppl 1):S8–15.
2. Horne JA, Reyner LA. Sleep related vehicle accidents. BMJ 1995;310(6979):565–7.
3. Axelsson J, Sundelin T, Ingre M, et al. Beauty sleep: experimental study on the perceived health and attractiveness of sleep deprived people. BMJ 2010;341:c6614.
4. Goel N, Rao H, Durmer JS, et al. Neurocognitive consequences of sleep deprivation. Semin Neurol 2009;29(4):320–39.
5. Palma JA, Urrestarazu E, Iriarte J. Sleep loss as risk factor for neurologic disorders: a review. Sleep Med 2013;14(3):229–36.
6. Hossain JL, Shapiro CM. The prevalence, cost implications, and management of sleep disorders: an overview. Sleep Breath 2002;6(2):85–102.
7. Tarasiuk A, Reuveni H. The economic impact of obstructive sleep apnea. Curr Opin Pulm Med 2013;19(6):639–44.
8. Jennum P, Kjellberg J. Health, social and economical consequences of sleep-disordered breathing: a controlled national study. Thorax 2011;66(7):560–6.
9. Diaz K, Faverio P, Hospenthal A, et al. Obstructive sleep apnea is associated with higher healthcare utilization in elderly patients. Ann Thorac Med 2014;9(2):92–8.
10. Leger D, Guilleminault C, Bader G, et al. Medical and socio-professional impact of insomnia. Sleep 2002;25(6):625–9.
11. Metlaine A, Leger D, Choudat D. Socioeconomic impact of insomnia in working populations. Ind Health 2005;43(1):11–9.
12. Spiegel K, Leproult R, L'hermite-Balériaux M, et al. Leptin levels are dependent on sleep duration: relationships with sympathovagal balance, carbohydrate regulation, cortisol, and thyrotropin. J Clin Endocrinol Metab 2004;89(11):5762–71.
13. Spiegel K, Tasali E, Leproult R, et al. Effects of poor and short sleep on glucose metabolism and obesity risk. Nat Rev Endocrinol 2009;5(5):253–61.
14. Spiegel K, Knutson K, Leproult R, et al. Sleep loss: a novel risk factor for insulin resistance and Type 2 diabetes. J Appl Physiol (1985) 2005;99(5):2008–19.
15. Manenschijn L, van Kruysbergen RG, de Jong FH, et al. Shift work at young age is associated with elevated long-term cortisol levels and body mass index. J Clin Endocrinol Metab 2011;96(11):E1862–5.
16. Gangwisch JE, Heymsfield SB, Boden-Albala B, et al. Short sleep duration as a risk factor for hypertension: analyses of the first National Health and Nutrition Examination Survey. Hypertension 2006;47(5):833–9.
17. Brondel L, Romer MA, Nougues PM, et al. Acute partial sleep deprivation increases food intake in healthy men. Am J Clin Nutr 2010;91(6):1550–9.
18. Benedict C, Brooks SJ, O'Daly OG, et al. Acute sleep deprivation enhances the brain's response to hedonic food stimuli: an fMRI study. J Clin Endocrinol Metab 2012;97(3):E443–7.
19. Laugsand LE, Vatten LJ, Platou C, et al. Insomnia and the risk of acute myocardial infarction: a population study. Circulation 2011;124(19):2073–81.
20. Vyas MV, Garg AX, Iansavichus AV, et al. Shift work and vascular events: systematic review and meta-analysis. BMJ 2012;345:e4800.
21. Institute of Medicine Committee on Sleep, M. and Research, Colten HR, Altevogt BM, editors. Sleep disorders and sleep deprivation: an unmet public health problem. Washington, DC: National Academies Press (US) National Academy of Sciences; 2006. The National Academies Collection: Reports funded by National Institutes of Health.
22. Kapur VK, Redline S, Nieto FJ, et al. The relationship between chronically disrupted sleep and healthcare use. Sleep 2002;25(3):289–96.
23. Wolfe CD. The impact of stroke. Br Med Bull 2000;56(2):275–86.
24. Rosamond W, Flegal K, Furie K, et al. Heart disease and stroke statistics–2008 update: a report from the American Heart Association Statistics Committee and Stroke Statistics Subcommittee. Circulation 2008;117(4):e25–146.

25. Di Carlo A. Human and economic burden of stroke. Age Ageing 2009;38(1):4–5.

26. Daniel K, Wolfe CD, Busch MA, et al. What are the social consequences of stroke for working-aged adults? A systematic review. Stroke 2009;40(6): e431–40.

27. Walters AS, Rye DB. Review of the relationship of restless legs syndrome and periodic limb movements in sleep to hypertension, heart disease, and stroke. Sleep 2009;32(5):589–97.

28. Yaggi HK, Concato J, Kernan WN, et al. Obstructive sleep apnea as a risk factor for stroke and death. N Engl J Med 2005;353(19):2034–41.

29. Shahar E, Whitney CW, Redline S, et al. Sleep-disordered breathing and cardiovascular disease: cross-sectional results of the Sleep Heart Health Study. Am J Respir Crit Care Med 2001;163(1):19–25.

30. Nieto FJ, Young TB, Lind BK, et al. Association of sleep-disordered breathing, sleep apnea, and hypertension in a large community-based study. Sleep Heart Health Study. JAMA 2000;283(14): 1829–36.

31. Arzt M, Young T, Finn L, et al. Association of sleep-disordered breathing and the occurrence of stroke. Am J Respir Crit Care Med 2005;172(11):1447–51.

32. Kufoy E, Palma JA, Lopez J, et al. Changes in the heart rate variability in patients with obstructive sleep apnea and its response to acute CPAP treatment. PLoS One 2012;7(3):e33769.

33. Somers VK, Dyken ME, Clary MP, et al. Sympathetic neural mechanisms in obstructive sleep apnea. J Clin Invest 1995;96(4):1897–904.

34. Patil SP, Schneider H, Schwartz AR, et al. Adult obstructive sleep apnea: pathophysiology and diagnosis. Chest 2007;132(1):325–37.

35. Hudgel DW. Mechanisms of obstructive sleep apnea. Chest 1992;101(2):541–9.

36. Barone DA, Krieger AC. Stroke and obstructive sleep apnea: a review. Curr Atheroscler Rep 2013;15(7):334.

37. Attal P, Chanson P. Endocrine aspects of obstructive sleep apnea. J Clin Endocrinol Metab 2010; 95(2):483–95.

38. Das AM, Khan M. Obstructive sleep apnea and stroke. Expert Rev Cardiovasc Ther 2012;10(4):525–35.

39. Helbig AK, Stöckl D, Heier M, et al. Symptoms of insomnia and sleep duration and their association with incident strokes: findings from the population-based MONICA/KORA Augsburg cohort study. PLoS One 2015;10(7):e0134480.

40. Sofi F, Cesari F, Casini A, et al. Insomnia and risk of cardiovascular disease: a meta-analysis. Eur J Prev Cardiol 2014;21(1):57–64.

41. Hsu CY, Chen YT, Chen MH, et al. The association between insomnia and increased future cardiovascular events: a nationwide population-based study. Psychosom Med 2015;77(7):743–51.

42. Headache Classification Subcommittee of the International Headache Society. The International classification of headache disorders: 2nd edition. Cephalalgia 2004;24(Suppl 1):9–160.

43. Classification and diagnostic criteria for headache disorders, cranial neuralgias and facial pain. Headache Classification Committee of the International Headache Society. Cephalalgia 1988;8(Suppl 7): 1–96.

44. Gobel H, Petersen-Braun M, Soyka D. The epidemiology of headache in Germany: a nationwide survey of a representative sample on the basis of the headache classification of the International Headache Society. Cephalalgia 1994;14(2): 97–106.

45. Henry P, Michel P, Brochet B, et al. A nationwide survey of migraine in France: prevalence and clinical features in adults. GRIM. Cephalalgia 1992; 12(4):229–37 [discussion: 186].

46. Scher AI, Stewart WF, Lipton RB. Migraine and headache: a meta-analytic approach. In: Crombie IK, editor. The epidemiology of pain. Seattle (WA): IASP Press; 1999. p. 159–70.

47. Pryse-Phillips W, Findlay H, Tugwell P, et al. A Canadian population survey on the clinical, epidemiologic and societal impact of migraine and tension-type headache. Can J Neurol Sci 1992; 19(3):333–9.

48. Rasmussen BK. Epidemiology of headache. Cephalalgia 1995;15(1):45–68.

49. Stewart WF, Simon D, Shechter A, et al. Population variation in migraine prevalence: a meta-analysis. J Clin Epidemiol 1995;48(2):269–80.

50. Steiner TJ, Scher AI, Stewart WF, et al. The prevalence and disability burden of adult migraine in England and their relationships to age, gender and ethnicity. Cephalalgia 2003;23(7):519–27.

51. Selekler MH, Gokmen G, Steiner TJ. Productivity impact of headache on a heavy-manufacturing workforce in Turkey. J Headache Pain 2013;14:88.

52. Lipton RB, Stewart WF, Celentano DD, et al. Undiagnosed migraine headaches. A comparison of symptom-based and reported physician diagnosis. Arch Intern Med 1992;152(6):1273–8.

53. Celentano DD, Stewart WF, Lipton RB, et al. Medication use and disability among migraineurs: a national probability sample survey. Headache 1992; 32(5):223–8.

54. Lipton RB, Stewart WF, Simon D. Medical consultation for migraine: results from the American Migraine Study. Headache 1998;38(2):87–96.

55. Lipton RB, Stewart WF, Diamond S, et al. Prevalence and burden of migraine in the United States: data from the American Migraine Study II. Headache 2001;41(7):646–57.

56. Rains JC, Poceta JS, Penzien DB. Sleep and headaches. Curr Neurol Neurosci Rep 2008;8(2):167–75.

57. Jennum P, Jensen R. Sleep and headache. Sleep Med Rev 2002;6(6):471–9.

58. Andress-Rothrock D, King W, Rothrock J. An analysis of migraine triggers in a clinic-based population. Headache 2010;50(8):1366–70.

59. Gilman DK, Palermo TM, Kabbouche MA, et al. Primary headache and sleep disturbances in adolescents. Headache 2007;47(8):1189–94.

60. Haque B, Rahman KM, Hoque A, et al. Precipitating and relieving factors of migraine versus tension type headache. BMC Neurol 2012;12:82.

61. Park JW, Chu MK, Kim JM, et al. Analysis of trigger factors in episodic migraineurs using a smartphone headache diary applications. PLoS One 2016; 11(2):e0149577.

62. Kelman L, Rains JC. Headache and sleep: examination of sleep patterns and complaints in a large clinical sample of migraineurs. Headache 2005; 45(7):904–10.

63. Spierings EL, Ranke AH, Honkoop PC. Precipitating and aggravating factors of migraine versus tension-type headache. Headache 2001;41(6): 554–8.

64. Scher AI, Lipton RB, Stewart WF. Habitual snoring as a risk factor for chronic daily headache. Neurology 2003;60(8):1366–8.

65. Chen PK, Fuh JL, Lane HY, et al. Morning headache in habitual snorers: frequency, characteristics, predictors and impacts. Cephalalgia 2011; 31(7):829–36.

66. Johnson KG, Ziemba AM, Garb JL. Improvement in headaches with continuous positive airway pressure for obstructive sleep apnea: a retrospective analysis. Headache 2013;53(2):333–43.

67. Ong JC, Park M. Chronic headaches and insomnia: working toward a biobehavioral model. Cephalalgia 2012;32(14):1059–70.

68. Houle TT, Butschek RA, Turner DP, et al. Stress and sleep duration predict headache severity in chronic headache sufferers. Pain 2012;153(12): 2432–40.

69. Fuh JL, Chung MY, Yao SC, et al. Susceptible genes of restless legs syndrome in migraine. Cephalalgia 2016;36(11):1028–37.

70. Osterhaus JT, Gutterman DL, Plachetka JR. Healthcare resource and lost labour costs of migraine headache in the US. Pharmacoeconomics 1992; 2(1):67–76.

71. de Lissovoy G, Lazarus SS. The economic cost of migraine. Present state of knowledge. Neurology 1994;44(6 Suppl 4):S56–62.

72. Solomon GD, Price KL. Burden of migraine. A review of its socioeconomic impact. Pharmacoeconomics 1997;11(Suppl 1):1–10.

73. Hu XH, Markson LE, Lipton RB, et al. Burden of migraine in the United States: disability and economic costs. Arch Intern Med 1999;159(8):813–8.

74. Moldofsky H. Sleep and pain. Sleep Med Rev 2001;5(5):385–96.

75. Smith MT, Edwards RR, McCann UD, et al. The effects of sleep deprivation on pain inhibition and spontaneous pain in women. Sleep 2007;30(4): 494–505.

76. Roehrs T, Hyde M, Blaisdell B, et al. Sleep loss and REM sleep loss are hyperalgesic. Sleep 2006; 29(2):145–51.

77. Haack M, Mullington JM. Sustained sleep restriction reduces emotional and physical well-being. Pain 2005;119(1–3):56–64.

78. Harrison L, Wilson S, Heron J, et al. Exploring the associations shared by mood, pain-related attention and pain outcomes related to sleep disturbance in a chronic pain sample. Psychol Health 2016;31(5):565–77.

79. Atkinson JH, Ancoli-Israel S, Slater MA, et al. Subjective sleep disturbance in chronic back pain. Clin J Pain 1988;4:225–32.

80. Smith MT, Perlis ML, Smith MS, et al. Sleep quality and presleep arousal in chronic pain. J Behav Med 2000;23(1):1–13.

81. Pilowsky I, Crettenden I, Townley M. Sleep disturbance in pain clinic patients. Pain 1985;23(1):27–33.

82. Morin CM, Gibson D, Wade J. Self-reported sleep and mood disturbance in chronic pain patients. Clin J Pain 1998;14(4):311–4.

83. Smith MT, Haythornthwaite JA. How do sleep disturbance and chronic pain inter-relate? Insights from the longitudinal and cognitive-behavioral clinical trials literature. Sleep Med Rev 2004;8(2): 119–32.

84. Loncaric-Katusin M, Milošević M, Žilić A, et al. Practical chronic pain assessment tools in clinical practice. Acta Clin Croat 2016;55(Suppl 1):19–26.

85. Zammit GK, Weiner J, Damato N, et al. Quality of life in people with insomnia. Sleep 1999;22(Suppl 2):S379–85.

86. Skevington SM, Carse MS, Williams AC. Validation of the WHOQOL-100: pain management improves quality of life for chronic pain patients. Clin J Pain 2001;17(3):264–75.

87. Smith MT, Carmody TP, Smith MS. Quality of well-being scale and chronic low back pain. J Clin Psychol Med Settings 2000;7:175–84.

88. Ford DE, Kamerow DB. Epidemiologic study of sleep disturbances and psychiatric disorders. An opportunity for prevention? JAMA 1989;262(11): 1479–84.

89. Wilson KG, Mikail SF, D'Eon JL, et al. Alternative diagnostic criteria for major depressive disorder in patients with chronic pain. Pain 2001;91(3): 227–34.

90. Katz DA, McHorney CA. Clinical correlates of insomnia in patients with chronic illness. Arch Intern Med 1998;158(10):1099–107.

91. Kuppermann M, Lubeck DP, Mazonson PD, et al. Sleep problems and their correlates in a working population. J Gen Intern Med 1995;10(1):25–32.

92. Katz WA. Musculoskeletal pain and its socioeconomic implications. Clin Rheumatol 2002;21(Suppl 1): S2–4.

93. Latham J, Davis BD. The socioeconomic impact of chronic pain. Disabil Rehabil 1994;16(1):39–44.

94. Gatchel RJ. A biopsychosocial overview of pretreatment screening of patients with pain. Clin J Pain 2001;17(3):192–9.

95. Stoller MK. Economic effects of insomnia. Clin Ther 1994;16(5):873–97 [discussion: 854].

96. Wilson KG, Eriksson MY, D'Eon JL, et al. Major depression and insomnia in chronic pain. Clin J Pain 2002;18(2):77–83.

97. Maniadakis N, Gray A. The economic burden of back pain in the UK. Pain 2000;84(1):95–103.

98. Katz JN. Lumbar disc disorders and low-back pain: socioeconomic factors and consequences. J Bone Joint Surg Am 2006;88(Suppl 2):21–4.

99. Loddenkemper T, Lockley SW, Kaleyias J, et al. Chronobiology of epilepsy: diagnostic and therapeutic implications of chrono-epileptology. J Clin Neurophysiol 2011;28(2):146–53.

100. Mattson RH, Pratt KL, Calverley JR. Electroencephalograms of epileptics following sleep deprivation. Arch Neurol 1965;13(3):310–5.

101. Manni R, Terzaghi M. Comorbidity between epilepsy and sleep disorders. Epilepsy Res 2010; 90(3):171–7.

102. de Weerd A, de Haas S, Otte A, et al. Subjective sleep disturbance in patients with partial epilepsy: a questionnaire-based study on prevalence and impact on quality of life. Epilepsia 2004;45(11): 1397–404.

103. de Boer HM, Mula M, Sander JW. The global burden and stigma of epilepsy. Epilepsy Behav 2008;12(4): 540–6.

104. Frucht MM, Quigg M, Schwaner C, et al. Distribution of seizure precipitants among epilepsy syndromes. Epilepsia 2000;41(12):1534–9.

105. Haut SR, Hall CB, Masur J, et al. Seizure occurrence: precipitants and prediction. Neurology 2007;69(20):1905–10.

106. Kreuzer P, Langguth B, Popp R, et al. Reduced intra-cortical inhibition after sleep deprivation: a transcranial magnetic stimulation study. Neurosci Lett 2011;493(3):63–6.

107. Malow BA, Passaro E, Milling C, et al. Sleep deprivation does not affect seizure frequency during inpatient video-EEG monitoring. Neurology 2002; 59(9):1371–4.

108. Malow BA, Levy K, Maturen K, et al. Obstructive sleep apnea is common in medically refractory epilepsy patients. Neurology 2000;55(7): 1002–7.

109. Legros B, Bazil CW. Effects of antiepileptic drugs on sleep architecture: a pilot study. Sleep Med 2003;4(1):51–5.

110. Chihorek AM, Abou-Khalil B, Malow BA. Obstructive sleep apnea is associated with seizure occurrence in older adults with epilepsy. Neurology 2007;69(19):1823–7.

111. Malow BA. The interaction between sleep and epilepsy. Epilepsia 2007;48(Suppl 9):36–8.

112. Malow BA, Foldvary-Schaefer N, Vaughn BV, et al. Treating obstructive sleep apnea in adults with epilepsy: a randomized pilot trial. Neurology 2008; 71(8):572–7.

113. Walsh S, Donnan J, Fortin Y, et al. A systematic review of the risks factors associated with the onset and natural progression of epilepsy. Neurotoxicology 2016. [Epub ahead of print].

114. Im HJ, Park SH, Baek SH, et al. Associations of impaired sleep quality, insomnia, and sleepiness with epilepsy: a questionnaire-based case-control study. Epilepsy Behav 2016;57(Pt A):55–9.

115. Kwon OY, Park SP. Interictal fatigue and its predictors in epilepsy patients: a case-control study. Seizure 2016;34:48–53.

116. Lee SA, Han SH, No YJ, et al. Sleep hygiene and its association with mood and quality of life in people with epilepsy. Epilepsy Behav 2015;52(Pt A): 225–9.

117. Cockerell OC, Hart YM, Sander JW, et al. The cost of epilepsy in the United Kingdom: an estimation based on the results of two population-based studies. Epilepsy Res 1994;18(3):249–60.

118. Tang DH, Malone DC, Warholak TL, et al. Prevalence and incidence of epilepsy in an elderly and low-income population in the United States. J Clin Neurol 2015;11(3):252–61.

119. Abbott SM, Videnovic A. Chronic sleep disturbance and neural injury: links to neurodegenerative disease. Nat Sci Sleep 2016;8:55–61.

120. Walker MP. Cognitive consequences of sleep and sleep loss. Sleep Med 2008;9(Suppl 1):S29–34.

121. Diekelmann S, Wilhelm I, Born J. The whats and whens of sleep-dependent memory consolidation. Sleep Med Rev 2009;13(5):309–21.

122. Havekes R, Vecsey CG, Abel T. The impact of sleep deprivation on neuronal and glial signaling pathways important for memory and synaptic plasticity. Cell Signal 2012;24(6):1251–60.

123. Miller MA. The role of sleep and sleep disorders in the development, diagnosis, and management of neurocognitive disorders. Front Neurol 2015;6:224.

124. Lin CC, Chou CH, Fan YM, et al. Increased risk of dementia among sleep-related movement disorders: a population-based longitudinal study in Taiwan. Medicine (Baltimore) 2015;94(51):e2331.

125. Diem SJ, Blackwell TL, Stone KL, et al. Measures of sleep-wake patterns and risk of mild cognitive

impairment or dementia in older women. Am J Geriatr Psychiatry 2016;24(3):248–58.

126. Blackwell T, Yaffe K, Ancoli-Israel S, et al. Poor sleep is associated with impaired cognitive function in older women: the study of osteoporotic fractures. J Gerontol A Biol Sci Med Sci 2006;61(4): 405–10.

127. Leissring MA. Abeta-degrading proteases: therapeutic potential in Alzheimer disease. CNS Drugs 2016;30(8):667–75.

128. Mucke L. Neuroscience: Alzheimer's disease. Nature 2009;461(7266):895–7.

129. Prince M, Wimo A, Guerchet M, et al. World Alzheimer's Report 2015. The global impact of dementia: an analysis of prevalence, incidence, cost and trends. London: Alzheimer's Disease International; 2015.

130. Alzheimer's Association. 2015 Alzheimer's disease facts and figures. Alzheimers Dement 2015;11(3): 332–84.

131. Harper DG, Stopa EG, Kuo-Leblanc V, et al. Dorsomedial SCN neuronal subpopulations subserve different functions in human dementia. Brain 2008;131(Pt 6):1609–17.

132. Harper DG, Volicer L, Stopa EG, et al. Disturbance of endogenous circadian rhythm in aging and Alzheimer disease. Am J Geriatr Psychiatry 2005; 13(5):359–68.

133. Xie L, Kang H, Xu Q, et al. Sleep drives metabolite clearance from the adult brain. Science 2013; 342(6156):373–7.

134. Roh JH, Huang Y, Bero AW, et al. Disruption of the sleep-wake cycle and diurnal fluctuation of beta-amyloid in mice with Alzheimer's disease pathology. Sci Transl Med 2012;4(150):150ra122.

135. Cricco M, Simonsick EM, Foley DJ. The impact of insomnia on cognitive functioning in older adults. J Am Geriatr Soc 2001;49(9):1185–9.

136. Lobo A, López-Antón R, de-la-Cámara C, et al. Non-cognitive psychopathological symptoms associated with incident mild cognitive impairment and dementia, Alzheimer's type. Neurotox Res 2008;14(2–3):263–72.

137. Benito-Leon J, Bermejo-Pareja F, Vega S, et al. Total daily sleep duration and the risk of dementia: a prospective population-based study. Eur J Neurol 2009;16(9):990–7.

138. Foley D, Monjan A, Masaki K, et al. Daytime sleepiness is associated with 3-year incident dementia and cognitive decline in older Japanese-American men. J Am Geriatr Soc 2001;49(12):1628–32.

139. Tworoger SS, Lee S, Schernhammer ES, et al. The association of self-reported sleep duration, difficulty sleeping, and snoring with cognitive function in older women. Alzheimer Dis Assoc Disord 2006;20(1):41–8.

140. Mander BA, Marks SM, Vogel JW, et al. Beta-amyloid disrupts human NREM slow waves and related hippocampus-dependent memory consolidation. Nat Neurosci 2015;18(7):1051–7.

141. Tranah GJ, Blackwell T, Stone KL, et al. Circadian activity rhythms and risk of incident dementia and mild cognitive impairment in older women. Ann Neurol 2011;70(5):722–32.

142. Spira AP, Blackwell T, Stone KL, et al. Sleep-disordered breathing and cognition in older women. J Am Geriatr Soc 2008;56(1):45–50.

143. Haley WE. The family caregiver's role in Alzheimer's disease. Neurology 1997;48(5 Suppl 6):S25–9.

144. Max W, Webber P, Fox P. Alzheimer's disease. The unpaid burden of caring. J Aging Health 1995;7(2): 179–99.

145. Moritz DJ, Kasl SV, Berkman LF. The health impact of living with a cognitively impaired elderly spouse: depressive symptoms and social functioning. J Gerontol 1989;44(1):S17–27.

146. Bosanquet N. The socioeconomic impact of Alzheimer's disease. Int J Geriatr Psychiatry 2001; 16(3):249–53.

147. Bulpitt CJ, Shaw K, Clifton P, et al. The symptoms of patients treated for Parkinson's disease. Clin Neuropharmacol 1985;8(2):175–83.

148. Findley L, Aujla M, Bain PG, et al. Direct economic impact of Parkinson's disease: a research survey in the United Kingdom. Mov Disord 2003;18(10): 1139–45.

149. Thannickal TC, Lai YY, Siegel JM. Hypocretin (orexin) cell loss in Parkinson's disease. Brain 2007;130(Pt 6):1586–95.

150. Comella CL. Sleep disturbances and excessive daytime sleepiness in Parkinson disease: an overview. J Neural Transm Suppl 2006;(70):349–55.

151. Chen H, Schernhammer E, Schwarzschild MA, et al. A prospective study of night shift work, sleep duration, and risk of Parkinson's disease. Am J Epidemiol 2006;163(8):726–30.

152. Gao J, Huang X, Park Y, et al. Daytime napping, nighttime sleeping, and Parkinson disease. Am J Epidemiol 2011;173(9):1032–8.

153. Abbott RD, Ross GW, White LR, et al. Excessive daytime sleepiness and subsequent development of Parkinson disease. Neurology 2005; 65(9):1442–6.

154. Park M, Comella CL, Leurgans SE, et al. Association of daytime napping and Parkinsonian signs in Alzheimer's disease. Sleep Med 2006;7(8): 614–8.

155. Kowal SL, Dall TM, Chakrabarti R, et al. The current and projected economic burden of Parkinson's disease in the United States. Mov Disord 2013;28(3): 311–8.

156. Dodel RC, Singer M, Köhne-Volland R, et al. Cost of illness in Parkinson disease. A retrospective 3-month analysis of direct costs. Nervenarzt 1997; 68(12):978–84 [in German].

157. Chrischilles EA, Rubenstein LM, Voelker MD, et al. The health burdens of Parkinson's disease. Mov Disord 1998;13(3):406–13.

158. Rubenstein LM, Chrischilles EA, Voelker MD. The impact of Parkinson's disease on health status, health expenditures, and productivity. Estimates from the National Medical Expenditure Survey. Pharmacoeconomics 1997;12(4):486–98.

159. Hewer RL. The economic impact of neurological illness on the health and wealth of the nation and of individuals. J Neurol Neurosurg Psychiatry 1997;63(Suppl 1):S19–23.

Social and Economic Impacts of Managing Sleep Hypoventilation Syndromes

Dianne M. Augelli, MD*, Ana C. Krieger, MD, MPH

KEYWORDS

- Obesity hypoventilation • Sleep hypoventilation • COPD with hypercapnia • Obesity
- Sleep-disordered breathing • Noninvasive ventilation

KEY POINTS

- Sleep hypoventilation is associated with significant societal and individual economic burdens.
- Early identification and diagnosis of sleep hypoventilation is imperative to prevent untoward outcomes.
- Implementation of treatment with positive airway pressure and noninvasive ventilation is crucial to improving morbid and mortality.

INTRODUCTION

Nocturnal hypoventilation is often the harbinger of multiple medical comorbidities and the development of hypercapnic respiratory failure. The emergence of hypoventilation is first noted during rapid eye movement (REM) sleep, before progressing to involve non-REM periods and later manifesting during the day. Failure to diagnose and treat sleep hypoventilation leads to decreased quality of life, increased morbidity, and mortality with marked societal impacts in terms of health care use.[1–8] The ability to intercede with approaches to treat or attenuate this condition has significant potential benefits.[2,5,9–18]

This article discusses the impact of the most common hypoventilatory disorders: obesity hypoventilation syndrome (OHS), chronic obstructive pulmonary disease (COPD), and the broader category of neuromuscular disorders (NMDs). Although not discussed here in detail, causes of hypoventilation also include restrictive thoracic cage disorders, acquired and congenital central breathing disorders, obstructive lung diseases, and respiratory suppressants.

OBESITY HYPOVENTILATION

Obesity hypoventilation is defined as the presence of daytime hypercapnia ($Pco_2 \geq 45$ mm Hg) in a patient with a body mass index (BMI) greater than or equal to 30 kg/m^2. The mechanisms leading to OHS are complex, relating to an interaction of change in lung mechanics and respiratory control that impairs normal gas exchange.[19–23] Restriction of the diaphragmatic excursion results in changes in breathing efficacy, and atelectasis from compressed lung volumes may further decrease tidal volume. In addition, there is an impairment of central chemosensitivity to decreased oxygen and increased carbon dioxide levels.[24–26] Leptin resistance associated with obesity may also reduce ventilation.[27] Nonetheless, not all obese patients develop OHS, and the pathophysiology between eucapnic obese patients and those with OHS is an area of emerging research.[28]

Although most of the OHS population have obstructive sleep apnea (OSA), it is not a required condition for diagnosis. Among the large population with OSA, 17% are estimated to have OHS.[1,29–33] However, this prevalence is highly

Disclosures: The authors have no disclosures or conflicts to report.
Department of Medicine, Center for Sleep Medicine, Weill Cornell Medical College, Cornell University, 425 East 61st Street, 5th Floor, New York, NY 10065, USA
* Corresponding author.
E-mail address: dma9013@med.cornell.edu

Sleep Med Clin 12 (2017) 87–98
http://dx.doi.org/10.1016/j.jsmc.2016.10.010
1556-407X/17/© 2016 Elsevier Inc. All rights reserved.

dependent on the level of obesity because patients with a BMI greater than or equal to 50 kg/m^2 could have an OHS prevalence greater than 50%.[34] Note that approximately 10% of patients with OHS do not have underlying OSA.[35]

Gender also has an effect on OHS: Despite men being more likely to have OSA, a higher prevalence of OHS is seen among obese women. One study showed OHS prevalence to be 3.5 times higher in women, with a delay in diagnosis of about a decade compared with men, as well as higher incidences of hypertension, diabetes, and hypothyroidism.[36] Among the US population, African Americans have higher rates of obesity and are therefore at higher risk for OSA and OHS.[37] The gender and racial differences may have a severe impact on comorbidities and socioeconomic factors, because it has been established that patients with OHS have increased health care costs and higher unemployment rates.[2] More information regarding differences in presentation and treatment of these populations is needed.

Patients with OHS often go unnoticed until they present in acute respiratory failure.[1,38] In one study, nearly a third of hospitalized obese (BMI ≥35 kg/m^2) patients, most of whom were previously undiagnosed, had OHS.[1] However, only 13% of those diagnosed were discharged with treatment. Compared with their obese peers, patients with OHS are more likely to require invasive ventilation and be admitted to the intensive care unit.[1] Postoperative complications are also more common in patients with hypercapnic OSA originating from COPD or OHS.[39] Quality-of-life indicators are worse in patients with OHS versus patients with eucapnic OSA and those with COPD.[8] In addition to increased morbidity, persons with OHS also have higher mortality.[1,2,40] Mortality for patients with OHS was 23% compared with 9% for their obese counterparts in the Nowbar and colleagues[1] study. Similarly, Jennum and colleagues[2] found mortalities of OHS at 25% versus 7% in patients with snoring alone. Treatment can confer significant benefit. Mortalities in a retrospective analysis of 126 patients showed that use of noninvasive ventilation (NIV) had survival rates of 97% at 1 year and 92% at 2 years.[7] However, patients with OHS fared worse than their counterparts with OSA, with one study of 330 subjects finding a 2-fold increase in mortality even in patients receiving treatment.[40] Adequate and timely intervention has the potential to reduce morbidity and mortality in OHS; however, major obstacles in treating OHS relate to delayed and incorrect diagnoses.[41]

Diagnosis

The onset of OHS is often insidious. Daytime fatigue, excessive sleepiness, dyspnea, morning headaches, cognitive impairment, sleep fragmentation, unexplained polycythemia, and cor pulmonale may be seen in patients with OHS.[42] Dyspnea and lower extremity edema may be more pronounced in OHS,[35] but many symptoms are similar to those found in OSA, making it difficult to identify these patients by clinical indicators alone. In the case of OHS, other causes of hypoventilation, such as NMD, severe obstructive lung disease, restrictive thoracic deformities, interstitial lung disease, congenital central hypoventilation, and thyroid disorders, must be excluded before the diagnosis.[43]

An arterial blood gas (ABG) level is needed to confirm the diagnosis of OHS by documenting a P_{CO_2} greater than or equal to 45 mm Hg. This method, although definitive, is not practical for repeated testing outside a hospital setting. A commonly accepted work-up includes pulmonary function tests (PFTs), which are important in the evaluation of OHS to rule out other lung diseases that may lead to hypercapnia.[44] PFTs may show a restrictive defect in patients with OHS. However, PFTs are not a reliable way to differentiate eucapnic patients with OSA from patients with OHS.[45,46]

Although there are no other specific biomarkers for OHS, serum bicarbonate levels greater than or equal to 27 mEq/L have been shown to have a high sensitivity (86%–92%[30,32]) for identifying patients at high risk of OHS.[30,32,47] When using serum bicarbonate level for screening of patients with OSA with potential OHS, it is important to exclude other causes of alkalosis, such as dehydration and use of steroids or loop diuretics.

Overnight oximetry data can serve as surrogate markers of hypoventilation and are often helpful in following patients after treatment. In a study of 152 patients with a BMI greater than or equal to 35 kg/m^2, an oxygen saturation (S_{PO_2}) nadir less than or equal to 80% during overnight polysomnography (PSG) showed a sensitivity of 83% in predicting OHS.[47] Although time with S_{PO_2} less than 90% is higher in patients with OHS,[31,34,35,43,45,47,48] no clear cutoff has been established. In conjunction with other measures for screening, a proposed consideration is S_{PO_2} less than 90% for greater than or equal to 20% of total sleep time (TST) to promp further investigation and in-lab testing. In addition, resting pulse oximetry of less than 93% in an obese patient while awake may suggest the need for further testing[31,34,49] (**Box 1**).

Attended PSG is the gold standard for assessing, monitoring, and treating hypoventilation. All patients with suspected hypoventilation are recommended to undergo an attended in-laboratory test to characterize and identify sleep-disordered breathing.[50] Besides providing a more accurate evaluation of respiratory events and oximetry

Box 1
Symptoms and indicators of hypoventilation

Clinical symptoms of OHS

- Sleep fragmentation
- Excessive daytime sleepiness
- Morning headaches
- Dyspnea/orthopnea
- Lower extremity edema
- Polycythemia
- Cor pulmonale

Potential indicators of hypoventilation in obese patients

- Serum bicarbonate level greater than or equal to 27 mEq/L
- Resting pulse oximetry less than 93% on room air
- SpO_2 less than 90% and greater than 20% of TST
- SpO_2 less than 80% in patients with BMI greater than or equal to 35 kg/m^2

during sleep, concomitant capnography allows better characterization of the disease. Transcutaneous and end-tidal CO_2 in-laboratory testing are helpful tools to identify sleep hypoventilation. End-tidal monitors can be attached to nasal flow meters but require frequent calibration and monitoring. A major downfall of this technique is that it cannot be used during titration studies. Transcutaneous CO_2 can be used during PSG in patients on oxygen or positive airway pressure (PAP) and NIV. Equipment expense is of concern because individual units can cost up to US$15,000. Attended PSG in patients with suspected OHS is essential for proper diagnosis, because treatment can be promptly initiated if needed.

Because of the burden of OSA, the use of portable home testing has increased significantly in the general population. Although there are benefits associated with its use, careful assessment of patients is advised. Portable testing is not recommended in patients at risk for OHS or other hypoventilatory disorders because of its inability to accurately detect hypoventilation. Furthermore, the Sleep Heart Health Study found that technical failure rates were higher with obese patients. A 1-unit increase in BMI increased the odds of failure by a factor of 1,[51] which may lead to an increase in costs, delay treatment, and result in the discontinuation of care. The widespread use of portable home testing in patients with suspected OHS is of major concern. Careful selection of testing is critical with these patients, because the use of portable sleep testing might lead to false-negative results based solely on Apnea-Hypopnea Index (AHI) estimates.

Treatment

Nocturnal treatment can improve sleep and quality of life, and increase nocturnal ventilation in patients with OHS. Improvement in gas exchange during sleep in patients with OHS leads to reduced hospitalizations, morbidity, and mortality.

Positive airway pressure

Options for OHS treatment include continuous PAP (CPAP), bilevel PAP (BPAP), or use of volume-assured pressure support (VAPS). These modalities should be titrated during attended PSG to ensure adequate treatment with improved ventilation during sleep. However, treatment should not be delayed in patients presenting with acute or chronic respiratory failure in the hospital (**Box 2**), because empiric or bedside treatment during acute care is often required. After initiation of treatment and stabilization of a patient's condition, PSG is recommended to optimize settings.[50]

CPAP is the most commonly used treatment modality and, in many cases, is sufficient. CPAP leads to positive outcomes in patients without severe nocturnal hypoxemia (arterial oxygen saturation [SaO_2] $\leq$80%)[9] and is likely to show a better response in obese patients with lower BMIs.[34,52,53] CPAP's role in OHS may be limited

Box 2
Respiratory assist device criteria for hypoventilation

1. Documentation of hypoventilation disorder and the associated symptoms

2. ABG shows $PaCO_2$ while awake greater than or equal to 45 mm Hg at usual fraction of inspired oxygen (FIO_2)

3. Spirometry forced expiratory volume in 1 second (FEV$_1$)/forced vital capacity (FVC) greater than or equal to 70% and FEV$_1$ greater than or equal to 50% of predicted

4. One of the following on the patient's usual FIO_2:

   a. ABG during sleep or after awakening shows PCO_2 increased by greater than 7 mm Hg

      Or:

   b. PSG shows oxygen saturation less than or equal to 88% for greater than 5 minutes with AHI less than 5[a]

[a] A minimum 2 hours of recording time is required.

by multiple circumstances. For example, Banerjee and colleagues[34] showed that, despite adequately treating apnea with CPAP, 43% of extremely obese subjects continued to desaturate with SpO_2 less than or equal to 90% for greater than or equal to 20% of TST. Those with significant hypoxemia may be considered for initial treatment with BPAP.[9] In addition, it has been recognized that patients without significant apnea have an inadequate response to CPAP and may have better success on BPAP at first.[12,14] BPAP confers additional benefits, because it is often more effective at resolving hypoventilation during REM sleep and in a supine position, leading to improved sleep quality and quality of life.[9–11] When started on CPAP, indications for switching patients to BPAP include continued desaturations of less than 90% after resolution of apnea, failure to correct gas exchange with CPAP within 1 to 2 months,[54] and intolerance to treatment. When critically ill, patients with OHS have a better response when started on empiric BPAP with a goal pressure support around 8 to 10 cm H_2O.[55] The spontaneous-timed (ST) mode should be used if central apneas develop.

VAPS is a newer modality of interest, used with the goal of providing stable tidal volumes. However, the absolute benefit of this treatment mode versus CPAP or BPAP has not been fully determined. In a small crossover study with 10 patients with OHS who failed CPAP therapy, treatment with VAPS showed a more pronounced reduction in PCO_2 than treatment with BPAP ST, without significant improvement in quality of life.[16] In a study of 12 patients previously stable on BPAP, Janssens and colleagues[56] found significant improvement in PCO_2 with VAPS compared with BPAP, although the patients on VAPS experienced more frequent awakenings and worse sleep quality. No significant differences were noted between BPAP and VAPS after 3 months in a randomized controlled trial with 50 patients.[10] Volume-targeted ventilation may be appropriate for patients who have failed CPAP and BPAP or have underlying obstructive lung disease. However, its role as a first-line treatment of OHS requires further research. Note that adaptive servoventilation (ASV) should be avoided in patients with OHS or other sleep-related hypoventilation, because it is not designed to enhance ventilation.

Oxygen

Oxygen therapy, when used in isolation, has been shown to worsen hypercapnia in patients with OHS.[57] For example, one study of 24 patients with OHS given 100% oxygen for 20 minutes showed worsening of hypercapnia as a result of the oxygen administration. PCO_2 increased by 5 mm Hg, with 3 patients discontinuing treatment because of an increase of PCO_2 greater than or equal to 10 mm Hg.[58] Although oxygen may initially be used during acute respiratory failure, the goal should be a reduction and then an elimination of oxygen once stable, if tolerated. Oxygen may be added as supplemental therapy when NIV alone fails to correct hypoxemia.

Weight reduction

Weight loss is a key component of the treatment plan in patients with OHS. However, a concerted effort needs to be present along with proper education in order to prioritize weight loss. Dietary and surgical weight loss approaches may lead to improved nocturnal ventilation in OHS, and pressure settings may need to be adjusted after weight loss.[59] It is critical to discuss strategies for weight reduction in all patients with OHS and guide patients toward appropriate evaluation and management. Patients should be advised that the use of PAP or NIV itself does not lead to weight reduction.

Pharmacotherapy

The use of medications to improve ventilation has been proposed in the past but has fallen out of favor because of safety concerns and lack of sufficient evidence of efficacy to recommend as a viable treatment option for chronic use.[60]

Impact

The obesity pandemic continues to be a global health concern. In some areas of the world, such as Tonga and Samoa, obesity is present in more than 50% of the population.[37] In the United States, a third of Americans are estimated to be obese (BMI $\geq$30 kg/m^2), comprising a disproportionate 13% of the world's obese population.[37] As the world's obese population ages, the scale of the problem strains resources and contributes to individual suffering. Compared with their eucapnic peers, people with OHS have decreased quality of life and higher incidence of pulmonary hypertension, diabetes type II, and heart failure.[2] Information is now emerging on the costs and consequences associated with untreated OHS. In 2012, the costs associated with OHS in the United States were estimated at approximately $200 billion annually.[61]

Jennum and colleagues[2,62] compared patient data from the Danish National Patient Registry (1998–2006) using patients with snoring, OSA, and OHS. Direct health care costs and indirect social costs were calculated using controls matched for age, sex, and socioeconomic status. Patients with OHS had costs 7.5 times higher than their control-matched peers and 2.5 times higher than patients with eucapnic OSA. The study also found lower rates of employment in patients with OHS, which affected pension rates. In the 8 years leading up to diagnosis, patients with OHS used more social services and medications.[2,62] In addition, spouses of patients with untreated OHS also incurred higher health care costs and received decreased overall income.[62] Clearly, this disease has widespread individual and societal consequences.

CHRONIC OBSTRUCTIVE PULMONARY DISEASE

COPD is projected to be the third leading cause of death worldwide by 2030,[63] with an estimated global prevalence of 65 million people. Sleep complaints in this population are common, although patients with COPD are not necessarily more likely to have OSA.[64] However, those with overlap syndrome (OS) have health implications that are much more pronounced.[65] Patients with OSA and COPD have a 7-fold increase in mortality compared with OSA alone.[66] Sleep-related hypoventilation in COPD/OS is characterized by a reduced ventilatory drive, worsened ventilation-perfusion mismatch, alterations in respiratory muscle activation, increased airflow obstruction, and decreased diaphragmatic contractility. Although not exclusive to COPD with sleep-related hypoventilation, patients with both COPD and poor sleep quality have been shown to have increased hospitalization and an increased risk of mortality.[67]

Identifying and screening patients with COPD for nocturnal hypoventilation is of key importance. The use of clinical symptoms and other screening measures, including overnight oximetry, can help identify appropriate patients for treatment, which could improve quality of life and prevent excessive use of health care resources.

Diagnosis

Complaints such as snoring, gasping for breath, daytime sleepiness, morning headaches, dyspnea, and cor pulmonale should all prompt further investigation for sleep-disordered breathing. Patients with COPD with hypercapnia should be viewed with a high degree of suspicion, because more than 40% of these patients are known to have nocturnal hypoventilation.[68,69]

Diagnostic tools include the use of ABG levels to identify hypercapnia and overnight oximetry to identify patients who need further evaluation. Continuous overnight pulse oximetry may show desaturations, suggesting sleep-disordered breathing, REM sleep-related hypoventilation, or sustained hypoxemia. Although pulse oximetry may be used for screening, caution must be

advised, because there is an absence of body position or sleep stage monitoring including REM sleep, which can be absent or diminished during a particular night of testing. Although PFTs are important for evaluation and management of COPD, they have not been shown to be predictive of nocturnal desaturations.

Treatment

Oxygen

Long-term oxygen therapy (LTOT) has long been a mainstay of treatment of patients with stable COPD and hypoxemia. The use of LTOT has shown a decrease in hospitalizations and an increase in survival rate, quality of life, and exercise capacity.[70–74] However, the use of nocturnal oxygen therapy in COPD may worsen hypoventilation, and needs to be carefully monitored because it does not improve ventilation.[75–77] Correction of nocturnal Pco_2 improves survival,[15,78] and additional strategies for enhancing ventilation during sleep might be useful in COPD. It remains unclear whether supplemental oxygen leads to long-term benefits in patients with COPD with nocturnal hypoventilation, and further research and guidelines are warranted.

Positive airway pressure

The use of PAP therapy may provide multiple benefits to patients with COPD. Ventilation may improve gas exchange and provide respiratory muscle rest. Patients with COPD and OS are known to receive the most benefit from PAP, but improvements may be seen in patients with hypercapnia.[4] In a cohort study including 213 patients with COPD/OS not treated with CPAP and 228 patients with COPD/OS treated with CPAP, Marin and colleagues[79] found that patients in the latter group had a lower mortality and reduced occurrences of COPD exacerbations leading to hospitalization.

CPAP is not a ventilatory mode and is typically eschewed for NIV. Most studies have focused on NIV, given its use for a wide spectrum of COPD complications, including acute respiratory failure. However, NIV studies with COPD have resulted in mixed outcomes.[5,80] A meta-analysis from the Cochrane Collaboration stated that NIV in hypercapnic patients with COPD had "no clinically or statistically significant effect on gas exchange, exercise tolerance, quality of life, lung function, respiratory muscle strength or sleep efficiency."[81] NIV with oxygen has been shown to reduce mortality compared with oxygen alone; however, quality of life was reduced.[78] Another study found a 1-year mortality risk reduction from 33% to 12% in patients with severe stable COPD (Gold class IV) and hypercapnia when treated with NIV.[82] A retrospective analysis of 166 patients by Galli and colleagues[83] showed reduced rehospitalizations in patients given NIV versus standard medical therapy after hospitalization. In addition, in a retrospective analysis, reduced rehospitalization was noted when VAPS was combined with a multifaceted treatment approach.[84] Multiple studies have shown equal improvement in gas exchange and compliance using either BPAP or VAPS.[85–88] However, in 2 crossover trials with BPAP and VAPS, sleep efficiency was superior in the VAPS groups.[85,86] In addition, compliance was higher in VAPS in a randomized crossover study with 23 patients using VAPS versus BPAP, although gas exchange and sleep quality were not significantly different.[89]

Asynchrony between NIV and the patient can affect compliance and comfort. Asynchrony can result from improper flow delivery, ineffective triggering, and cycle timing. Dynamic hyperinflation can be seen in patients with COPD and can lead to further asynchrony. Some modalities allow for inspiratory, expiratory, and rise times to be manually adjusted. Each treatment modality must be customized for individual patients. Patients with severe COPD and hypercapnia may qualify for a respiratory assist device (RAD), and PSG to confirm appropriate treatment after initiation is suggested[50] (Box 3).

Pharmacotherapy

From a pharmacotherapy standpoint, safety concerns regarding the use of respiratory stimulants have limited their application, keeping them from being considered a feasible option for long-term use.[90]

Impact

The economic implications of this disease are enormous. In 2010, the cost of COPD was US$36 billion, with projections of $50 billion by 2020.[6] The Continuing to Confront COPD International Patient Survey, which included direct and indirect costs, found that total societal costs per individual with COPD ranged from a low of US$1721 per patient in Russia to a high of $30,826 per patient in the United States, with most of the cost coming from hospitalizations and oxygen therapy.[91] In 3 of 12 countries surveyed, oxygen therapy was the largest contributor to direct costs. These costs are not specific to nocturnal hypoventilation but show the high impact and amount of resources required to manage COPD. Improved management of COPD should target cost-saving strategies to prevent exacerbations and hospitalizations and improve quality of life. Alternatives to costly and indiscriminate use of oxygen therapy, such as NIV, might be a way to improve care.

NEUROMUSCULAR DISORDERS

NMDs encompass a wide range of both slowly and rapidly progressive disease conditions, including Duchenne muscular dystrophy, amyotrophic lateral sclerosis (ALS), myopathies, motor neuron diseases, spinal cord injury, congenital myopathies and dystrophies, and postpolio syndrome. Although there are many types of NMD, they share a common pathway leading to hypoventilation. Respiratory muscle weakness, especially of the diaphragm, is a manifestation of progressive NMD. Hypoventilation has been shown to alter chemoresponsiveness,[24–26] contributing to abnormal ventilation as the disease state progresses. In addition, weakness of upper airway muscles may lead to airway obstruction in NMD. The presence of underlying obesity may also place patients at risk for concomitant OSA. The eventual progression of NMD leads to respiratory failure. Decreased hospitalizations as well as prolonged survival may be achieved with appropriate timing of intervention and treatment.[18,89,92–94]

Diagnosis

Sleep hypoventilation may be present months to years before respiratory failure ensues.[95–97] Hypoventilation first appears in REM before progressing to non-REM sleep and then to wakefulness.

> **Box 3**
> **Respiratory assist device criteria for chronic obstructive pulmonary disease**
>
> Two of the following criteria must be met:
>
> 1. Hypercapnia
>
>   a. ABG while awake shows $Paco_2$ greater than or equal to 52 mm Hg at usual Fio_2
>
>   Or:
>
>   b. ABG while awake shows $Paco_2$ greater than or equal to 52 mm Hg at usual Fio_2 after 61 days on CPAP if OSA present
>
>   And:
>
> 2. Sleep oximetry shows oxygen saturation less than or equal to 88% for greater than or equal to 5 continuous minutes on oxygen at 2 L/min or patient's usual Fio_2 with AHI less than 5[a]
>
> [a] A minimum 2 hours of recording time is required.

Patients may complain of dyspnea, orthopnea, sleep fragmentation, morning headaches, or fatigue. Paradoxic movement of the thorax and abdomen, use of accessory muscles of inspiration, and shallow breathing may be noted on the clinical examination. However, these clinical features are typically late signs of disease. Hypoventilation in sleep is often asymptomatic and presents before any abnormality in daytime blood gas levels are noted,[98–100] limiting the effectiveness of using ABG alone. Assessments of respiratory muscle strength and pulmonary functions are important indicators of nocturnal hypoventilation and are best used in combination for identifying patients at risk and monitoring disease progression.

PFTs are an important assessment tool for NMD. A typical pattern of restriction is found on PFTs, with forced vital capacity (FVC) and vital capacity (VC) being important markers. Evidence of hypoventilation in REM sleep has been shown in patients with NMDs with a VC of less than or equal to 60%, with a VC less than or equal to 40% being predictive of hypoventilation in 50% of patients.[101] Current treatment guidelines suggest initiation of treatment when FVC is less than or equal to 50%. However, a study of 72 patients with ALS showed increased survival and decreased decline in FVC percentage when intervention was started at an FVC less than or equal to 75%.[18] Inspiratory muscle and diaphragmatic strength are assessed by maximum inspiratory pressure (MIP). MIP less than or equal to 60 cm H_2O is used to identify patients with ALS with hypoventilation.[102] Changes in expiratory muscle strength can also contribute to hypoventilation, because the work of breathing increases due to the inability to clear secretions. Maximum expiratory pressure (MEP) less than or equal to 40 cm H_2O indicates the need for ventilatory support.[103] A suggested clinical measure to initiate NIV using the 20 to 30 to 40 rule has been proposed for NMD: VC less than or equal to 20 mL/kg, MIP less than 30 cm H_2O, or MEP less than or equal to 40 cm H_2O.[104–106] Sniff nasal inspiratory pressure (SNIP) can be used in conjunction with MIP and VC, which together show global inspiratory strength versus diaphragmatic strength. SNIP less than 30 cm H_2O was shown to be more sensitive in predicting initiation of treatment than VC or MIP in patients with ALS.[98]

Treatment

Treatment is often based on RAD guidelines established for NMD (**Box 4**). Hospitalized inpatients are started on empiric NIV therapy, and attended PSG for ventilation titration is

---

> **Box 4**
> **Respiratory assist device criteria for neuromuscular disorders**
>
> Documentation of neuromuscular disorder and 1 of the following:
>
> A. ABG while awake shows $Paco_2$ greater than or equal to 45 mm Hg at usual Flo_2
>
> Or:
>
> B. Sleep oximetry shows oxygen saturation less than or equal to 88% for greater than or equal to 5 minutes on room air with AHI less than 5[a]
>
> Or:
>
> C. Progressive NMD only
>
>   ○ MIP less than or equal to 60 cm H_2O
>
>   ○ FVC less than or equal to 50% of predicted
>
> [a] A minimum 2 hours of recording time is required.

---

recommended to ensure optimal treatment. The use of $TcPco_2$ is helpful for evaluating gas exchange, and it can be used for diagnostic testing, as well as monitoring once NIV is initiated. The cost of $TcPco_2$ often limits its use at home, because the device is not reimbursed by insurance companies. Treatment of hypoventilation in NMD has been shown to improve chemoresponsiveness even in the absence of improvements in muscle strength.[107] Nonetheless, intervention before the presence of daytime hypercapnia in NIV is recommended.

Positive airway pressure

CPAP and automatic PAP modalities are generally avoided in patients with progressive NMD unless OSA is a prominent feature earlier in the disease process.

NIV is the preferred PAP modality for patients with NMD. Multiple studies have shown that NIV reduces dyspnea, improves quality of life, and increases survival for patients with NMD.[18,92,93] NIV and mechanical-assisted coughing prolong survival and permit extubation in patients with Duchenne muscular dystrophy.[94] Carratu and colleagues[18] showed that early intervention in patients with ALS reduced decline in FVC and prolonged survival.

Studies have shown conflicting evidence regarding VAPS superiority to BPAP or BPAP ST. However, volume-targeted pressure may be useful in patients who have the need for progressive changes in ventilator settings. As with patients with COPD, ventilator asynchrony may decrease comfort and compliance in patients with NMD. One study found better compliance in PAP-naive patients given VAPS versus PAP.[89] VAPS was shown to reduce patient-ventilator asynchrony in those with NMD versus those treated with BPAP.[108] The use of VAPS in NMD continues to be studied because different algorithms exist and the progressive nature of the disease offers a major limitation in research methodology for device comparison.

Oxygen

Oxygen may be used if adequate ventilation is achieved and hypoxemia persists, although a work-up for underlying cardiopulmonary disorders is suggested in these patients.[102]

SUMMARY

Nocturnal hypoventilation is an underlying disturbance in ventilation that often does not manifest apparent daytime symptoms. Increased awareness is key to properly diagnose and treat sleep-related hypoventilation, leading to improvement in patients' quality of life, morbidity, and mortality, and clear impacts in health care use. The proper use of diagnostic approaches, including attended PSG and adjunctive capnography, is critical to the identification of this condition. Home sleep testing is not a recommended strategy for the evaluation or treatment of nocturnal hypoventilation. Treatment options include traditional and newer PAP modalities, including VAPS. Treatment efficacy needs to be closely monitored and settings adjusted based on changes in the underlying medical condition. Note that ASV is not indicated in patients with hypoventilation because of its inability to enhance ventilatory support.

Using quality-adjusted life years (QALY) as a marker, PAP therapy has a cost of US$2100/QALY compared with US$81,000/QALY for generic statins and US$11,000/QALY for ED.[109-111] The cost, including attended PSG testing, is small given the significant health benefits and long-term economic savings. Early diagnosis and treatment of sleep hypoventilation disorders offers a unique opportunity to avoid complex comorbidities and reduce health care costs. Guidelines to provide a clear route for allowing appropriate and optimal treatment of patients with hypoventilation are needed.

REFERENCES

1. Nowbar S, Burkart KM, Gonzales R, et al. Obesity-associated hypoventilation in hospitalized patients: prevalence, effects, and outcome. Am J Med 2004; 116(1):1–7.

2. Jennum P, Kjellberg J. Health, social and economical consequences of sleep-disordered breathing: a controlled national study. Thorax 2011;66(7): 560–6.

3. Lewis CA, Fergusson W, Eaton T, et al. Isolated nocturnal desaturation in COPD: prevalence and impact on quality of life and sleep. Thorax 2009; 64(2):133–8.

4. Machado MC, Vollmer WM, Togeiro SM, et al. CPAP and survival in moderate-to-severe obstructive sleep apnoea syndrome and hypoxaemic COPD. Eur Respir J 2010;35(1):132–7.

5. Casanova C, Celli BR, Tost L, et al. Long-term controlled trial of nocturnal nasal positive pressure ventilation in patients with severe COPD. Chest 2000;118(6):1582–90.

6. Ford ES, Murphy LB, Khavjou O, et al. Total and state-specific medical and absenteeism costs of COPD among adults aged ≥ 18 years in the United States for 2010 and projections through 2020. Chest 2015;147(1):31–45.

7. Budweiser S, Riedl SG, Jorres RA, et al. Mortality and prognostic factors in patients with obesity-hypoventilation syndrome undergoing noninvasive ventilation. J Intern Med 2007;261(4):375–83.

8. Budweiser S, Hitzl AP, Jorres RA, et al. Health-related quality of life and long-term prognosis in chronic hypercapnic respiratory failure: a prospective survival analysis. Respir Res 2007;8:92.

9. Piper AJ, Wang D, Yee BJ, et al. Randomised trial of CPAP vs bilevel support in the treatment of obesity hypoventilation syndrome without severe nocturnal desaturation. Thorax 2008;63(5):395–401.

10. Murphy PB, Davidson C, Hind MD, et al. Volume targeted versus pressure support non-invasive ventilation in patients with super obesity and chronic respiratory failure: a randomised controlled trial. Thorax 2012;67(8):727–34.

11. Borel JC, Tamisier R, Gonzalez-Bermejo J, et al. Noninvasive ventilation in mild obesity hypoventilation syndrome: a randomized controlled trial. Chest 2012;141(3):692–702.

12. Berg G, Delaive K, Manfreda J, et al. The use of health-care resources in obesity-hypoventilation syndrome. Chest 2001;120(2):377–83.

13. Masa JF, Corral J, Caballero C, et al. Non-invasive ventilation in obesity hypoventilation syndrome without severe obstructive sleep apnoea. Thorax 2016;71:899–906.

14. Masa JF, Celli BR, Riesco JA, et al. The obesity hypoventilation syndrome can be treated with noninvasive mechanical ventilation. Chest 2001;119(4): 1102–7.

15. Windisch W, Haenel M, Storre JH, et al. High-intensity non-invasive positive pressure ventilation for stable hypercapnic COPD. Int J Med Sci 2009; 6(2):72–6.

16. Storre JH, Seuthe B, Fiechter R, et al. Average volume-assured pressure support in obesity hypoventilation: a randomized crossover trial. Chest 2006;130(3):815–21.

17. Storre JH, Matrosovich E, Ekkernkamp E, et al. Home mechanical ventilation for COPD: high-intensity versus target volume noninvasive ventilation. Respir Care 2014;59(9):1389–97.

18. Carratu P, Spicuzza L, Cassano A, et al. Early treatment with noninvasive positive pressure ventilation prolongs survival in amyotrophic lateral sclerosis patients with nocturnal respiratory insufficiency. Orphanet J Rare Dis 2009;4:10.

19. Chlif M, Keochkerian D, Choquet D, et al. Effects of obesity on breathing pattern, ventilatory neural drive and mechanics. Respir Physiol Neurobiol 2009;168(3):198–202.

20. Wannamethee SG, Shaper AG, Whincup PH. Body fat distribution, body composition, and respiratory function in elderly men. Am J Clin Nutr 2005; 82(5):996–1003.

21. Javaheri S, Colangelo G, Lacey W, et al. Chronic hypercapnia in obstructive sleep apnea-hypopnea syndrome. Sleep 1994;17(5):416–23.

22. Lee MY, Lin CC, Shen SY, et al. Work of breathing in eucapnic and hypercapnic sleep apnea syndrome. Respiration 2009;77(2):146–53.

23. Zavorsky GS, Hoffman SL. Pulmonary gas exchange in the morbidly obese. Obes Rev 2008; 9(4):326–39.

24. Becker HF, Piper AJ, Flynn WE, et al. Breathing during sleep in patients with nocturnal desaturation. Am J Respir Crit Care Med 1999;159(1):112–8.

25. Goldring RM, Turino GM, Heinemann HO. Respiratory-renal adjustments in chronic hypercapnia in man. Extracellular bicarbonate concentration and the regulation of ventilation. Am J Med 1971; 51(6):772–84.

26. Goldring RM, Heinemann HO, Turino GM. Regulation of alveolar ventilation in respiratory failure. Am J Med Sci 1975;269(2):160–70.

27. O'Donnell CP, Schaub CD, Haines AS, et al. Leptin prevents respiratory depression in obesity. Am J Respir Crit Care Med 1999;159(5 Pt 1):1477–84.

28. Masa JF, Corral J, Romero A, et al. Protective cardiovascular effect of sleep apnea severity in obesity hypoventilation syndrome. Chest 2016; 150:68–79.

29. Balachandran JS, Masa JF, Mokhlesi B. Obesity hypoventilation syndrome epidemiology and diagnosis. Sleep Med Clin 2014;9(3):341–7.

30. Macavei VM, Spurling KJ, Loft J, et al. Diagnostic predictors of obesity-hypoventilation syndrome in patients suspected of having sleep disordered breathing. J Clin Sleep Med 2013;9(9):879–84.

31. Resta O, Foschino-Barbaro MP, Bonfitto P, et al. Prevalence and mechanisms of diurnal hypercapnia in a sample of morbidly obese subjects with obstructive sleep apnoea. Respir Med 2000;94(3):240–6.

32. Mokhlesi B, Tulaimat A, Faibussowitsch I, et al. Obesity hypoventilation syndrome: prevalence and predictors in patients with obstructive sleep apnea. Sleep Breath 2007;11(2):117–24.

33. Kawata N, Tatsumi K, Terada J, et al. Daytime hypercapnia in obstructive sleep apnea syndrome. Chest 2007;132(6):1832–8.

34. Banerjee D, Yee BJ, Piper AJ, et al. Obesity hypoventilation syndrome: hypoxemia during continuous positive airway pressure. Chest 2007;131(6): 1678–84.

35. Kessler R, Chaouat A, Schinkewitch P, et al. The obesity-hypoventilation syndrome revisited: a prospective study of 34 consecutive cases. Chest 2001;120(2):369–76.

36. BaHammam AS, Pandi-Perumal SR, Piper A, et al. Gender differences in patients with obesity hypoventilation syndrome. J Sleep Res 2016;25:445–53.

37. Ng M, Fleming T, Robinson M, et al. Global, regional, and national prevalence of overweight and obesity in children and adults during 1980-2013: a systematic analysis for the Global Burden of Disease Study 2013. Lancet 2014;384(9945): 766–81.

38. Lee WY, Mokhlesi B. Diagnosis and management of obesity hypoventilation syndrome in the ICU. Crit Care Clin 2008;24(3):533–49, vii.

39. Kaw R, Bhateja P, Paz YMH, et al. Postoperative complications in patients with unrecognized obesity hypoventilation syndrome undergoing elective noncardiac surgery. Chest 2016;149(1): 84–91.

40. Castro-Añón O, Pérez de Llano LA, De la Fuente Sánchez S, et al. Obesity-hypoventilation syndrome: increased risk of death over sleep apnea syndrome. PLoS One 2015;10(2):e0117808.

41. Marik PE, Desai H. Characteristics of patients with the "malignant obesity hypoventilation syndrome" admitted to an ICU. J Intensive Care Med 2013; 28(2):124–30.

42. Ahmed Q, Chung-Park M, Tomashefski JF Jr. Cardiopulmonary pathology in patients with sleep apnea/obesity hypoventilation syndrome. Hum Pathol 1997;28(3):264–9.

43. Mokhlesi B. Obesity hypoventilation syndrome: a state-of-the-art review. Respir Care 2010;55(10): 1347–62 [discussion: 1363–5].

44. Piper AP, Yee B, Badr S, et al. Clinical manifestations and diagnosis of obesity hypoventilation syndrome. UptoDate; 2016. Available at: http://wwwupto datecom/contents/clinical-manifestations-and-diag nosis-of-obesity-hypoventilation-syndrome?source =search_result&search=hypoventilation&selected Title=3~150#H6259511.

45. Kaw R, Hernandez AV, Walker E, et al. Determinants of hypercapnia in obese patients with obstructive sleep apnea: a systematic review and metaanalysis of cohort studies. Chest 2009; 136(3):787–96.

46. Akashiba T, Kawahara S, Kosaka N, et al. Determinants of chronic hypercapnia in Japanese men with obstructive sleep apnea syndrome. Chest 2002;121(2):415–21.

47. Bingol Z, Pihtili A, Cagatay P, et al. Clinical predictors of obesity hypoventilation syndrome in obese subjects with obstructive sleep apnea. Respir Care 2015;60(5):666–72.

48. Mokhlesi B, Tulaimat A, Parthasarathy S. Oxygen for obesity hypoventilation syndrome: a double-edged sword? Chest 2011;139(5):975–7.

49. Piper AJ. Obesity hypoventilation syndrome–the big and the breathless. Sleep Med Rev 2011; 15(2):79–89.

50. Berry RB, Chediak A, Brown LK, et al. Best clinical practices for the sleep center adjustment of noninvasive positive pressure ventilation (NPPV) in stable chronic alveolar hypoventilation syndromes. J Clin Sleep Med 2010;6(5):491–509.

51. Kapur VK, Rapoport DM, Sanders MH, et al. Rates of sensor loss in unattended home polysomnography: the influence of age, gender, obesity, and sleep-disordered breathing. Sleep 2000;23(5): 682–8.

52. Piper A. Obesity hypoventilation syndrome: weighing in on therapy options. Chest 2016;149(3):856–68.

53. Perez de Llano LA, Golpe R, Piquer MO, et al. Clinical heterogeneity among patients with obesity hypoventilation syndrome: therapeutic implications. Respiration 2008;75(1):34–9.

54. Mokhlesi B, Tulaimat A. Recent advances in obesity hypoventilation syndrome. Chest 2007; 132(4):1322–36.

55. Jones SF, Brito V, Ghamande S. Obesity hypoventilation syndrome in the critically ill. Crit Care Clin 2015;31(3):419–34.

56. Janssens JP, Metzger M, Sforza E. Impact of volume targeting on efficacy of bi-level non-invasive ventilation and sleep in obesity-hypoventilation. Respir Med 2009;103(2):165–72.

57. Hollier CA, Harmer AR, Maxwell LJ, et al. Moderate concentrations of supplemental oxygen worsen hypercapnia in obesity hypoventilation syndrome: a randomised crossover study. Thorax 2014;69(4): 346–53.

58. Wijesinghe M, Williams M, Perrin K, et al. The effect of supplemental oxygen on hypercapnia in subjects with obesity-associated hypoventilation: a randomized, crossover, clinical study. Chest 2011;139(5):1018–24.

59. Sugerman HJ, Fairman RP, Sood RK, et al. Long-term effects of gastric surgery for treating respiratory insufficiency of obesity. Am J Clin Nutr 1992;55(2 Suppl):597s–601s.

60. Mason M, Welsh EJ, Smith I. Drug therapy for obstructive sleep apnoea in adults. Cochrane Database Syst Rev 2013;(5):CD003002.

61. Cawley J, Meyerhoefer C. The medical care costs of obesity: an instrumental variables approach. J Health Econ 2012;31(1):219–30.

62. Jennum P, Ibsen R, Kjellberg J. Social consequences of sleep disordered breathing on patients and their partners: a controlled national study. Eur Respir J 2014;43(1):134–44.

63. Organization WH. Chronic respiratory disease: burden of COPD Web site. 2015. Available at: http://www.who.int/respiratory/copd/burden/en/. Accessed June 23, 2016.

64. Sanders MH, Newman AB, Haggerty CL, et al. Sleep and sleep-disordered breathing in adults with predominantly mild obstructive airway disease. Am J Respir Crit Care Med 2003;167(1): 7–14.

65. Chaouat A, Weitzenblum E, Krieger J, et al. Association of chronic obstructive pulmonary disease and sleep apnea syndrome. Am J Respir Crit Care Med 1995;151(1):82–6.

66. Lavie P, Herer P, Lavie L. Mortality risk factors in sleep apnoea: a matched case–control study. J Sleep Res 2007;16(1):128–34.

67. Omachi TA, Blanc PD, Claman DM, et al. Disturbed sleep among COPD patients is longitudinally associated with mortality and adverse COPD outcomes. Sleep Med 2012;13(5):476–83.

68. O'Donoghue FJ, Catcheside PG, Ellis EE, et al. Sleep hypoventilation in hypercapnic chronic obstructive pulmonary disease: prevalence and associated factors. Eur Respir J 2003;21(6):977–84.

69. Budhiraja R, Siddiqi TA, Quan SF. Sleep disorders in chronic obstructive pulmonary disease: etiology, impact, and management. J Clin Sleep Med 2015; 11(3):259–70.

70. Eaton T, Lewis C, Young P, et al. Long-term oxygen therapy improves health-related quality of life. Respir Med 2004;98(4):285–93.

71. Clini E, Vitacca M, Foglio K, et al. Long-term home care programmes may reduce hospital admissions in COPD with chronic hypercapnia. Eur Respir J 1996;9(8):1605–10.

72. Haidl P, Clement C, Wiese C, et al. Long-term oxygen therapy stops the natural decline of endurance in COPD patients with reversible hypercapnia. Respiration 2004;71(4):342–7.

73. Continuous or nocturnal oxygen therapy in hypoxemic chronic obstructive lung disease: a clinical trial. Nocturnal Oxygen Therapy Trial Group. Ann Intern Med 1980;93(3):391–8.

74. Long term domiciliary oxygen therapy in chronic hypoxic cor pulmonale complicating chronic

bronchitis and emphysema. Report of the Medical Research Council Working Party. Lancet 1981; 1(8222):681–6.

75. Schneider HM, Stoller J, Badr S, et al. Sleep-related breathing disorders in COPD. UptoDate; 2016. Available at: http://wwwuptodatecom/contents/sleep-related-breathing-disorders-in-copd?source=search_result&search=copd&selectedTitle=23~150.

76. Pathogenesis and outcomes of sleep disordered breathing in chronic obstructive pulmonary disease (COPD). NCT 01764165. Available: https://clinicaltrials.gov/ct2/results?term=01764165&Search=Search. Accessed November 02, 2015.

77. Tarrega J, Anton A, Guell R, et al. Predicting nocturnal hypoventilation in hypercapnic chronic obstructive pulmonary disease patients undergoing long-term oxygen therapy. Respiration 2011; 82(1):4–9.

78. McEvoy RD, Pierce RJ, Hillman D, et al. Nocturnal non-invasive nasal ventilation in stable hypercapnic COPD: a randomised controlled trial. Thorax 2009;64(7):561–6.

79. Marin JM, Soriano JB, Carrizo SJ, et al. Outcomes in patients with chronic obstructive pulmonary disease and obstructive sleep apnea: the overlap syndrome. Am J Respir Crit Care Med 2010;182(3): 325–31.

80. Struik FM, Lacasse Y, Goldstein R, et al. Nocturnal non-invasive positive pressure ventilation for stable chronic obstructive pulmonary disease. Cochrane Database Syst Rev 2013;(6):CD002878.

81. Struik FM, Lacasse Y, Goldstein RS, et al. Nocturnal noninvasive positive pressure ventilation in stable COPD: a systematic review and individual patient data meta-analysis. Respir Med 2014;108(2):329–37.

82. Kohnlein T, Windisch W, Kohler D, et al. Non-invasive positive pressure ventilation for the treatment of severe stable chronic obstructive pulmonary disease: a prospective, multicentre, randomised, controlled clinical trial. Lancet Respir Med 2014; 2(9):698–705.

83. Galli JA, Krahnke JS, James Mamary A, et al. Home non-invasive ventilation use following acute hypercapnic respiratory failure in COPD. Respir Med 2014;108(5):722–8.

84. Coughlin S, Liang WE, Parthasarathy S. Retrospective assessment of home ventilation to reduce rehospitalization in chronic obstructive pulmonary disease. J Clin Sleep Med 2015;11(6):663–70.

85. Battisti A, Tassaux D, Bassin D, et al. Automatic adjustment of noninvasive pressure support with a bilevel home ventilator in patients with acute respiratory failure: a feasibility study. Intensive Care Med 2007;33(4):632–8.

86. Crisafulli E, Manni G, Kidonias M, et al. Subjective sleep quality during average volume assured pressure support (AVAPS) ventilation in patients with hypercapnic COPD: a physiological pilot study. Lung 2009;187(5):299–305.

87. Oscroft NS, Chadwick R, Davies MG, et al. Volume assured versus pressure preset non-invasive ventilation for compensated ventilatory failure in COPD. Respir Med 2014;108(10):1508–15.

88. Oscroft NS, Ali M, Gulati A, et al. A randomised crossover trial comparing volume assured and pressure preset noninvasive ventilation in stable hypercapnic COPD. COPD 2010;7(6):398–403.

89. Kelly JL, Jaye J, Pickersgill RE, et al. Randomized trial of 'intelligent' autotitrating ventilation versus standard pressure support non-invasive ventilation: impact on adherence and physiological outcomes. Respirology 2014;19(4):596–603.

90. Sevilla Berrios RA, Gay PC. Advances and new approaches to managing sleep-disordered breathing related to chronic pulmonary disease. Sleep Med Clin 2016;11:257–64.

91. Foo J, Landis SH, Maskell J, et al. Continuing to Confront COPD International Patient Survey: economic impact of COPD in 12 countries. PLoS One 2016;11(4):e0152618.

92. Terzano C, Romani S. Early use of non invasive ventilation in patients with amyotrophic lateral sclerosis: what benefits? Eur Rev Med Pharmacol Sci 2015;19(22):4304–13.

93. Raphael JC, Chevret S, Chastang C, et al. Randomised trial of preventive nasal ventilation in Duchenne muscular dystrophy. French Multicentre Cooperative Group on Home Mechanical Ventilation Assistance in Duchenne de Boulogne Muscular Dystrophy. Lancet 1994;343(8913):1600–4.

94. Gomez-Merino E, Bach JR. Duchenne muscular dystrophy: prolongation of life by noninvasive ventilation and mechanically assisted coughing. Am J Phys Med Rehabil 2002;81(6):411–5.

95. Piper A. Sleep abnormalities associated with neuromuscular disease: pathophysiology and evaluation. Semin Respir Crit Care Med 2002;23(3): 211–9.

96. Carre PC, Didier AP, Tiberge YM, et al. Amyotrophic lateral sclerosis presenting with sleep hypopnea syndrome. Chest 1988;93(6):1309–12.

97. Fromm GB, Wisdom PJ, Block AJ. Amyotrophic lateral sclerosis presenting with respiratory failure. Diaphragmatic paralysis and dependence on mechanical ventilation in two patients. Chest 1977; 71(5):612–4.

98. Lyall RA, Donaldson N, Polkey MI, et al. Respiratory muscle strength and ventilatory failure in amyotrophic lateral sclerosis. Brain 2001;124(Pt 10):2000–13.

99. Piper AJ, Gonzalez-Bermejo J, Janssens J-P. Sleep hypoventilation. Sleep Med Clin 2014;9(3): 301–13.

100. Ward S, Chatwin M, Heather S, et al. Randomised controlled trial of non-invasive ventilation (NIV) for nocturnal hypoventilation in neuromuscular and chest wall disease patients with daytime normocapnia. Thorax 2005;60(12):1019–24.

101. Ragette R, Mellies U, Schwake C, et al. Patterns and predictors of sleep disordered breathing in primary myopathies. Thorax 2002;57(8):724–8.

102. Hill NM, Kramer N, Shefner J, et al. Practical aspects of nocturnal noninvasive ventilation in neuromuscular and chest wall disease. UptoDate; 2016. Available at: http://wwwuptodatecom/contents/practical-aspects-of-nocturnal-noninvasive-ventilation-in-neuromuscular-and-chest-wall-disease?source=search_result&search=neurmuscular+niv&selected Title=2~134.

103. Adamson JP, Lewis L, Stein JD. Application of abdominal pressure for artificial respiration. J Am Med Assoc 1959;169(14):1613–7.

104. Bach JM, King T Jr, Morrison S, et al. Continuous noninvasive ventilatory support for patients with neuromuscular or chest wall disease. UptoDate; 2016. Available at: http://wwwuptodatecom/contents/continuous-noninvasive-ventilatory-support-for-patients-with-neuromuscular-or-chest-wall-disease?source=search_result&search=clinical+manifestations+nmd&selectedTitle=1~1.

105. Lawn ND, Fletcher DD, Henderson RD, et al. Anticipating mechanical ventilation in Guillain-Barre syndrome. Arch Neurol 2001;58(6):893–8.

106. Mehta S. Neuromuscular disease causing acute respiratory failure. Respir Care 2006;51(9):1016–21 [discussion: 1021–3].

107. Annane D, Quera-Salva MA, Lofaso F, et al. Mechanisms underlying effects of nocturnal ventilation on daytime blood gases in neuromuscular diseases. Eur Respir J 1999;13(1):157–62.

108. Crescimanno G, Marrone O, Vianello A. Efficacy and comfort of volume-guaranteed pressure support in patients with chronic ventilatory failure of neuromuscular origin. Respirology 2011;16(4):672–9.

109. Kim RD, Kapur VK, Redline-Bruch J, et al. An economic evaluation of home versus laboratory-based diagnosis of obstructive sleep apnea. Sleep 2015;38(7):1027–37.

110. Pandya A, Sy S, Cho S, et al. Cost-effectiveness of 10-year risk thresholds for initiation of statin therapy for primary prevention of cardiovascular disease. JAMA 2015;314(2):142–50.

111. Martin AL, Huelin R, Wilson D, et al. A systematic review assessing the economic impact of sildenafil citrate (Viagra) in the treatment of erectile dysfunction. J Sex Med 2013;10(5):1389–400.

Screening for Obstructive Sleep Apnea in Patients with Atrial Fibrillation

Pedro R. Genta, MD, PhD[a], Luciano F. Drager, MD, PhD[b],
Geraldo Lorenzi Filho, MD, PhD[a],*

KEYWORDS

• Obstructive sleep apnea • Atrial fibrillation • Screening • Questionnaires • Home sleep testing

KEY POINTS

- Atrial fibrillation (AF) is a common arrhythmia associated with adverse health outcomes and elevated health costs. Obstructive sleep apnea (OSA) is common among AF patients.
- OSA may contribute to the occurrence and recurrence of AF. Screening for OSA among AF patients is justified by the adverse impact OSA may cause.
- Appropriate screening strategies should be used due to the high prevalence of OSA among AF subjects and variable symptomatology.
- OSA questionnaires may have limited performance among patients with high pretest probability, such as the AF population.
- Home sleep testing (HST) is a promising alternative for screening and diagnosing OSA in AF patients. The cost-effectiveness of such approach, however, needs to be studied.

INTRODUCTION

OSA is characterized by repetitive upper airway obstruction during sleep. The most common symptoms of OSA are snoring, fatigue, disrupted sleep, and excessive daytime sleepiness.[1] Obesity, male gender, and increasing age are the most important risk factors for OSA.[2] There is growing evidence, however, that a significant proportion of OSA patients are minimally symptomatic and frequently also not obese. OSA may present several distinct phenotypes,[3] which points to the potential necessity of simple and cost-effective diagnostic methods.

OSA is common in the general population and strikingly common among patients with established cardiovascular disease. The high prevalence of OSA is largely due to OSA and cardiovascular disease sharing several risk factors, including male gender, obesity, sedentary life, and increasing age. In addition, OSA may independently contribute to poor cardiovascular outcome.[4] Obstructive events during sleep cause (1) large swings in intrathoracic pressure during the futile efforts to breathe, (2) arousals from sleep, and (3) intermittent hypoxia.[5] These 3 primary mechanisms occurring during sleep trigger a cascade of intermediate mechanisms, which may ultimately contribute to the development or recurrence of AF. There is no definitive evidence, however, that the diagnosis and treatment of OSA reduce the incidence of AF or conversely that the recognition and

The authors have nothing to disclose.
a Pulmonary Division, Heart Institute (InCor), Hospital das Clínicas, University of São Paulo School of Medicine, Av Dr. Eneas de Carvalho Aguiar, 44, 8th Floor, São Paulo, São Paulo 05403-000, Brasil; b Hypertension Unit of the Renal Division and Heart Institute (InCor), Hospital das Clínicas, University of São Paulo School of Medicine, Av Dr. Eneas de Carvalho Aguiar, 44, 8th Floor, São Paulo, São Paulo 05403-000, Brasil
* Corresponding author.
E-mail address: geraldo.lorenzi@gmail.com

sleep.theclinics.com

treatment of OSA among patients with established AF have a positive impact on the cardiovascular outcome. On the other hand, the recognition and treatment of OSA may also have a positive impact on quality of life.[6] In clinical practice, OSA remains largely under-recognized among patients with established cardiovascular disease.[7] The reasons for such low recognition include the possibility that several symptoms associated with OSA may overlap with symptoms associated with the underlying cardiovascular disease. In addition, the diagnosis of OSA has traditionally been restricted to full sleep studies, creating a potential barrier. This observation raises the question of how to recognize OSA among patients with AF.

To provide a clinical rationale to justify the screening of OSA among AF patients, the epidemiology of OSA and AF and the mechanisms by which OSA may contribute to AF are reviewed. Possible strategies to screen for OSA are then reviewed and discussed.

PREVALENCE OF ATRIAL FIBRILLATION

AF is a common arrhythmia associated with adverse consequences and high health-related cost. The clinical risk factors for AF include advancing age, diabetes, hypertension, congestive heart failure, valve disease, and myocardial infarction.[8] The prevalence of AF in the general population is between 1% and 2% and is higher in men than in women.[9] The risk of developing AF increases dramatically with age, and the estimated lifetime risk of developing AF is 1 in 4 for men and women ages 40 years and above.[9] AF is the most common arrhythmia in patients older than 65 years.[10] For instance, data from a cross-sectional study of adults ages 20 years or older who were enrolled in a large health maintenance organization in California estimated that the prevalence of AF increased from 0.1% among adults younger than 55 years to 9.0% in persons ages 80 years or older.[10] Aging heart, characterized by myocardial fibrosis and atrial dilation, is a main risk factor for AF. Structural heart disease enforces atrial chamber abnormality, and this explains the higher prevalence of AF in patients with underlying cardiovascular conditions.[11] Other risk factors for AF, such as obesity and diabetes, are also steadily increasing in society. AF not only is a marker of an underlying cardiovascular disease but also, once established, an independent risk factor for stroke as well as increased mortality. The high lifetime risk of AF and increased longevity underscore the important public health burden posed worldwide.[12] The cost of AF is escalating. A systematic review of recent literature estimated the direct costs of AF at $2,000 to $14,200 per patient-year in the United States and €450 to €3000 per patient-year in Europe.[13] This is comparable to costs associated with other chronic conditions, such as diabetes. Hospitalizations were the main contributors to the high direct cost of AF.[13]

PREVALENCE OF OBSTRUCTIVE SLEEP APNEA AND ASSOCIATION WITH ATRIAL FIBRILLATION

OSA is common in the general population. A landmark Wisconsin cohort initially reported that the estimated prevalence of OSA syndrome in the general population, as defined by an apnea-hypopnea index above 5 events per hour of sleep determined by full polysomnography plus symptoms of excessive daytime sleepiness, was 2% and 4% in adult women and men, respectively.[14] Several factors, however, including the increased capacity to recognize hypopneas with the use of pressure cannula, the recognition that several patients do not have symptoms of excessive daytime sleepiness, and the increasing rates of obesity of the population have led to the recognition that OSA is more common than initially imagined. For instance, the estimated prevalence of OSA among adults of the city of São Paulo, Brazil, and Lausanne, Switzerland, was estimated to be approximately 30% to 50%.[2,15]

The prevalence of unrecognized OSA among patients with established cardiovascular disease is strikingly high. For instance, 1 study evaluated 500 consecutive outpatients from a tertiary cardiovascular university hospital and found that although only 3.1% had a previous diagnosis of OSA, more than half of the population (51.6%) had symptoms suggestive of OSA as evaluated by the Berlin questionnaire. The high prevalence of OSA was further confirmed by HST in a subset of 50 patients.[7]

The prevalence of AF among OSA patients is approximately 5%,[16] which is higher than the prevalence of AF in the general population (1%–2%).[9] On the other hand, studies that assessed the prevalence of OSA in patients with AF showed prevalence ranging from 21% to 81%.[17–20] The impact of OSA on AF incidence, however, remains controversial. One study showed an independent association between OSA and increased AF incidence,[21] whereas another study found an association of AF and central sleep apnea but not with OSA.[22]

THE IMPACT OF OBSTRUCTIVE SLEEP APNEA ON ATRIAL FIBRILLATION

Although the precise mechanisms by which OSA is linked to arrhythmias are not fully elucidated, several studies showed an increase propensity of OSA patients to develop AF. As discussed previously, obstructive events during sleep promote reductions in the intrathoracic pressure, intermittent hypoxia, and sleep fragmentation.[5] One or more of the OSA-related components elicits sympathetic surges, atrial distension (due to the increase in atrial transmural pressure gradients), surges in blood pressure, increased systemic inflammation, and oxidative stress. Chronically, these repetitive events may promote structural cardiac changes, including atrial enlargement and fibrosis.[23] Two main factors may contribute to atrial remodeling in OSA: (1) chronic atrial dilation by repetitive changes in intrathoracic pressure[24] and (2) surges in blood pressure. In addition, OSA has been shown to increase aorta stiffness that in turn contributes to increased heart afterload and atrial and ventricular remodeling.[25,26]

In the past 2 decades, growing evidence has suggested the potential role of OSA in the genesis of AF occurrence and recurrence.[27,28] The increased risk of AF among OSA patients seems independent of potential confounding factors, such as age and obesity. The increased risk of recurrence of AF has been also observed in patients who have had catheter ablation.[29] In line with this evidence, one observational study showed that patients with untreated OSA have a higher recurrence of AF after ablation. Appropriate treatment of OSA with continuous positive airway pressure (CPAP) was associated with a lower recurrence of AF.[30] In the Outcomes Registry for Better Informed Treatment of Atrial Fibrillation study, patients with OSA were more symptomatic and more often on rhythm control therapy than patients with AF without OSA.[31] In adjusted analyses, patients with OSA had higher risk of hospitalization. Supporting the impact of OSA, patients with OSA on CPAP treatment were less likely to progress to more permanent forms of AF compared with patients without CPAP.[31]

Circadian Variation of Atrial Fibrillation

Data from the Sleep Heart Health Study also evaluated paroxysmal AF.[32] The investigators found that the relative risk of paroxysmal AF during sleep was markedly increased shortly after a respiratory event.[32] These results support a direct temporal link between OSA events and the development of AF. The potential implications for these findings rely on OSA associated with increased risk for stroke, and this may be partially explained by the higher occurrence of AF in this population. Patients with OSA who had a stroke had higher rates

of AF even after accounting for potential confounders.[33] Further studies in this important research field are warranted.

SCREENING OBSTRUCTIVE SLEEP APNEA IN PATIENTS WITH ATRIAL FIBRILLATION USING QUESTIONNAIRES

It is well established that standard overnight polysomnography is the recommended method for the overall diagnosis of OSA. It is expensive, however, and may not be readily available in many places. To simplify and improve the access to OSA diagnosis, screening questionnaires and simplified diagnostic methods performed at home have been proposed. OSA screening questionnaires have been used to screen for OSA among AF patients, to predict the postoperative occurrence of AF, and to predict the recurrence of AF among subjects undergoing catheter ablation and (described later). The characteristics of the most commonly used OSA screening questionnaires are summarized in **Table 1**.

Epworth Sleepiness Scale

Sleepiness can be subjectively assessed through several questionnaires. The most commonly used is the Epworth Sleepiness Scale.[34] Sleepiness is an important symptom of OSA due to its impact on health-related quality of life, accident risk, and productivity. Sleepiness is also associated with adherence to CPAP treatment,[35] although this relationship has not been found in several studies.[36] On the other hand, sleepiness is a common symptom among adults, with several differential diagnoses that include sleep deprivation, major depression, hypothyroidism, and medication side effects. Moreover, sleepiness assessed by the Epworth Sleepiness Scale is only present in approximately 30% of OSA subjects.[37] Sleepiness has been shown to be less prevalent among OSA patients with comorbid cerebrovascular and heart disease.[38,39] Similarly, in a study by Albuquerque and colleagues,[17] the proportion of patients with excessive daytime sleepiness among 151 patients with AF was not different between those with and without OSA. Therefore, active search for excessive daytime sleepiness is not a valid approach to screen for OSA among AF patients.

Berlin Questionnaire

The Berlin questionnaire was designed and tested in a primary care setting and showed reasonable performance (sensitivity of 86% and specificity of 77%).[40] The Berlin questionnaire assesses the

Table 1
Obstructive sleep apnea questionnaires used among atrial fibrillation patients

Questionnaire	Description	Advantages/Disadvantages
Epworth Sleepiness Scale	Chance of dozing is graded in 8 daily activities to determine sleepiness severity.	<1/3 of OSA patients are sleepy. Sleepiness is common in other disorders.
Berlin questionnaire	Has 3 domains (snoring, tiredness, and presence of obesity or arterial hypertension)	Somewhat complicated to score Low specificity in populations with a high prevalence of OSA
STOP-Bang	8 Questions with a dichotomous (yes/no) format	Simple to answer and score Low specificity

The accuracy of these questionnaires has not been adequately studied among AF patients.

risk of OSA through 3 domains that focus on snoring, tiredness, and the presence of diagnosed arterial hypertension and obesity. The performance of the Berlin questionnaire, however, was shown to be suboptimal in populations with a higher prevalence of OSA. The Berlin questionnaire has been tested in patients with cardiovascular disorders, such as hypertension, coronary artery disease, and hypertrophic cardiomyopathy,[41–43] with sensitivities ranging from 40% to 93% and specificities ranging from 30% to 59%. Tang and colleagues[44] tested the validity of the Berlin questionnaire among 30 patients undergoing radiofrequency ablation for AF compared with polysomnography with a portable device. The investigators reported a sensitivity of 100% but a specificity of 30%. Larger studies are necessary to confirm the Berlin questionnaire as a sensitive screening tool for OSA. Based on the performance of the Berlin questionnaire in other populations with a high prevalence of OSA, however, such as those with other cardiovascular disorders, the specificity most likely is not enough to rule out a diagnosis of OSA.

STOP-Bang Questionnaire

The STOP-Bang questionnaire was derived from the Berlin questionnaire and initially tested in the surgical population, showing a sensitivity of 84% and specificity of 56%.[45] The STOP-Bang questionnaire assesses the risk of OSA based on the positive or negative answer to 8 different questions (presence of loud snore, tiredness, observed apneas, body mass index ≥ 35 kg/m^2, age >50 years, neck circumference >16 inches, and male gender). Despite its simplicity, subsequent studies in different patient groups confirmed that the STOP-Bang has a low specificity and, therefore, confirmation of OSA with a sleep test will still be necessary.[46]

Neck Circumference, Obesity, Snoring, Age, and Sex Score

The NoSAS (neck circumference, obesity, snoring, age, and sex) score has been recently described as a promising OSA screening questionnaire.[47] The NoSAS score was developed using the HypnoLaus cohort and independently validated in the EPISONO cohort and showed better performance than the Berlin and STOP-Bang questionnaires.[47] The NoSAS score has not been tested in populations with high OSA prevalence, however, such as in patients with cardiovascular disorders or AF.

Occurrence of Postoperative Atrial Fibrillation

Mungan and colleagues[48] tested the Berlin questionnaire and Epworth Sleepiness Scale in 73 patients undergoing coronary artery bypass grafting. Increased subjective sleepiness and a higher percentage of high-risk Berlin questionnaire were found among the 33 patients who developed AF compared with those who did not develop AF.[48] van Oosten and colleagues[49] used a modified Berlin questionnaire (in which subjects with a previous confirmed diagnosis of OSA were considered high-risk) to identify subjects at a higher risk for developing AF after coronary artery bypass graft. The investigators showed a 2-fold increased risk for the development of postoperative AF among patients with high-risk or confirmed OSA.[49] Therefore, patients with high risk of having OSA as determined by the Berlin questionnaire are at increased risk for developing AF. These findings are in line with studies that diagnosed OSA preoperatively using polysomnography and showed that OSA was a risk factor for postoperative AF.[50,51] The significance of being at high risk for OSA in the preoperative setting is limited, however, due to the low specificity of the screening questionnaires to detect OSA and the need to further confirm the diagnosis and implement therapy.

Recurrence of Atrial Fibrillation After Catheter Ablation

OSA diagnosed through standard polysomnography has been shown to be an independent predictor of AF recurrence after radiofrequency ablation.[30,52] OSA screening questionnaires have been used to identify patients with an increased risk of AF recurrence due to OSA. Both the Berlin and STOP-Bang questionnaires have been tested as predictors of AF recurrence after radiofrequency ablation. A high-risk score for OSA at the STOP-Bang questionnaire was associated with a 3.7-fold increased risk of AF recurrence.[53] Conflicting results have been reported on the performance of the Berlin questionnaire to predict AF recurrence after catheter ablation. Tang and colleagues[44] used the Berlin questionnaire among 178 AF patients undergoing catheter ablation. A high OSA risk was not associated with AF recurrence. In contrast, Chilukuri and colleagues[54] used the Berlin questionnaire and showed that high-risk OSA was independently associated with increased AF recurrence after catheter ablation. Screening using questionnaires to predict those who are more likely to have AF recurrence after catheter ablation can be useful to select those who should undergo confirmation using HST or polysomnography.

HOME SLEEP TESTING

The utility of screening questionnaires for OSA among populations with a known high prevalence of OSA has been questioned.[55,56] HST is becoming increasingly cheaper and more readily available. Devices that only have respiratory channels (nasal pressure cannula, chest and abdominal respiratory effort belts, and oximetry) can be assembled by patients at home with instructions that are simple to follow. Skomro and colleagues[57] showed that the outcomes of HST followed by CPAP titration using an auto-CPAP at home were similar to the traditional laboratory-based approach. HST has become an attractive single-step approach to detect OSA among populations known to have a high OSA prevalence.

FUTURE DIRECTIONS

OSA is a common comorbidity of AF patients and has been shown to adversely influence health outcome and quality of life. Detecting OSA among AF patients seems to decrease AF recurrence after cardioversion or catheter ablation. Apart from the prevention of AF recurrence, however, it is not clear who among patients with AF and OSA benefits from OSA treatment. Randomized studies on the impact of OSA among AF patients are lacking.

OSA screening questionnaires among AF patients have been used in several studies. The validity of such questionnaires, however, is limited. Additional studies using more accurate diagnostic methods are necessary. One possibility is using a 2-step approach, beginning with screening questionnaires (eg, Berlin and STOP-Bang questionnaires) followed by confirmatory HST (for those identified as at high risk). Conversely, HST alone should be considered an alternative to diagnosing OSA in the AF population. The cost-effectiveness of such approaches, however, needs to be studied.

REFERENCES

1. Jordan AS, McSharry DG, Malhotra A. Adult obstructive sleep apnoea. Lancet 2014;383:736–47.
2. Heinzer R, Vat S, Marques-Vidal P, et al. Prevalence of sleep-disordered breathing in the general population: the HypnoLaus study. Lancet Respir Med 2015; 3:310–8.
3. Ye L, Pien GW, Ratcliffe SJ, et al. The different clinical faces of obstructive sleep apnoea: a cluster analysis. Eur Respir J 2014;44:1600–7.
4. Marin J, Carrizo S, Vicente E, et al. Long-term cardiovascular outcomes in men with obstructive sleep apnoea-hypopnoea with or without treatment with continuous positive airway pressure: an observational study. Lancet 2005;365:1046–53.
5. Drager LF, Togeiro SM, Polotsky VY, et al. Obstructive sleep apnea: a cardiometabolic risk in obesity and the metabolic syndrome. J Am Coll Cardiol 2013;62:569–76.
6. McEvoy RD, Antic NA, Heeley E, et al. CPAP for prevention of cardiovascular events in obstructive sleep apnea. N Engl J Med 2016;375:919–31.
7. Costa LE, Uchoa CH, Harmon RR, et al. Potential underdiagnosis of obstructive sleep apnoea in the cardiology outpatient setting. Heart 2015;101:1288–92.
8. Psaty BM, Manolio TA, Kuller LH, et al. Incidence of and risk factors for atrial fibrillation in older adults. Circulation 1997;96:2455–61.
9. Go AS, Hylek EM, Phillips KA, et al. Prevalence of diagnosed atrial fibrillation in adults: national implications for rhythm management and stroke prevention: the anticoagulation and risk factors in atrial fibrillation (ATRIA) Study. JAMA 2001;285: 2370–5.
10. Lakshminarayan K, Solid CA, Collins AJ, et al. Atrial fibrillation and stroke in the general medicare population: a 10-year perspective (1992 to 2002). Stroke 2006;37:1969–74.

11. Burstein B, Nattel S. Atrial fibrosis: mechanisms and clinical relevance in atrial fibrillation. J Am Coll Cardiol 2008;51:802–9.

12. Camm AJ, Savelieva I, Potpara T, et al. The changing circumstance of atrial fibrillation - progress towards precision medicine. J Intern Med 2016;279:412–27.

13. Wolowacz SE, Samuel M, Brennan VK, et al. The cost of illness of atrial fibrillation: a systematic review of the recent literature. Europace 2011;13:1375–85.

14. Young T, Palta M, Dempsey J, et al. The occurrence of sleep-disordered breathing among middle-aged adults. N Engl J Med 1993;328:1230–5.

15. Tufik S, Santos-Silva R, Taddei J, et al. Obstructive sleep apnea syndrome in the Sao Paulo epidemiologic sleep study. Sleep Med 2010;11:441–6.

16. Mehra R, Benjamin EJ, Shahar E, et al. Association of nocturnal arrhythmias with sleep-disordered breathing: the sleep heart health study. Am J Respir Crit Care Med 2006;173:910–6.

17. Albuquerque FN, Calvin AD, Sert Kuniyoshi FH, et al. Sleep-disordered breathing and excessive daytime sleepiness in patients with atrial fibrillation. Chest 2012;141:967–73.

18. Bitter T, Langer C, Vogt J, et al. Sleep-disordered breathing in patients with atrial fibrillation and normal systolic left ventricular function. Dtsch Arztebl Int 2009;106:164–70.

19. Patel D, Mohanty P, Di Biase L, et al. Safety and efficacy of pulmonary vein antral isolation in patients with obstructive sleep apnea: the impact of continuous positive airway pressure. Circ Arrhythm Electrophysiol 2010;3:445–51.

20. Gami AS, Pressman G, Caples SM, et al. Association of atrial fibrillation and obstructive sleep apnea. Circulation 2004;110:364–7.

21. Cadby G, McArdle N, Briffa T, et al. Severity of OSA is an independent predictor of incident atrial fibrillation hospitalization in a large sleep-clinic cohort. Chest 2015;148:945–52.

22. May AM, Blackwell T, Stone PH, et al. Central sleep-disordered breathing predicts incident atrial fibrillation in older men. Am J Respir Crit Care Med 2016;193:783–91.

23. Linz D, Linz B, Hohl M, et al. Atrial arrhythmogenesis in obstructive sleep apnea: therapeutic implications. Sleep Med Rev 2016;26:87–94.

24. Orban M, Bruce CJ, Pressman GS, et al. Dynamic changes of left ventricular performance and left atrial volume induced by the mueller maneuver in healthy young adults and implications for obstructive sleep apnea, atrial fibrillation, and heart failure. Am J Cardiol 2008;102:1557–61.

25. Drager LF, Bortolotto LA, Pedrosa RP, et al. Left atrial diameter is independently associated with arterial stiffness in patients with obstructive sleep apnea: potential implications for atrial fibrillation. Int J Cardiol 2010;144:257–9.

26. Drager LF, Bortolotto LA, Figueiredo AC, et al. Obstructive sleep apnea, hypertension, and their interaction on arterial stiffness and heart remodeling. Chest 2007;131:1379–86.

27. Gami AS, Hodge DO, Herges RM, et al. Obstructive sleep apnea, obesity, and the risk of incident atrial fibrillation. J Am Coll Cardiol 2007;49:565–71.

28. Kanagala R, Murali NS, Friedman PA, et al. Obstructive sleep apnea and the recurrence of atrial fibrillation. Circulation 2003;107:2589–94.

29. Li L, Wang ZW, Li J, et al. Efficacy of catheter ablation of atrial fibrillation in patients with obstructive sleep apnoea with and without continuous positive airway pressure treatment: a meta-analysis of observational studies. Europace 2014;16:1309–14.

30. Naruse Y, Tada H, Satoh M, et al. Concomitant obstructive sleep apnea increases the recurrence of atrial fibrillation following radiofrequency catheter ablation of atrial fibrillation: clinical impact of continuous positive airway pressure therapy. Heart Rhythm 2013;10:331–7.

31. Holmqvist F, Guan N, Zhu Z, et al. Impact of obstructive sleep apnea and continuous positive airway pressure therapy on outcomes in patients with atrial fibrillation-results from the outcomes registry for better informed treatment of atrial fibrillation (ORBIT-AF). Am Heart J 2015;169:647–54.e2.

32. Monahan K, Storfer-Isser A, Mehra R, et al. Triggering of nocturnal arrhythmias by sleep-disordered breathing events. J Am Coll Cardiol 2009;54:1797–804.

33. Mansukhani MP, Calvin AD, Kolla BP, et al. The association between atrial fibrillation and stroke in patients with obstructive sleep apnea: a population-based case-control study. Sleep Med 2013;14:243–6.

34. Johns MW. A new method for measuring daytime sleepiness: the Epworth sleepiness scale. Sleep 1991;14:540–5.

35. Waldhorn RE, Herrick TW, Nguyen MC, et al. Long-term compliance with nasal continuous positive airway pressure therapy of obstructive sleep apnea. Chest 1990;97:33–8.

36. Weaver TE, Sawyer AM. Adherence to continuous positive airway pressure treatment for obstructive sleep apnoea: implications for future interventions. Indian J Med Res 2010;131:245–58.

37. Gottlieb D, Whitney C, Bonekat W, et al. Relation of sleepiness to respiratory disturbance index. Am J Respir Crit Care Med 1999;159:502–7.

38. Arzt M, Young T, Finn L, et al. Sleepiness and sleep in patients with both systolic heart failure and obstructive sleep apnea. Arch Intern Med 2006;166:1716–22.

39. Arzt M, Young T, Peppard PE, et al. Dissociation of obstructive sleep apnea from hypersomnolence and obesity in patients with stroke. Stroke 2010;41:e129–34.

40. Netzer N, Stoohs R, Netzer C, et al. Using the Berlin Questionnaire to identify patients at risk for the sleep apnea syndrome. Ann Intern Med 1999;131:485–91.

41. Danzi-Soares ND, Genta PR, Nerbass FB, et al. Obstructive sleep apnea is common among patients referred for coronary artery bypass grafting and can be diagnosed by portable monitoring. Coron Artery Dis 2012;23:31–8.

42. Drager LF, Genta PR, Pedrosa RP, et al. Characteristics and predictors of obstructive sleep apnea in patients with systemic hypertension. Am J Cardiol 2010;105:1135–9.

43. Nerbass FB, Pedrosa RP, Genta PR, et al. Lack of reliable clinical predictors to identify obstructive sleep apnea in patients with hypertrophic cardiomyopathy. Clinics (Sao Paulo) 2013;68:992–6.

44. Tang RB, Dong JZ, Liu XP, et al. Obstructive sleep apnoea risk profile and the risk of recurrence of atrial fibrillation after catheter ablation. Europace 2009;11:100–5.

45. Chung F, Yegneswaran B, Liao P, et al. STOP questionnaire: a tool to screen patients for obstructive sleep apnea. Anesthesiology 2008;108:812–21.

46. Nagappa M, Liao P, Wong J, et al. Validation of the STOP-bang questionnaire as a screening tool for obstructive sleep apnea among different populations: a systematic review and meta-analysis. PLoS One 2015;10:e0143697.

47. Marti-Soler H, Hirotsu C, Marques-Vidal P, et al. The NoSAS score for screening of sleep-disordered breathing: a derivation and validation study. Lancet Respir Med 2016;4:742–8.

48. Mungan U, Ozeke O, Mavioglu L, et al. The role of the preoperative screening of sleep apnoea by Berlin Questionnaire and epworth sleepiness scale for postoperative atrial fibrillation. Heart Lung Circ 2013;22:38–42.

49. van Oosten EM, Hamilton A, Petsikas D, et al. Effect of preoperative obstructive sleep apnea on the frequency of atrial fibrillation after coronary artery bypass grafting. Am J Cardiol 2014;113:919–23.

50. Mooe T, Gullsby S, Rabben T, et al. Sleep-disordered breathing: a novel predictor of atrial fibrillation after coronary artery bypass surgery. Coron Artery Dis 1996;7:475–8.

51. Uchoa CH, Danzi-Soares Nde J, Nunes FS, et al. Impact of OSA on cardiovascular events after coronary artery bypass surgery. Chest 2015;147:1352–60.

52. Fein AS, Shvilkin A, Shah D, et al. Treatment of obstructive sleep apnea reduces the risk of atrial fibrillation recurrence after catheter ablation. J Am Coll Cardiol 2013;62:300–5.

53. Farrehi PM, O'Brien LM, Bas HD, et al. Occult obstructive sleep apnea and clinical outcomes of radiofrequency catheter ablation in patients with atrial fibrillation. J Interv Card Electrophysiol 2015;43:279–86.

54. Chilukuri K, Dalal D, Marine JE, et al. Predictive value of obstructive sleep apnoea assessed by the Berlin Questionnaire for outcomes after the catheter ablation of atrial fibrillation. Europace 2009;11:896–901.

55. Oldenburg O, Teerlink JR. Screening for sleep-disordered breathing in patients hospitalized for heart failure. JACC Heart Fail 2015;3:732–3.

56. Westlake K, Polak J. Screening for obstructive sleep apnea in type 2 diabetes patients – questionnaires are not good enough. Front Endocrinol (Lausanne) 2016;7:124.

57. Skomro RP, Gjevre J, Reid J, et al. Outcomes of home-based diagnosis and treatment of obstructive sleep apnea. Chest 2010;138:257–63.

Management of Sleep Apnea Syndromes in Heart Failure

 CrossMark

Bernardo J. Selim, MD*, Kannan Ramar, MD

KEYWORDS

- Heart failure • Central sleep apnea • Obstructive sleep apnea • Cheyne-Stokes breathing
- Sleep-disordered breathing • Positive airway pressure • Oxygen • Positional therapy

KEY POINTS

- Obstructive sleep apnea (OSA) and central sleep apnea (CSA) are prevalent in heart failure (HF) and associated with worse prognosis.
- Continuous positive airway pressure (CPAP) therapy for OSA may improve mortality in patients with HF with reduced ejection fraction (HFrEF), and it may be beneficial in those with preserved ejection fraction (HFpEF).
- CPAP therapy may improve hemodynamics (left ventricular ejection fraction [LVEF]), and exercise capacity in HFrEF with CSA, although mortality benefit is unknown.
- Adaptive servo ventilation (ASV) therapy is contraindicated in patients with symptomatic HFrEF (EF ≤ 45%.) with predominant CSA due to increased risk of all-cause mortality and cardiovascular mortality.
- Nocturnal oxygen therapy can decrease CSA events, sympathetic tone, and improve LVEF. Mortality benefit is unknown.

INTRODUCTION

Heart failure (HF) is a complex clinical syndrome that results from any structural or functional impairment of ventricular filling or ejection of blood. Classified based on left ventricular (LV) functionality, patients with HF may be divided into those with predominantly normal LV size and preserved ejection fraction (EF) (diastolic HF or HFpEF), and those with severe dilatation and/or markedly reduced EF (systolic HF or HFrEF).[1] Due to an aging US population, the prevalence of HF continues to increase.[2] Although guideline-driven pharmacologic interventions in patients with HF have improved outcomes, the mortality rate in this population continues to be excessively high (the absolute mortality rates for HF are approximately 50% within 5 years of diagnosis).[3,4] Thus, in the search of additional comorbidities that contribute to HF progression and impair prognosis, sleep-related breathing disorders (SRBDs) have been identified as novel reversible risk factors. The American College of Cardiology Foundation and the American Heart Association in their most recent published guidelines for the management of heart failure recommend continuous positive airway pressure (CPAP) therapy for obstructive sleep apnea (OSA) in patients with HF, giving it a recommendation class IIa ("benefits > > risks").[1] Contrary to OSA, the treatment of central sleep apnea (CSA) in patients with HF, with or without Cheyne-Stokes breathing (CSA-CSB) pattern, remains controversial.

Dr B.J. Selim and Dr K. Ramar have no commercial or financial conflicts of interest.
Division of Pulmonary and Critical Care Medicine, Mayo Clinic Center for Sleep Medicine, Mayo Clinic, 200 First Street Southwest, Rochester, MN 55905, USA
* Corresponding author.
E-mail address: Selim.bernardo@mayo.edu

sleep.theclinics.com

EPIDEMIOLOGY

The association between HF and SRBD is complex, and their interaction can be obscured by shared cardiovascular comorbidities (eg, hypertension, diabetes, coronary disease, and obesity).[5] Two primary types of SRBD occur and may coexist in patients with HF: OSA and CSA, with or without Cheyne-Stokes breathing (CSA-CSB). Likely representing 2 different pathophysiologic mechanistic pathways in patients with HF, OSA may contribute to the development and progression of HF, whereas CSA likely arises as a consequence of it (see the following section on pathophysiology).[5,6] However, OSA and CSA should not be considered as separate processes, but may be part of the spectrum of periodic breathing, the predominant type of which can transform over time in response to alterations in cardiac function.[7,8] Furthermore, both OSA and CSA-Cheyne-Stokes respiration (CSR) have been shown to be markers of disease severity and predictors of increased mortality in chronic HF as well as in patients with decompensated HF.[9–13]

Patients with HFpEF tend to have OSA in comparison with patients with HFrEF who tend to have CSA to a greater extent.[14] Regarding gender, men with HF are more likely to have SRBD compared with women, and its severity may be higher.[15] Sharing similar predictors (eg, older age, male gender), HF and SRBD (predominately OSA) are highly prevalent.[16] In the general population (unselected population), and based on data from the Sleep Heart Health Study, OSA occurred in approximately 1 of 5 subjects (46% had apnea-hypopnea index [AHI] $\geq$5/h; 18% had AHI $\geq$15/h and 6% had AHI $\geq$30/h) whereas CSA-CSB was rare (<1%).[17] However, in the referral HF population, the prevalence of OSA and CSA is higher. In a seminal study of patients with HFrEF (LVEF $\leq$45%), the prevalence of moderate to severe (AHI $\geq$15/h of sleep) OSA and CSA was 26% and 21%, respectively, remaining unchanged in time despite reaching optimal pharmacologic therapy as per current guidelines (eg, use of beta-blockers and spironolactone).[15,16,18–25] Similarly, recent publications on the HFrEF population receiving also optimally dosed medical management with both β-blockade and renin-angiotensin system antagonists also have shown high prevalence of moderate-severe SRBD in different Western countries (United States, 30% OSA and 31% CSA; Canada, 32% OSA and 29% CSA; and Germany, 19% OSA and 32% CSA).[20,22,26] In those patients with predominant HFpEF, the prevalence of OSA and CSA was 36.0% and 6.0% in moderate SRBD, and 24.0% and 16.3% in severe SRBD, respectively (**Fig. 1, Table 1**). Furthermore, there is a proportional increase in predominant CSA with increasing impairment of diastolic function.[27] Despite the high prevalence of SRBD in the HF population, SRBD continues to be underdiagnosed in current clinical practice for various

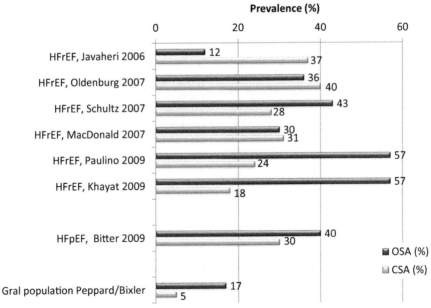

Fig. 1. Prevalence of SRBD in the HF population (referral) and general population (unselected). (*Data from* Refs.[15,19–25,27])

Table 1
Prevalence of SRBD in referral HF population

First Author, Year	Population Type/Center	Sample Size, n	Age, y, Mean	Mean EF, %	SDB, %	OSA, %	CSA, %
Javaheri,[19] 2006	HFrEF/Single center	100	62–69	21–25	49	12	37
Oldenburg et al,[20] 2007	HFrEF/Single center	700	61–65	27–29	76	36	40
Schulz et al,[21] 2007	HFrEF/ Multicenter	203	65–66	28–29	71	43	28
MacDonald et al,[22] 2008	HFrEF/Single center	108	57–58	20	61	30	31
Paulino et al,[15] 2009	HFrEF/Single center	316	55–60	30–31	81	57	24
Khayat et al,[23] 2009	HFrEF/Single center	395	57–60	32–35	75	57	18
Bitter et al,[27] 2009	HFpEF/Single center	244	61–66	> 55%	69	40	30

Abbreviations: CSA, central sleep apnea; EF, ejection fraction; HF, heart failure; HFpEF, heart failure with preserved ejection fraction; HFrEF, heart failure with reduced ejection fraction; OSA, obstructive sleep apnea; SDB, sleep-disordered breathing; SRBD, sleep-related breathing disorders.

reasons. This is likely because patients with HF, including those with documented sleep disorders, rarely report excessive daytime sleepiness to their health providers.[28,29]

PATHOPHYSIOLOGY: LINKING OBSTRUCTIVE SLEEP APNEA AND CENTRAL SLEEP APNEA WITH HEART FAILURE, A LIKELY BIDIRECTIONAL RELATIONSHIP
Mechanistic Pathways Linking Obstructive Sleep Apnea–Heart Failure

There are several pathophysiologic pathways that predispose and perpetuate HFrEF in patients with OSA.[6,30,31] Obstructive apnea and hypopnea are associated with repeated inspiratory efforts against the collapsed upper airway associated with large swings in the intrathoracic pressure (ITP), which may be as high as 60 to 80 mm Hg. During each obstructive apnea and hypopnea, the negative intrathoracic pressure exerts a direct distending force on the intrathoracic vascular system (aorta and vena cava) and heart, which in turn increases venous return, right heart volume, and pressure overload.[32] Cardiac wall stress (afterload) is additionally augmented by considerable acute changes in ventricular transmural pressure of LV during obstructive apnea events.[33,34] Apneas and hypopneas (by cyclical arousals) also activate the sympathetic nervous system, associated with swings in blood pressure and heart rate, which in turn generates shear stress on the vascular endothelium and, in combination with

recurrent hypoxemia, may lead to endothelial dysfunction.[35,36] These stressors, repeated during each apneic-hypopneic phase, may lead in the long-term to the electrical and mechanical remodeling of both atria and ventricles, thereby possibly explaining the high prevalence of congestive HF in patients with OSA[37] (**Table 2**)

The relationship of OSA with HF may be bidirectional, with recent data supporting the role of rostral fluid redistribution as a potential mechanistic pathway linking HF as a predisposing factor for OSA. When patients with HF sleep in the supine position, fluid accumulates in the legs while upright (high venous return) will shift rostrally overnight while supine. By redistribution into the jugular vein and peri-pharyngeal neck's soft tissue, it may predispose to OSA.[38,39] Supporting this hypothesis, relief of congestion through diuresis has been shown to attenuate OSA in patients with HF.[40]

The Impact of Positive Airway Pressure Therapy in Obstructive Sleep Apnea–Heart Failure Relationship

Because the heart is a pressure chamber within another pressure chamber (the thorax), changes in ITP during the ventilatory cycle will affect the venous return to the right ventricle (RV), and the systemic outflow of the LV, independent of the cardiac function.

By pneumatic splinting of upper airway, positive airway pressure (PAP) will diminish or eliminate the

Table 2
Pathophysiologic stressors on the heart associated with OSA

Physiologic Stressors	CV Impact	Electro-Mechanical Effects
Cyclical swing in intrathoracic pressure (up to 60 cm H_2O)	RV dilation with left septal deviation, impairing LV filling (ventricular interdependency)[33,128–130]	Increased RV preload Decreased LV preload
	Increased LV transmural pressures by Laplace law[a] (by which the afterload is determined by the cardiac wall stress)[131–133]	Increased LV afterload
	Recurrent atrial stretching, increased LV hypertrophy and diastolic dysfunction[133–136]	Enlarged LA
	Vagal nerve activation[137]	Increased effective refractory period (propensity for tachyarrhythmias, atrial fibrillation)
ICH	Hypoxic pulmonary vasoconstriction	Increased RV afterload RV diastolic failure
	ICH induced stimulation of the carotid body (glomus)	Increased sympathetic surge Increased systemic blood pressure
	Systemic vasoconstriction[138] Increased oxidative stress	Increased LV afterload Microvascular endothelial dysfunction

Abbreviations: CV, cardiovascular; ICH, intermittent chronic hypoxia; LA, left atrium; LV, left ventricular; OSA, obstructive sleep apnea; RV, right ventricular.
[a] Laplace law: cardiac wall stress (σ) is proportional to: Δ P, transmural pressure; r, ventricular radius; h, wall thickness.

markedly negative swings in ITP of patients with OSA, with subsequent stabilization of the cardiac wall stress (afterload), and cardiac volumes. In hypervolemic patients (patients with HF), abolishing negative swings of ITP will decrease LV afterload and will augment LVEF, with subsequent increase in cardiac output and decrease in myocardial oxygen demand.[31,41–44] Furthermore, by decreasing the number of arousals and recurrent hypoxia, CPAP therapy decreases the sympathetic nervous system surge, with subsequent improvement of its associated vasoconstriction, peripheral resistance, and heart rate variability.[31,35,45,46]

Mechanistic Pathways Linking Central Sleep Apnea and Central Sleep Apnea–Cheyne-Stokes Breathing with Heart Failure

CSA-CSB is a prevalent form of CSA in patients with HF, predominately in those with HFrEF.[14] It arises as a consequence of multiple hemodynamic changes observed in patients with HF. This particular periodic respiratory disturbance pattern (crescendo-decrescendo hyperventilation followed by central apnea) is explained by the engineer model of loop gain. Briefly, loop gain is defined as the response of the ventilatory control system

to a disturbance in ventilation (the ratio of the size of a response to the size of a disturbance). In systems controlled by negative feedback mechanisms, high loop gain is associated with rapid but often unstable respiratory responses to perturbations.[47] The higher the loop gain, the higher the overventilation or underventilation response, resulting in respiratory instability.[48–50] Noteworthy, a decrease in upper airway tone also can occur at the end of a central apnea.[51] Thus, obstruction of the upper airway is part of the mechanism of central apnea in addition to increased chemosensitivity to $Paco_2$ (**Fig. 2**).

Similar to OSA in patients with HF, rostral fluid shift from legs to lung may stimulate pulmonary vagal irritant receptors (by pulmonary congestion) with subsequent reflex hyperventilation, dropping $Paco_2$ below the apnea threshold, as a mechanistic pathway to increase the loop gain with subsequent development of CSA.[39]

Several reports have demonstrated a spontaneous conversion from predominately CSA to OSA associated with LVEF improvement, including patients undergoing cardiac transplantation.[7,8] Therefore, CSA and OSA may not be considered 2 separate entities in patients with HF, but part of the spectrum of periodic breathing, the predominant type of which can transform over

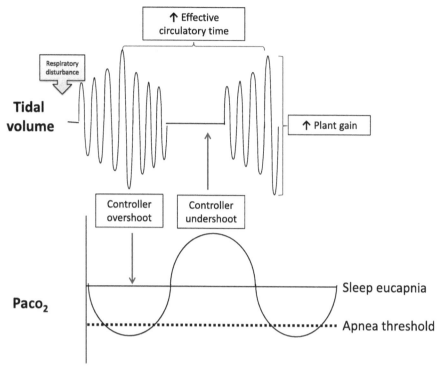

Fig. 2. Schematic of respiratory control response in CSB. The loop gain is the respiratory control system's degree of response to a ventilatory disturbance. It is composed of (1) the controller gain, (2) the plant gain, and (3) the mixing gain (effective circulatory time).

time in response to alterations in cardiac function. As mentioned previously, the mechanisms involved in this transformation may include alteration of ventilatory drive, which is elevated in association with pulmonary congestion and increased chemosensitivity. With the improvement in cardiac dysfunction, these inciting factors may be relieved, leading to a shortened circulation time and alleviation of SRBD.

TREATMENT OPTIONS FOR PATIENTS WITH SLEEP-RELATED BREATHING DISORDERS AND HEART FAILURE

Shared Therapeutic Management of Obstructive Sleep Apnea and Central Sleep Apnea in Patients with Heart Failure

The main objectives in treating SRBD in HF are to slow the progression of disease, reduce the need for hospitalization, and increase the length or quality of life. The evidence for this, until recently, has largely been confined to observational data or small, short-term randomized trials with surrogate endpoints, such as EF, plasma B-type natriuretic peptide concentration, and quality-of-life assessments. Few randomized controlled trials are available in this area. The following recommendations are based on current literature in

the management of OSA and CSA in patients with HF.

Lifestyle modifications

In several studies published to date, body mass index (BMI) and LVEF are consistently identified as clinical predictors for increased prevalence of OSA in patients with HFrEF.[16,22,26,52] Therefore, lifestyle modifications should be targeted to improve weight (BMI), the most common risk factor for OSA, with goal of being within 10% of ideal body weight.[53] In patients with HFpEF, predominately those with obese phenotype, supervised exercise training and caloric restriction have been also shown to be beneficial.[54–56] Regarding LVEF, a common predictor of CSA, a strict adherence to a low-salt diet (low-salt diet of 2–3 g/d) may be beneficial to control high blood pressure and volume overload.

Cardiovascular pharmacologic therapy

Optimization of cardiovascular pharmacotherapy should be counted among the first interventions in the management of SRBD in patients with HFrEF. The use of β-blockers, angiotensin-converting enzyme (ACE) inhibitors, angiotensin II receptor blockers (ARB), aldosterone antagonists, and diuretics have salutary effects in the hemodynamics of HF, with potential benefits in OSA and CSA-CSB. For example, β-blockers may influence hypoxemic chemosensitivity (controller gain), whereas ACE inhibitors and diuretic therapy may decrease the intracardiac filling pressures.[57–60] Furthermore, based on the hypothesis of rostral fluid shift in patients with HF, relief of congestion through diuresis has been shown to also attenuate OSA in this population.[40] However, current small observational studies have not been able to detect changes in prevalence of CSA-CSB in those patients with severe HFrEF on guideline-driven pharmacologic therapy in comparison with those on suboptimal pharmacologic regimens.[61]

Although HFpEF counts for approximately 50% of all HF cases and has an outcome similar to that of systolic HF, an effective pharmacologic treatment impacting mortality has yet to be established.[62,63] The use of β-blockers, ACE inhibitors, ARBs, and aldosterone antagonists might improve exercise capacity; however, none of these treatments has convincingly shown to improve long-term cardiovascular (CV) outcomes in this population[64] (**Fig. 3**).

Continuous positive airway pressure therapy
Continuous positive airway pressure therapy in patients with heart failure (heart failure with reduced ejection fraction or heart failure with preserved ejection fraction) with obstructive sleep apnea Regarding CPAP therapy in patients with HFrEF with OSA, several studies have provided consistent data to support beneficial hemodynamic effects.[31,65] In general, chronic CPAP therapy preferentially improves LV systolic function, even in stable patients receiving optimal medical therapy, including β-blocker medications. In particular, CPAP therapy results in increased stroke volume, and increased LVEF (13% relative increase, 5% absolute increase) by lowering systemic vascular resistance.[66] Current observational studies also support mortality benefits from CPAP therapy in patients with HFrEF with OSA, as well as in the general OSA population (middle-aged and elderly patients with OSA) at risk for fatal and nonfatal cardiovascular events, including HF.[9,11,29,67–69] This issue will be further addressed by the Sleep Apnea cardioVascular Endpoints (SAVE) study (NCT00738179), an ongoing multicenter, randomized controlled trial designed to

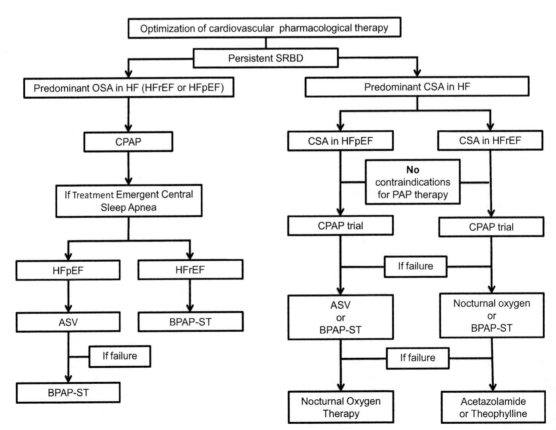

Fig. 3. Treatment pathway in sleep apnea syndromes in patients with HF.

determine whether treatment of OSA with CPAP can reduce the risk of serious CV events in patients with established CV disease.[70]

The benefit of CPAP therapy in patients with HFpEF with OSA is less well documented, with studies showing contradictory results.[71,72] In the only currently available randomized controlled trial, patients with moderate to severe OSA with HFpEF (LVEF >50%) treated with optimal pharmacologic regimen and while on CPAP showed improvement of right heart function (by echocardiography), pulmonary function, and exercise capacity (by cardiopulmonary exercise testing) in comparison with those without CPAP therapy. Furthermore, mortality was significantly lower (0% vs 12.8%; log rank *P* = .014) in the PAP group than in the non-PAP group at 6 months of follow-up.[71] On the contrary, a recently published small observational study showed that even when treated appropriately with CPAP, long-term cardiac function and outcomes remained unchanged in patients with HFpEF with OSA in comparison with those without OSA.[72] However, caution should be applied in drawing definitive conclusions from this study based on the small sample size[72] (see **Fig. 3**).

Continuous positive airway pressure therapy in patients with heart failure with reduced ejection fraction with central sleep apnea–Cheyne-Stokes breathing Although generally accepted that CPAP therapy benefits patients with HFrEF with OSA, the impact of CPAP in patients with HFrEF with CSA-CSB remains controversial. In 2005, the Canadian Continuous Positive Airway Pressure for Patients with Central Sleep Apnea and Heart Failure trial (CANPAP trial) failed to show survival benefit with CPAP treatment despite attenuation of CSA, improvement of nocturnal oxygenation, and an increase in the EF.[73] This negative result in survival benefit could have been attributed to a lack of PAP titration to achieve a therapeutic reduction of AHI or limited compliance with the device. In a subsequent post hoc subgroup analysis of the same trial, CPAP showed positive effect on LVEF and transplant-free survival when CPAP therapy was able to normalize the AHI to fewer than 15 events per hour.[74] Subsequent studies and meta-analyses have consistently shown CPAP therapy to increase the LVEF by 6%, and decrease the AHI between 21/h (95% confidence interval [CI] 17–25) and 30/h (95% CI 23–37), and a trend toward decreasing combined mortality-cardiac transplantation rate in those patients with HF with CSR-CSA who comply with therapy.[75,76]

In summary, the available data suggest CPAP therapy benefits patients with HFrEF with OSA

and patients with HFpEF with OSA (predominately HFpEF obese phenotype). On the contrary, the use of any positive airway modality for CSA in patients with HFrEF must be approached with caution based on the patient's hemodynamics. Current guidelines on treatment of CSA syndromes from the American Academy of Sleep Medicine states that "CPAP therapy targeted to normalize the AHI is indicated for the initial treatment of CSA related to CHF."[75] In these patients, CPAP may improve hemodynamics (LVEF) and survival if titrated to achieve a therapeutic reduction of AHI of fewer than 15 events per hour (see **Fig. 3**).

Positional therapy
It has long been recognized that sleeping in the supine position increases the frequency and severity of obstructive respiratory events in patients with OSA.[77] In patients with moderate to severe optimally treated HFrEF, positional sleep apnea was observed in 76% of patients with OSA and 53% of patients with CSA.[78] Similar to OSA, CSA-CSR severity is worse in the supine position and it is alleviated when the nonsupine position is reached or when the head of the bed is raised.[79,80] However, as cardiac dysfunction progresses in patients with HFrEF, the severity of CSA increases and positional CSA may become position-independent. Still, intensive pharmacologic treatment for HF may change CSA from nonpositional back to positional.[81] In a recent study comparing the impact of body position on the severity of sleep apnea in patients with OSA with HFrEF and patients with CSA with HFrEF, lateral sleeping position was shown to have a major beneficial effect on the severity of SRBD in patients with HF, and that this improvement was greater in subjects with OSA than in those with CSA.[78]

In conclusion, positional therapy should be considered as monotherapy only in those patients with exclusive positional OSA or CSA sleep apnea determined by polysomnography; otherwise, positional therapy should be a supplemental therapeutic intervention in patients with suboptimal control of their SRBD by therapies mentioned as follows.

SPECIFIC MANAGEMENT OF CENTRAL SLEEP APNEA AND CENTRAL SLEEP APNEA–CHEYNE-STOKES BREATHING IN PATIENTS WITH HEART FAILURE

There is no widely accepted treatment modality or approach for CSA and CSA-CSR treatment. Following is a review of treatment options for CSA. Although several interventions have been used, none have demonstrated efficacy or safety today to become broadly accepted.

Cardiovascular Pharmacologic Therapy Targeting Central Sleep Apnea in Patients with Heart Failure

Even though not commonly used in daily clinical practice, other pharmacologic therapies used in CSA-CSB are acetazolamide and theophylline. Acetazolamide, by respiratory stimulation and diuretic effect, may reduce AHI and improve a patient's perception of sleep quality.[82] However, side effects associated with acetazolamide, such as paresthesias, tinnitus, metabolic acidosis, electrolyte imbalance, and dizziness, should be considered. Theophylline, by competing with adenosine at a central level, stimulates respiratory centers, resulting in a 51% reduction in the AHI, mostly because of a reduction in the number of episodes of central apneas. It also shows a decrease in the duration of arterial oxyhemoglobin desaturation during sleep.[83] However, the benefits of theophylline should be weighed against the narrow therapeutic range safety and its side-effect profile.

Gas Therapy

Carbon dioxide supplementation and dead space therapy

The pathophysiology of CSR-HF is currently explained by changes in $Paco_2$ above or below the apneic threshold, a tightly regulated level of $Paco_2$ above or below which chemoreceptor response results in unstable breathing in presence of high loop gain. Therefore, avoiding relative hypocapnia (drop of $Paco_2$ below the apneic threshold) may stabilize the respiratory system. This can be reached by CO2 supplementation (gas modulator) or by increasing anatomic dead space (DS). Low CO2 supplementation can be bled from a PAP gas modulator into a PAP device. However, limitations related to cost of the gas modulator, supply of CO2, and side effects of treatment have affected the practical application of this therapy in the clinical field.[84] Increasing physiologic DS during positive pressure therapy has been reported to control CSAs in those with HF.[85] This is achieved by the sequential connection of a nonvented oronasal mask to 4 to 6 inches of tubing (rebreathing space), an exhalation valve, and a conventional positive pressure circuit. This expiratory rebreathing reservoir represents an increase of $Paco_2$ in the order of 2 to 3 mm Hg. Unfortunately, pressure leaks and sleep fragmentation are common.[86] When compared with adaptive servo ventilation (ASV) therapy (discussed later) in patients with congestive HF, DS and ASV caused a similar reduction in the AHI, but total sleep time was significantly decreased by DS, attributed to a high arousal index and disruption of sleep architecture.[87]

Nocturnal oxygen therapy

Publications regarding the role of nocturnal oxygen therapy (NOT) in patients with HF with CSA are limited, lacking large-scale randomized controlled trials. Most uncontrolled studies of NOT via nasal cannula (NC; 2–3 L per minute) reported significant improvements in oxygen saturation index, AHI, LVEF, and specific activity scale at 3 to 12 months of follow-up without clinically significant adverse effects.[88–91] At the same time, there was a reduction in the sympathetic nervous system activity and in serum B-type natriuretic peptide levels; however, without a change in quality of life.[89,92,93] Furthermore, cost-effective analysis of NOT in patients with HF with CSA have shown a possible cost-benefit from reductions in hospitalization and emergency visits, and also time-saving benefits from an increase in expected days free from hospital care.[94]

Hypoxemic burden (T <90 – time with oxygen saturation <90%) is a robust and independent predictor of all-cause mortality in chronic stable patients with HFrEF.[95] The mechanistic pathways from which NOT benefits patients with CSA-CSR are not yet well understood; however, data exist to support that NOT reduces sympathetic drive by increasing nocturnal saturation in patients with CSA with HF.[93] Other benefits may be reached by reducing the hypersensitivity from chemoreceptors/respiratory drive (controller gain), and changing $Paco_2$ levels.[96,97]

In summary, NOT seemed effective in approximately 50% of CSA cases alongside a 50% AHI decrease in CSA-CSR. However, NOT has no effect on OSA. Even though oxygen supplementation cannot replace CPAP treatment benefits, NOT could be considered in those patients with HF with predominant CSA-CSR and safety concerns regarding PAP implementation.[75,98] Whether or not targeting nocturnal hypoxemia is associated with beneficial effects on mortality remains to be determined.

Assist Devices

Several assist device modalities have been studied in patients with HF. CPAP, bilevel positive airway pressure without backup rate (BPAP-S) and with respiratory backup rate (BPAP-ST), and ASV have been researched (see **Fig. 3**).

Bilevel positive airway pressure therapy

There is paucity of publications regarding the impact of bilevel positive pressure ventilation in patients with HF. The data available up to now discourages the use of BPAP-S mode in this population, as it may aggravate central apneas/periodic breathing by hyperventilation. It has been shown that CPAP and BPAP-ST are equally effective in lowering the AHI and New York Heart Association (NYHA) class.[99] BPAP-ST could be an effective alternative to those patients with high residual AHI while on CPAP, benefiting from an increase in LVEF of up to 12.7% ± 10.0%.[100]

Adaptive servo ventilation therapy

Based on sophisticated negative feedback control systems (servomechanism), ASV has the capability to self-adjust its respiratory controlled variables (eg, PAP, respiratory rate), by adapting to patient's respiratory fluctuations in real time. During a period of respiratory instability (eg, central apnea), the ASV mode may provide a higher respiratory support (ie, minute ventilation or peak flow) by increasing inspiratory pressure support and/or respiratory rate when the patient's airflow is waning, and a lower (or none) respiratory support when the patient returns to a more stable breathing pattern or during hyperventilation in CSR. Also called anticyclical ventilation, this particular "on-demand" support of a patient's breathing allows a dampening effect of a patient's drive to respiratory fluctuations. This is particularly useful in patients with CSB secondary to a highly unstable respiratory drive system.[101–103]

ASV has proven an effective noninvasive ventilation mode to decrease the number of CSA events in patients with HFrEF with CSB.[104–108] Furthermore, some studies have established the superiority of ASV in suppressing CSB when compared with CPAP, BPAP, and oxygen supplementation (AHI declined from 44.5 ± 3.4/h in untreated CSA, to 28.2 ± 3.4/h on oxygen, 26.8 ± 4.6/h on CPAP, 14.8 ± 2.3/h on BPAP, and 6.3 ± 0.9/h on ASV).[104,109] ASV mode has also proven to have a beneficial impact on surrogate markers of cardiac failure (eg, N-terminal pro brain natriuretic peptide, neurohormonal activation), functional status (NYHA functional class, cardiopulmonary exercise tolerance parameters), and cardiorenal function in patients with CHF and chronic kidney disease.[104,110,111] Similar improvements were also shown in patients with HFpEF with CSA-CSB on ASV, as well as in patients with HFrEF with OSA and CSA occurring concurrently within the same night, independent of the severity of the sleep-disordered breathing.[112–114] However, reduction in CSA events and improvement of intermediate CV end points and improvement of intermediate CV end points have not translated necessarily into lower mortality. Recently published results of the SERVE-HF trial, which assessed the effects of treatment of CSA with ASV on mortality and morbidity in patients with symptomatic chronic HF (NYHA 2–4)

with reduced EF (LVEF ≤45%), showed an increased risk of CV mortality for those treated with ASV in comparison with those with best medical care alone. The increased risk appears to be greatest in those with pure CSA with more severe ventricular dysfunction, presumably related to sudden cardiac death.[115] Further analysis of the mode of death, and data from patients' implanted devices are ongoing, but initial results suggest that the excess mortality is driven by an increase in sudden death. This mechanism of harm may be supported by mortality reduction in those with an implanted defibrillator. Although the SERVE-HF trial results are currently under intense scrutiny, they have translated into a change in clinical practice in the United States until further data from post hoc analysis are available. Concerns about this article's population characterization (inclusion of patients with CHF with preserved EF), ASV adherence (44% of patients on ASV had an average use of ≤3 hours), and ASV control of sleep-disordered breathing (wide range in AHI control, and prolonged nocturnal hypoxemia in ASV group) have ignited an intense discussion about the validity of the results of SERVE-HF.[116] Further longitudinal prospective studies, including the ADVENT-HF (effect of ASV on survival and hospital admissions in heart failure; NCT01128816) and CAT-HF (Cardiovascular Improvements with MV ASV Therapy in Heart Failure; NCT01953874) are needed to accurately identify the long-term impact of ASV in CSA therapy of patients with HF.[117]

In summary, until data from the SERVE-HF post hoc analysis and other ongoing longitudinal studies (ADVENT-HF study, NCT01128816) are available, ASV should not be used for the treatment of CSAs in patients with HFrEF with an EF of 45% or less and moderate or severe CSA-predominant SRBD. However, this recommendation is not necessarily applicable to patients with HFpEF (LVEF >45%), or those with HFrEF with predominant OSA[118] (see **Fig. 3**).

Other devices and interventions Small case series have shown improvement in the AHI when atrial overdrive pacing (AOP) is used to improve cardiac function in patients with CSA-HF in comparison with those without AOP.[119] Although less robust that CPAP therapy, AOP reduction of AHI may be attributed to an increase in cardiac output with subsequent decrease in pulmonary wedge pressures and circulatory time.[120] Similar to AOP, cardiac resynchronization therapy (CRT) significantly reduces the AHI without altering sleep stages.[121,122] A meta-analysis of small, not randomized controlled trials investigating the effect of CRT on CSA reported a mean reduction of AHI of 13.05/h (95% CI −16.74 to −9.36, $P<.00001$), whereas CRT has no effect on AHI in patients with OSA.[121] When both AOP and CRT are combined, a minor additional improvement of AHI is obtained by a decrease in the central AHI.[123] A novel therapy for CSA currently under evaluation is the phrenic nerve stimulator, a pacemakerlike device that induces a breath by stimulation of phrenic nerve when no impulse is sent in a predetermined time. Preliminary data from ongoing trials with unilateral transvenous phrenic nerve stimulation in patients with CSB-CHF showed a trend toward stabilization of breathing and improvement in AHI (55% reduction in AHI from baseline to 3 months), central apnea index, oxygen saturation, and arousals at 3 months. Favorable effects on quality of life and sleepiness were also noted.[124] The ongoing Remedē System Pivotal Trial (NCT01816776) will provide more definitive data about the safety and efficacy of transvenous phrenic nerve stimulation in HF with CSA.[125]

In those patients with CSA secondary to impaired cardiac function from valvular disease, surgical treatment has been shown to improve sleep-disordered breathing. Even though improved, CSB may persist or even convert to OSA after posttransplant normalization of cardiac function, which could be explained by increased weight after heart transplantation.[8,126,127]

SUMMARY

The outcome metric (eg, AHI, vs oxygenation, vs arousal/sympathetic activation, vs quality of life, vs morbidity/mortality) to assess "success" in treating OSA and CSA in patients with HF is still debatable. Success in treatment of SRBD should focus on (1) treatment of underlying disease, (2) symptomatic benefit (eg, fatigue, insomnia, daytime sleepiness, poor concentration), and (3) treatment of the adverse pathophysiological effects of SRBD on patients with HF. These goals should be balanced against a strong safety profile.

CPAP, BPAP, and ASV may be considered to treat OSA or treatment-emergent sleep apnea in patients with HF. Treatment of OSA in patients with HF has shown to improve LVEF, blood pressure control, quality of life, and exercise tolerance. Despite equivocal conclusions from published literature, CPAP therapy in patients with HFrEF with predominately OSA may have mortality benefits.

Contrary to OSA, use of PAP devices for CSA in patients with HFrEF must be approached with caution. Multiple studies have been performed in the past aiming to find a therapy for this group of patients. None of these studies thus far has demonstrated reduced mortality or morbidity in patients with HF with CSA. As a result, there is currently no recommended therapy for CSA in patients with HF. However, if therapy is considered, CPAP implementation for CSA in patients with HF has been shown to reduce the frequency of respiratory events, and improve hemodynamics and exercise tolerance, but did not improve prognosis or the rate of HF-related hospitalizations. On the contrary, ASV used in patients with symptomatic HFrEF and predominantly CSA showed an increase in both all-cause and cardiovascular mortality. Therefore, ASV is not recommended in patients with HFrEF (EF ≤45%) and predominantly CSA.

The safety and efficacy of alternative novel approaches to treating CSA in patients with HFrEF, such as implantable phrenic nerve stimulation, are presently undergoing clinical investigation and may require additional long-term studies before it becomes routine clinical practice.

REFERENCES

1. Yancy CW, Jessup M, Bozkurt B, et al. 2013 ACCF/AHA guideline for the management of heart failure: a report of the American College of Cardiology Foundation/American Heart Association Task Force on practice guidelines. Circulation 2013;128(16):e240–327.
2. Go AS, Mozaffarian D, Roger VL, et al. Heart disease and stroke statistics–2013 update: a report from the American Heart Association. Circulation 2013;127(1):e6–245.
3. Roger VL, Weston SA, Redfield MM, et al. Trends in heart failure incidence and survival in a community-based population. JAMA 2004;292(3):344–50.
4. Levy D, Kenchaiah S, Larson MG, et al. Long-term trends in the incidence of and survival with heart failure. N Engl J Med 2002;347(18):1397–402.
5. Drager LF, Togeiro SM, Polotsky VY, et al. Obstructive sleep apnea: a cardiometabolic risk in obesity and the metabolic syndrome. J Am Coll Cardiol 2013;62(7):569–76.
6. Ljunggren M, Byberg L, Theorell-Haglow J, et al. Increased risk of heart failure in women with symptoms of sleep-disordered breathing. Sleep Med 2016;17:32–7.
7. Ryan CM, Floras JS, Logan AG, et al. Shift in sleep apnoea type in heart failure patients in the CANPAP trial. Eur Respir J 2010;35(3):592–7.
8. Mansfield DR, Solin P, Roebuck T, et al. The effect of successful heart transplant treatment of heart failure on central sleep apnea. Chest 2003;124(5):1675–81.

9. Wang H, Parker JD, Newton GE, et al. Influence of obstructive sleep apnea on mortality in patients with heart failure. J Am Coll Cardiol 2007;49(15): 1625–31.

10. Javaheri S, Shukla R, Zeigler H, et al. Central sleep apnea, right ventricular dysfunction, and low diastolic blood pressure are predictors of mortality in systolic heart failure. J Am Coll Cardiol 2007; 49(20):2028–34.

11. Jilek C, Krenn M, Sebah D, et al. Prognostic impact of sleep disordered breathing and its treatment in heart failure: an observational study. Eur J Heart Fail 2011;13(1):68–75.

12. Khayat R, Jarjoura D, Porter K, et al. Sleep disordered breathing and post-discharge mortality in patients with acute heart failure. Eur Heart J 2015;36(23):1463–9.

13. Khayat R, Abraham W, Patt B, et al. Central sleep apnea is a predictor of cardiac readmission in hospitalized patients with systolic heart failure. J Card Fail 2012;18(7):534–40.

14. Herrscher TE, Akre H, Overland B, et al. High prevalence of sleep apnea in heart failure outpatients: even in patients with preserved systolic function. J Card Fail 2011;17(5):420–5.

15. Paulino A, Damy T, Margarit L, et al. Prevalence of sleep-disordered breathing in a 316-patient French cohort of stable congestive heart failure. Arch Cardiovasc Dis 2009;102(3):169–75.

16. Yumino D, Wang H, Floras JS, et al. Prevalence and physiological predictors of sleep apnea in patients with heart failure and systolic dysfunction. J Card Fail 2009;15(4):279–85.

17. Nieto FJ, Young TB, Lind BK, et al. Association of sleep-disordered breathing, sleep apnea, and hypertension in a large community-based study. Sleep Heart Health Study. JAMA 2000;283(14): 1829–36.

18. Yancy CW, Jessup M, Bozkurt B, et al. 2016 ACC/AHA/HFSA focused update on new pharmacological therapy for heart failure: an update of the 2013 ACCF/AHA guideline for the management of heart failure: a report of the American College of Cardiology/American Heart Association task force on clinical practice guidelines and the Heart Failure Society of America. J Card Fail 2016; 68(13):1476–88.

19. Javaheri S. Sleep disorders in systolic heart failure: a prospective study of 100 male patients. The final report. Int J Cardiol 2006;106(1):21–8.

20. Oldenburg O, Lamp B, Faber L, et al. Sleep-disordered breathing in patients with symptomatic heart failure: a contemporary study of prevalence in and characteristics of 700 patients. Eur J Heart Fail 2007;9(3):251–7.

21. Schulz R, Blau A, Borgel J, et al. Sleep apnoea in heart failure. Eur Respir J 2007;29(6):1201–5.

22. MacDonald M, Fang J, Pittman SD, et al. The current prevalence of sleep disordered breathing in congestive heart failure patients treated with beta-blockers. J Clin Sleep Med 2008;4(1):38–42.

23. Khayat RN, Jarjoura D, Patt B, et al. In-hospital testing for sleep-disordered breathing in hospitalized patients with decompensated heart failure: report of prevalence and patient characteristics. J Card Fail 2009;15(9):739–46.

24. Peppard PE, Young T, Barnet JH, et al. Increased prevalence of sleep-disordered breathing in adults. Am J Epidemiol 2013;177(9):1006–14.

25. Bixler EO, Vgontzas AN, Ten Have T, et al. Effects of age on sleep apnea in men: I. Prevalence and severity. Am J Respir Crit Care Med 1998;157(1): 144–8.

26. Sin DD, Fitzgerald F, Parker JD, et al. Risk factors for central and obstructive sleep apnea in 450 men and women with congestive heart failure. Am J Respir Crit Care Med 1999;160(4):1101–6.

27. Bitter T, Faber L, Hering D, et al. Sleep-disordered breathing in heart failure with normal left ventricular ejection fraction. Eur J Heart Fail 2009;11(6):602–8.

28. Arzt M, Young T, Finn L, et al. Sleepiness and sleep in patients with both systolic heart failure and obstructive sleep apnea. Arch Intern Med 2006; 166(16):1716–22.

29. Javaheri S, Caref EB, Chen E, et al. Sleep apnea testing and outcomes in a large cohort of Medicare beneficiaries with newly diagnosed heart failure. Am J Respir Crit Care Med 2011;183(4):539–46.

30. Gottlieb DJ, Yenokyan G, Newman AB, et al. Prospective study of obstructive sleep apnea and incident coronary heart disease and heart failure: the sleep heart health study. Circulation 2010;122(4): 352–60.

31. Kaneko Y, Floras JS, Usui K, et al. Cardiovascular effects of continuous positive airway pressure in patients with heart failure and obstructive sleep apnea. N Engl J Med 2003;348(13):1233–41.

32. Stowhas AC, Namdar M, Biaggi P, et al. The effect of simulated obstructive apnea and hypopnea on aortic diameter and BP. Chest 2011;140(3):675–80.

33. Orban M, Bruce CJ, Pressman GS, et al. Dynamic changes of left ventricular performance and left atrial volume induced by the Mueller maneuver in healthy young adults and implications for obstructive sleep apnea, atrial fibrillation, and heart failure. Am J Cardiol 2008;102(11):1557–61.

34. Virolainen J, Ventila M, Turto H, et al. Effect of negative intrathoracic pressure on left ventricular pressure dynamics and relaxation. J Appl Physiol (1985) 1995;79(2):455–60.

35. Spaak J, Egri ZJ, Kubo T, et al. Muscle sympathetic nerve activity during wakefulness in heart failure patients with and without sleep apnea. Hypertension 2005;46(6):1327–32.

36. Kato M, Roberts-Thomson P, Phillips BG, et al. Impairment of endothelium-dependent vasodilation of resistance vessels in patients with obstructive sleep apnea. Circulation 2000; 102(21):2607–10.

37. Kasai T, Bradley TD. Obstructive sleep apnea and heart failure: pathophysiologic and therapeutic implications. J Am Coll Cardiol 2011;57(2):119–27.

38. Yumino D, Redolfi S, Ruttanaumpawan P, et al. Nocturnal rostral fluid shift: a unifying concept for the pathogenesis of obstructive and central sleep apnea in men with heart failure. Circulation 2010; 121(14):1598–605.

39. Kasai T, Motwani SS, Yumino D, et al. Contrasting effects of lower body positive pressure on upper airways resistance and partial pressure of carbon dioxide in men with heart failure and obstructive or central sleep apnea. J Am Coll Cardiol 2013; 61(11):1157–66.

40. Bucca CB, Brussino L, Battisti A, et al. Diuretics in obstructive sleep apnea with diastolic heart failure. Chest 2007;132(2):440–6.

41. Naughton MT, Rahman MA, Hara K, et al. Effect of continuous positive airway pressure on intrathoracic and left ventricular transmural pressures in patients with congestive heart failure. Circulation 1995;91(6):1725–31.

42. Lin M, Yang YF, Chiang HT, et al. Reappraisal of continuous positive airway pressure therapy in acute cardiogenic pulmonary edema. Short-term results and long-term follow-up. Chest 1995; 107(5):1379–86.

43. Buckle P, Millar T, Kryger M. The effect of short-term nasal CPAP on Cheyne-Stokes respiration in congestive heart failure. Chest 1992;102(1): 31–5.

44. Guyton AC, Lindsey AW, Abernathy B, et al. Venous return at various right atrial pressures and the normal venous return curve. Am J Physiol 1957;189(3):609–15.

45. Usui K, Bradley TD, Spaak J, et al. Inhibition of awake sympathetic nerve activity of heart failure patients with obstructive sleep apnea by nocturnal continuous positive airway pressure. J Am Coll Cardiol 2005;45(12):2008–11.

46. Ruttanaumpawan P, Gilman MP, Usui K, et al. Sustained effect of continuous positive airway pressure on baroreflex sensitivity in congestive heart failure patients with obstructive sleep apnea. J Hypertens 2008;26(6):1163–8.

47. Younes M, Ostrowski M, Thompson W, et al. Chemical control stability in patients with obstructive sleep apnea. Am J Respir Crit Care Med 2001; 163(5):1181–90.

48. Khoo MC. Determinants of ventilatory instability and variability. Respir Physiol 2000;122(2–3): 167–82.

49. Xie A, Skatrud JB, Puleo DS, et al. Apnea-hypopnea threshold for CO2 in patients with congestive heart failure. Am J Respir Crit Care Med 2002; 165(9):1245–50.

50. Javaheri S. A mechanism of central sleep apnea in patients with heart failure. N Engl J Med 1999; 341(13):949–54.

51. Badr MS, Toiber F, Skatrud JB, et al. Pharyngeal narrowing/occlusion during central sleep apnea. J Appl Physiol (1985) 1995;78(5):1806–15.

52. Arzt M, Woehrle H, Oldenburg O, et al. Prevalence and predictors of sleep-disordered breathing in patients with stable chronic heart failure: the SchlaHF Registry. JACC Heart Fail 2016;4(2): 116–25.

53. Araghi MH, Chen YF, Jagielski A, et al. Effectiveness of lifestyle interventions on obstructive sleep apnea (OSA): systematic review and meta-analysis. Sleep 2013;36(10):1553–62, 1562a-1562e.

54. Kitzman DW, Brubaker PH, Morgan TM, et al. Exercise training in older patients with heart failure and preserved ejection fraction: a randomized, controlled, single-blind trial. Circ Heart Fail 2010; 3(6):659–67.

55. Shah SJ, Katz DH, Selvaraj S, et al. Phenomapping for novel classification of heart failure with preserved ejection fraction. Circulation 2015;131(3): 269–79.

56. Kitzman DW, Brubaker P, Morgan T, et al. Effect of caloric restriction or aerobic exercise training on peak oxygen consumption and quality of life in obese older patients with heart failure with preserved ejection fraction: a randomized clinical trial. JAMA 2016;315(1):36–46.

57. Tamura A, Kawano Y, Naono S, et al. Relationship between beta-blocker treatment and the severity of central sleep apnea in chronic heart failure. Chest 2007;131(1):130–5.

58. Warner MM, Mitchell GS. Role of catecholamines and beta-receptors in ventilatory response during hypoxic exercise. Respir Physiol 1991;85(1):41–53.

59. Walsh JT, Andrews R, Starling R, et al. Effects of captopril and oxygen on sleep apnoea in patients with mild to moderate congestive cardiac failure. Br Heart J 1995;73(3):237–41.

60. Solin P, Jackson DM, Roebuck T, et al. Cardiac diastolic function and hypercapnic ventilatory responses in central sleep apnoea. Eur Respir J 2002;20(3):717–23.

61. Hagenah G, Zapf A, Schuttert JB. Cheyne-stokes respiration and prognosis in modern-treated congestive heart failure. Lung 2010; 188(4):309–13.

62. Owan TE, Hodge DO, Herges RM, et al. Trends in prevalence and outcome of heart failure with preserved ejection fraction. N Engl J Med 2006; 355(3):251–9.

63. Bhatia RS, Tu JV, Lee DS, et al. Outcome of heart failure with preserved ejection fraction in a population-based study. N Engl J Med 2006; 355(3):260–9.

64. Holland DJ, Kumbhani DJ, Ahmed SH, et al. Effects of treatment on exercise tolerance, cardiac function, and mortality in heart failure with preserved ejection fraction. A meta-analysis. J Am Coll Cardiol 2011;57(16):1676–86.

65. Mansfield DR, Gollogly NC, Kaye DM, et al. Controlled trial of continuous positive airway pressure in obstructive sleep apnea and heart failure. Am J Respir Crit Care Med 2004;169(3):361–6.

66. Johnson CB, Beanlands RS, Yoshinaga K, et al. Acute and chronic effects of continuous positive airway pressure therapy on left ventricular systolic and diastolic function in patients with obstructive sleep apnea and congestive heart failure. Can J Cardiol 2008;24(9):697–704.

67. Marin JM, Carrizo SJ, Vicente E, et al. Long-term cardiovascular outcomes in men with obstructive sleep apnoea-hypopnoea with or without treatment with continuous positive airway pressure: an observational study. Lancet 2005;365(9464): 1046–53.

68. Martinez-Garcia MA, Campos-Rodriguez F, Catalan-Serra P, et al. Cardiovascular mortality in obstructive sleep apnea in the elderly: role of long-term continuous positive airway pressure treatment: a prospective observational study. Am J Respir Crit Care Med 2012;186(9):909–16.

69. Kasai T, Narui K, Dohi T, et al. Prognosis of patients with heart failure and obstructive sleep apnea treated with continuous positive airway pressure. Chest 2008;133(3):690–6.

70. Antic NA, Heeley E, Anderson CS, et al. The sleep apnea cardiovascular endpoints (SAVE) trial: rationale, ethics, design, and progress. Sleep 2015; 38(8):1247–57.

71. Yoshihisa A, Suzuki S, Yamauchi H, et al. Beneficial effects of positive airway pressure therapy for sleep-disordered breathing in heart failure patients with preserved left ventricular ejection fraction. Clin Cardiol 2015;38(7):413–21.

72. Arikawa T, Toyoda S, Haruyama A, et al. Impact of obstructive sleep apnoea on heart failure with preserved ejection fraction. Heart Lung Circ 2016; 25(5):435–41.

73. Bradley TD, Logan AG, Kimoff RJ, et al. Continuous positive airway pressure for central sleep apnea and heart failure. N Engl J Med 2005;353(19): 2025–33.

74. Arzt M, Floras JS, Logan AG, et al. Suppression of central sleep apnea by continuous positive airway pressure and transplant-free survival in heart failure: a post hoc analysis of the Canadian Continuous Positive Airway Pressure for Patients with Central Sleep Apnea and Heart Failure Trial (CANPAP). Circulation 2007;115(25):3173–80.

75. Aurora RN, Chowdhuri S, Ramar K, et al. The treatment of central sleep apnea syndromes in adults: practice parameters with an evidence-based literature review and meta-analyses. Sleep 2012;35(1): 17–40.

76. Sin DD, Logan AG, Fitzgerald FS, et al. Effects of continuous positive airway pressure on cardiovascular outcomes in heart failure patients with and without Cheyne-Stokes respiration. Circulation 2000;102(1):61–6.

77. Oksenberg A, Silverberg DS, Arons E, et al. Positional vs nonpositional obstructive sleep apnea patients: anthropomorphic, nocturnal polysomnographic, and multiple sleep latency test data. Chest 1997;112(3):629–39.

78. Pinna GD, Robbi E, La Rovere MT, et al. Differential impact of body position on the severity of disordered breathing in heart failure patients with obstructive vs. central sleep apnoea. Eur J Heart Fail 2015;17(12):1302–9.

79. Szollosi I, Roebuck T, Thompson B, et al. Lateral sleeping position reduces severity of central sleep apnea/Cheyne-Stokes respiration. Sleep 2006; 29(8):1045–51.

80. Altschule MD, Iglauer A. The effect of position on periodic breathing in chronic cardiac decompensation. N Engl J Med 1958;259(22): 1064–6.

81. Joho S, Oda Y, Hirai T, et al. Impact of sleeping position on central sleep apnea/Cheyne-Stokes respiration in patients with heart failure. Sleep Med 2010;11(2):143–8.

82. Javaheri S. Acetazolamide improves central sleep apnea in heart failure: a double-blind, prospective study. Am J Respir Crit Care Med 2006;173(2): 234–7.

83. Javaheri S, Parker TJ, Wexler L, et al. Effect of theophylline on sleep-disordered breathing in heart failure. N Engl J Med 1996;335(8):562–7.

84. Thomas RJ, Daly RW, Weiss JW. Low-concentration carbon dioxide is an effective adjunct to positive airway pressure in the treatment of refractory mixed central and obstructive sleep-disordered breathing. Sleep 2005;28(1):69–77.

85. Khayat RN, Xie A, Patel AK, et al. Cardiorespiratory effects of added dead space in patients with heart failure and central sleep apnea. Chest 2003; 123(5):1551–60.

86. Gilmartin G, McGeehan B, Vigneault K, et al. Treatment of positive airway pressure treatment-associated respiratory instability with enhanced expiratory rebreathing space (EERS). J Clin Sleep Med 2010;6(6):529–38.

87. Szollosi I, O'Driscoll DM, Dayer MJ, et al. Adaptive servo-ventilation and deadspace: effects on

central sleep apnoea. J Sleep Res 2006;15(2): 199–205.

88. Sasayama S, Izumi T, Matsuzaki M, et al. Improvement of quality of life with nocturnal oxygen therapy in heart failure patients with central sleep apnea. Circ J 2009;73(7):1255–62.

89. Toyama T, Seki R, Kasama S, et al. Effectiveness of nocturnal home oxygen therapy to improve exercise capacity, cardiac function and cardiac sympathetic nerve activity in patients with chronic heart failure and central sleep apnea. Circ J 2009; 73(2):299–304.

90. Javaheri S, Ahmed M, Parker TJ, et al. Effects of nasal O2 on sleep-related disordered breathing in ambulatory patients with stable heart failure. Sleep 1999;22(8):1101–6.

91. Bordier P, Orazio S, Hofmann P, et al. Short- and long-term effects of nocturnal oxygen therapy on sleep apnea in chronic heart failure. Sleep Breath 2015;19(1):159–68.

92. Shigemitsu M, Nishio K, Kusuyama T, et al. Nocturnal oxygen therapy prevents progress of congestive heart failure with central sleep apnea. Int J Cardiol 2007;115(3):354–60.

93. Staniforth AD, Kinnear WJ, Starling R, et al. Effect of oxygen on sleep quality, cognitive function and sympathetic activity in patients with chronic heart failure and Cheyne-Stokes respiration. Eur Heart J 1998;19(6):922–8.

94. Seino Y, Imai H, Nakamoto T, et al. Clinical efficacy and cost-benefit analysis of nocturnal home oxygen therapy in patients with central sleep apnea caused by chronic heart failure. Circ J 2007; 71(11):1738–43.

95. Oldenburg O, Wellmann B, Buchholz A, et al. Nocturnal hypoxaemia is associated with increased mortality in stable heart failure patients. Eur Heart J 2016;37(21):1695–703.

96. Chowdhuri S, Sinha P, Pranathiageswaran S, et al. Sustained hyperoxia stabilizes breathing in healthy individuals during NREM sleep. J Appl Physiol (1985) 2010;109(5):1378–83.

97. Xie A, Skatrud JB, Puleo DS, et al. Exposure to hypoxia produces long-lasting sympathetic activation in humans. J Appl Physiol (1985) 2001;91(4): 1555–62.

98. Bordier P, Lataste A, Hofmann P, et al. Nocturnal oxygen therapy in patients with chronic heart failure and sleep apnea: a systematic review. Sleep Med 2016;17:149–57.

99. Kohnlein T, Welte T, Tan LB, et al. Assisted ventilation for heart failure patients with Cheyne-Stokes respiration. Eur Respir J 2002; 20(4):934–41.

100. Dohi T, Kasai T, Narui K, et al. Bi-level positive airway pressure ventilation for treating heart failure with central sleep apnea that is unresponsive to continuous positive airway pressure. Circ J 2008; 72(7):1100–5.

101. Selim BJ, Junna MR, Morgenthaler TI. Therapy for sleep hypoventilation and central apnea syndromes. Curr Treat Options Neurol 2012;14(5): 427–37.

102. Javaheri S, Dempsey JA. Central sleep apnea. Compr Physiol 2013;3(1):141–63.

103. Javaheri S, Brown LK, Randerath WJ. Positive airway pressure therapy with adaptive servoventilation: part 1: operational algorithms. Chest 2014; 146(2):514–23.

104. Sharma BK, Bakker JP, McSharry DG, et al. Adaptive servoventilation for treatment of sleep-disordered breathing in heart failure: a systematic review and meta-analysis. Chest 2012;142(5): 1211–21.

105. Asakawa N, Sakakibara M, Noguchi K, et al. Adaptive servo-ventilation has more favorable acute effects on hemodynamics than continuous positive airway pressure in patients with heart failure. Int Heart J 2015;56(5):527–32.

106. Yamada S, Sakakibara M, Yokota T, et al. Acute hemodynamic effects of adaptive servo-ventilation in patients with heart failure. Circ J 2013;77(5): 1214–20.

107. Haruki N, Takeuchi M, Kaku K, et al. Comparison of acute and chronic impact of adaptive servo-ventilation on left chamber geometry and function in patients with chronic heart failure. Eur J Heart Fail 2011;13(10):1140–6.

108. Haruki N, Takeuchi M, Yoshitani H, et al. Immediate amelioration of mechanical pulsus alternans by adaptive servo-ventilation therapy. Heart Lung Circ 2013;22(4):300–2.

109. Teschler H, Dohring J, Wang YM, et al. Adaptive pressure support servo-ventilation: a novel treatment for Cheyne-Stokes respiration in heart failure. Am J Respir Crit Care Med 2001;164(4):614–9.

110. Randerath WJ, Nothofer G, Priegnitz C, et al. Long-term auto-servoventilation or constant positive pressure in heart failure and coexisting central with obstructive sleep apnea. Chest 2012;142(2): 440–7.

111. Owada T, Yoshihisa A, Yamauchi H, et al. Adaptive servoventilation improves cardiorenal function and prognosis in heart failure patients with chronic kidney disease and sleep-disordered breathing. J Card Fail 2013;19(4):225–32.

112. Bitter T, Westerheide N, Faber L, et al. Adaptive servoventilation in diastolic heart failure and Cheyne-Stokes respiration. Eur Respir J 2010; 36(2):385–92.

113. Takama N, Kurabayashi M. Effectiveness of adaptive servo-ventilation for treating heart failure regardless of the severity of sleep-disordered breathing. Circ J 2011;75(5):1164–9.

114. Yoshihisa A, Suzuki S, Yamaki T, et al. Impact of adaptive servo-ventilation on cardiovascular function and prognosis in heart failure patients with preserved left ventricular ejection fraction and sleep-disordered breathing. Eur J Heart Fail 2013;15(5):543–50.

115. Cowie MR, Woehrle H, Wegscheider K, et al. Adaptive servo-ventilation for central sleep apnea in systolic heart failure. N Engl J Med 2015;373(12): 1095–105.

116. Javaheri S, Brown LK, Randerath W, et al. SERVE-HF: more questions than answers. Chest 2016; 149(4):900–4.

117. Gottlieb DJ, Craig SE, Lorenzi-Filho G, et al. Sleep apnea cardiovascular clinical trials—current status and steps forward: the International Collaboration of Sleep Apnea Cardiovascular Trialists. Sleep 2013;36(7):975–80.

118. Aurora RN, Bista SR, Casey KR, et al. Updated adaptive servo-ventilation recommendations for the 2012 AASM guideline: "the treatment of central sleep apnea syndromes in adults: practice parameters with an evidence-based literature review and meta-analyses". J Clin Sleep Med 2016;12(5):757–61.

119. Weng CL, Chen Q, Ma YL, et al. A meta-analysis of the effects of atrial overdrive pacing on sleep apnea syndrome. Pacing Clin Electrophysiol 2009; 32(11):1434–43.

120. Baranchuk A, Healey JS, Simpson CS, et al. Atrial overdrive pacing in sleep apnoea: a meta-analysis. Europace 2009;11(8):1037–40.

121. Lamba J, Simpson CS, Redfearn DP, et al. Cardiac resynchronization therapy for the treatment of sleep apnoea: a meta-analysis. Europace 2011; 13(8):1174–9.

122. Sinha AM, Skobel EC, Breithardt OA, et al. Cardiac resynchronization therapy improves central sleep apnea and Cheyne-Stokes respiration in patients with chronic heart failure. J Am Coll Cardiol 2004; 44(1):68–71.

123. Luthje L, Renner B, Kessels R, et al. Cardiac resynchronization therapy and atrial overdrive pacing for the treatment of central sleep apnoea. Eur J Heart Fail 2009;11(3):273–80.

124. Abraham WT, Jagielski D, Oldenburg O, et al. Phrenic nerve stimulation for the treatment of central sleep apnea. JACC Heart Fail 2015;3(5): 360–9.

125. Costanzo MR, Augostini R, Goldberg LR, et al. Design of the remede system pivotal trial: a prospective, randomized study in the use of respiratory rhythm management to treat central sleep apnea. J Card Fail 2015;21(11):892–902.

126. Thalhofer SA, Kiwus U, Dorow P. Influence of orthotopic heart transplantation on breathing pattern disorders in patients with dilated cardiomyopathy. Sleep Breath 2000;4(3):121–6.

127. Javaheri S, Abraham WT, Brown C, et al. Prevalence of obstructive sleep apnoea and periodic limb movement in 45 subjects with heart transplantation. Eur Heart J 2004;25(3):260–6.

128. Bradley TD, Hall MJ, Ando S, et al. Hemodynamic effects of simulated obstructive apneas in humans with and without heart failure. Chest 2001;119(6):1827–35.

129. Stoohs R, Guilleminault C. Cardiovascular changes associated with obstructive sleep apnea syndrome. J Appl Physiol (1985) 1992;72(2):583–9.

130. Brinker JA, Weiss JL, Lappe DL, et al. Leftward septal displacement during right ventricular loading in man. Circulation 1980;61(3):626–33.

131. Buda AJ, Pinsky MR, Ingels NB Jr, et al. Effect of intrathoracic pressure on left ventricular performance. N Engl J Med 1979;301(9):453–9.

132. Koshino Y, Villarraga HR, Orban M, et al. Changes in left and right ventricular mechanics during the Mueller maneuver in healthy adults: a possible mechanism for abnormal cardiac function in patients with obstructive sleep apnea. Circ Cardiovasc Imaging 2010;3(3):282–9.

133. Oliveira W, Campos O, Bezerra Lira-Filho E, et al. Left atrial volume and function in patients with obstructive sleep apnea assessed by real-time three-dimensional echocardiography. J Am Soc Echocardiogr 2008;21(12):1355–61.

134. Otto ME, Belohlavek M, Romero-Corral A, et al. Comparison of cardiac structural and functional changes in obese otherwise healthy adults with versus without obstructive sleep apnea. Am J Cardiol 2007;99(9):1298–302.

135. Kim SM, Cho KI, Kwon JH, et al. Impact of obstructive sleep apnea on left atrial functional and structural remodeling beyond obesity. J Cardiol 2012; 60(6):475–83.

136. Niroumand M, Kuperstein R, Sasson Z, et al. Impact of obstructive sleep apnea on left ventricular mass and diastolic function. Am J Respir Crit Care Med 2001;163(7):1632–6.

137. Linz D, Schotten U, Neuberger HR, et al. Negative tracheal pressure during obstructive respiratory events promotes atrial fibrillation by vagal activation. Heart Rhythm 2011;8(9):1436–43.

138. Buchner NJ, Quack I, Woznowski M, et al. Microvascular endothelial dysfunction in obstructive sleep apnea is caused by oxidative stress and improved by continuous positive airway pressure therapy. Respiration 2011;82(5):409–17.

The Benefits of Perioperative Screening for Sleep Apnea in Surgical Patients

Yamini Subramani, MD[a], Jean Wong, MD, FRCPC[a],
Mahesh Nagappa, MD, DNB[b],
Frances Chung, MBBS, FRCPC[a],*

KEYWORDS

- OSA • Screening • Postoperative complications • Cost

KEY POINTS

- Obstructive sleep apnea (OSA) is highly prevalent in the surgical population.
- Perioperative screening using simple tools like questionnaires is reasonable to identify high-risk patients and institute appropriate precautions, risk mitigation, and monitoring.
- The decision of further referral and management before surgery should be individualized based on the associated comorbidities in the patient, nature and urgency of the procedure, postoperative requirement for opioids, and institutional capabilities and protocols.
- Routine screening for OSA increases the preparedness for effective perioperative management, ensuring that appropriate risk stratification strategy and monitoring are in place.
- Subsequent diagnosis and treatment of OSA are associated with long-term health benefits for patients with OSA and indirectly minimize the health care burden on the society.

INTRODUCTION

Obstructive sleep apnea (OSA) is a prevalent sleep breathing disorder affecting 9% to 26% of the general adult population.[1] Its prevalence is higher in the surgical population, and it may be present in up to 70% of patients presenting for bariatric surgery.[2] Approximately 90% of surgical patients with moderate to severe OSA are undiagnosed and untreated at the time of surgery.[3]

OSA has important implications for anesthetic management because of the association with several systemic diseases such as cardiovascular disease, heart failure, arrhythmia, hypertension, cerebrovascular disease, and metabolic syndrome.[4–6] The care of surgical patients with OSA is often fraught with safety and liability concerns. Two meta-analyses found that the cardiac and pulmonary complications were increased by two to three fold in patients with OSA undergoing surgery.[7,8]

The literature on the association between OSA and perioperative mortality is less clear. A population-based database study found that OSA was associated with increased risk of in-hospital mortality in patients undergoing revision

Disclosure: The authors have nothing to disclose.
[a] Department of Anesthesiology, Toronto Western Hospital, University Health Network, University of Toronto, 399 Bathurst Street, Toronto, ON M5T 2S8, Canada; [b] Department of Anesthesia and Perioperative Medicine, London Health Science Centre, St. Joseph Health Care, Schulich School of Medicine and Dentistry, Western University, 339 Windermere Road, London, ON N6A 5A5, Canada
* Corresponding author.
E-mail address: frances.chung@uhn.ca

sleep.theclinics.com

total hip and knee arthroplasty.[9] Also, several studies reported increased mortality in patients with OSA versus patients without OSA undergoing cardiac surgeries.[10,11] Despite the evidence of increased mortality and morbidity, most patients with OSA presenting for surgery remain undiagnosed. The reasons may include lack of awareness among primary health care providers, limited access to diagnostic services, and reluctance among patients to get treatment after diagnosis. The American Society of Anesthesiologists practice guidelines and the recent Society of Anesthesia and Sleep Medicine guidelines strongly recommend the use of screening tools to identify surgical patients with suspected OSA in the preoperative period.[12,13] There are opportunities to improve the quality and safety of perioperative care by screening for OSA using simple questionnaires. In addition, a potential to improve long-term social and economic outcomes exists with the appropriate diagnosis and management of OSA in patients screened as high risk.[14]

This article discusses the perioperative and long-term implications of preoperative screening for OSA. The importance of OSA screening in decreasing the incidence of postoperative complications, current OSA screening methods, OSA screening in pregnancy, obesity hypoventilation syndrome (OHS), and long-term social and economic benefits of preoperative OSA screening are described in this article.

IMPORTANCE OF PREOPERATIVE OBSTRUCTIVE SLEEP APNEA SCREENING

Every year 250 million major surgical procedures are performed worldwide.[15] An increasing number of procedures are being performed in ambulatory settings and patients with OSA are likely to present for outpatient surgical procedures.

A recent survey found that most anesthesiologists do not rely on screening tools and continue to identify OSA by clinical suspicion alone, despite the growing evidence of postoperative complications associated with OSA.[16] Their preferred management strategies were constrained by hospital resources for preoperative work-up or postoperative monitoring.[13] Hospitals and ambulatory surgical units need to establish their own site-specific policies.

Patients with suspected OSA who experienced recurrent respiratory events like apnea, bradypnea, oxygen desaturation, and analgesic-sedation mismatch in the post-anesthesia care unit were found to have increased postoperative respiratory events.[17] These patients have a high probability of OSA. There should be a low threshold for use of postoperative monitoring of oxygenation and ventilation in these patients. A postoperative evaluation and follow-up with the primary health care provider should be arranged for referral, diagnosis, and long-term treatment.

The administration of sedatives, anesthetics, and analgesics can worsen airway collapse in patients with OSA. Some patients with OSA have a lower propensity to arouse from sleep and could possibly have a phenotype of high arousal threshold. These patients may be in a state of arousal-dependent survival. Sedatives and narcotics that further delay their arousal can precipitate a respiratory arrest, which can lead to sudden unexpected death.[18] However, there is no conventional clinical way to identify these patients preoperatively. Continuous postoperative monitoring has been recommended with high-resolution pulse oximetry[18] and capnography[19] to detect early desaturation and hypoventilation, and to initiate treatment. The choice of anesthetic may be important in these patients. Regional anesthesia, by an opioid-sparing effect, decreases the risk of airway collapsibility and respiratory depression.[20] In patients with OSA undergoing joint arthroplasty, neuraxial anesthesia may have potential benefits in terms of reducing perioperative morbidity, resource use, and cost compared with general anesthesia.[20]

In a study examining patient safety indicators for 40 million hospitalized patients, many deaths and permanent disabilities were found to be avoidable if health care systems adopted safe practice.[21] The preventable deaths are usually described as failure to rescue.[22] Screening for OSA preoperatively facilitates risk stratification and appropriate monitoring to detect early postoperative respiratory depression.[23]

PERIOPERATIVE MORBIDITY AND MORTALITY IN PATIENTS WITH OBSTRUCTIVE SLEEP APNEA AND BENEFITS OF PREOPERATIVE OBSTRUCTIVE SLEEP APNEA SCREENING

The presence of OSA represents a major clinical and economic challenge in the postoperative period. Postoperative complications are a significant source of morbidity and mortality. A recent systematic review on the postoperative outcomes in surgical patients with OSA included 61 studies with 413,304 patients with OSA and 8,556,279 patients without OSA. The presence of OSA was associated with an increased risk of postoperative pulmonary, cardiovascular, and combined complications after general anesthesia, neuraxial anesthesia, and sedation.[24] A nationwide retrospective database study in the orthopedic population showed that patients with OSA are 2 times more likely to have pulmonary and cardiac complications respectively.[25] Most cardiac complications were caused by atrial fibrillation, accounting for 8% of all complications. Patients with OSA have a 10-fold increased risk for ventilatory support, 2-fold increased risk for prolonged intensive care unit (ICU) stay, 1.6 times increased odds for step-down care, and 1.2 times increased odds for prolonged hospitalization.[25] A large database study in a tertiary care center concluded that OSA increased the hospital costs by 78% and the length of stay (LOS) by 114% because of postoperative complications, and the increases in hospital costs were attributable to prolonged hospital stay.[26]

In bariatric surgery, patients with OSA had a 50% higher risk for 30-day hospital readmission.[27] In cardiac surgery, OSA was associated with a higher incidence of encephalopathy, postoperative infection, and increased ICU LOS.[28] Although 2 studies that examined the association between postoperative mortality and OSA were inconclusive,[29,30] death cannot be ruled out as an unexpected sentinel event in surgical patients with OSA, especially when there are additional insults, such as opioid-related respiratory depression. A nationwide inpatient study on 258,455 patients who underwent revision total hip arthroplasty or total knee arthroplasty found that OSA was associated with a 2-fold increase in in-hospital mortality: OSA versus non-OSA 0.4% versus 0.2%. There was an association of OSA with pulmonary embolism (odds ratio [OR], 2.1; $P = .001$), and increased postoperative charges ($61,044 vs $58,813; $P = .001$).[9]

Another nationwide retrospective cohort study examined the effect of sleep disordered breathing (SDB) on outcomes such as in-hospital death, charges, and LOS after elective orthopedic, prostate, abdominal, and cardiovascular surgeries.[29] SDB was independently associated with a significantly increased OR of up to 14.3 for emergent intubation and 2.2 for atrial fibrillation across the surgical categories. There was a small increase in estimated mean LOS by 0.14 days and estimated mean total charges by $860 in the orthopedic surgery group in patients with SDB.[29] Note that SDB was independently associated with decreased odds for mortality. This lower postoperative mortality in patients with SDB could be caused by diagnosis and monitoring leading to early effective intervention and decreasing mortality.[29] Effective screening and appropriate measures may decrease the incidence of postoperative complications, making them avoidable with vigilance and meticulous monitoring.

EVIDENCE OF BENEFITS OF PERIOPERATIVE CONTINUOUS POSITIVE AIRWAY PRESSURE

At present, there is limited literature evaluating the efficacy of continuous positive airway pressure (CPAP) in the perioperative period. A randomized controlled trial investigating the effectiveness of perioperative CPAP in patients with OSA found that it significantly reduced postoperative apnea-hypopnea index (AHI) and improved oxygen saturation in patients with moderate and severe OSA.[31] Two recent large retrospective studies suggest potential efficacy of CPAP in patients with diagnosed OSA in reducing the postoperative cardiopulmonary complications. In one study, patients with diagnosed OSA with a CPAP prescription had decreased odds for developing cardiac arrest and shock (OR, 0.75) compared with patients with undiagnosed OSA (OR, 2.2).[32] The other cohort study showed that untreated OSA was independently associated with more cardiopulmonary complications (risk-adjusted rates 6.7% vs 4.0%; adjusted OR, 1.8; $P = .001$), particularly unplanned reintubations and myocardial infarction.[33]

A recent meta-analysis of 6 studies including 904 patients examined the effectiveness of CPAP therapy on postoperative outcomes. Patients using CPAP had significantly lower postoperative AHI (preoperative AHI vs postoperative AHI, 37 ± 19 vs 12 ± 16 events per hour; $P<.001$) and a trend toward shorter LOS in hospital (4.0 ± 4 vs 4.4 ± 8 days; $P = .05$).[34] Hence there are potential benefits in the use of CPAP during the perioperative period.

The concept of the perioperative surgical home, encompassing optimization of surgical patients' health statuses from the preoperative period to postoperative discharge care,[35] can be applied to patients with suspected or diagnosed OSA presenting for surgery. Perioperative physicians are in an ideal position to identify patients with OSA, optimize their perioperative management, and contribute to their long-term health and quality of life, which in turn reduces the economic burden on society.

PREOPERATIVE EVALUATION: PATIENT HISTORY

A preoperative evaluation of OSA should include a comprehensive review of medical records for a history of difficulty in airway management, problems with previous anesthetics, hypertension, stroke, myocardial infarction, diabetes mellitus, and congenital medical conditions like Down syndrome and acromegaly that may be associated with OSA.[36,37] It is useful to review the results of polysomnography (PSG) to confirm the diagnosis of OSA and evaluate the severity of the disease.

History should focus on the questions related to snoring, apneic episodes, frequent arousals from sleep, nocturia, gastroesophageal reflux disease, daytime headache, somnolence, and impaired memory.[12] Patients should be asked about the worsening of symptoms in the supine position. Supine position–related OSA is a dominant phenotype that can be treated by managing the patient in a semiupright or lateral position in the perioperative period.[38] The history of the current treatment modality of OSA, compliance with CPAP treatment, and previous surgery for OSA should be obtained.

PHYSICAL EXAMINATION

Physical examination includes evaluation of the nose, oral cavity, facial morphology, and oropharynx, and measurement of neck circumference and body mass index (BMI). Nasal septal deviation, turbinate hypertrophy, nasal polyps, and other masses can predispose to OSA.[39] The ratio of the tongue volume to the oral cavity volume is higher in patients with versus without OSA.[40]

Enlarged tonsils, uvula, and oropharyngeal tumors contribute to upper airway narrowing, predisposing the individual to OSA. A combination of BMI, pharyngeal anatomic abnormalities, and the modified Mallampati grade were related to the presence and severity of OSA.[41] For every 1-point increase in the Mallampati score, the odds of having OSA (AHI ≥5) increased more than 2-fold.[42] Neck circumference greater than 43 cm (17 in) in men and 41 cm (16 in) in women indicates the possibility of OSA.[43] Obesity is another major risk factor with moderate to severe sleep apnea (AHI cutoff, >30 events/h) present in 65% of men and 23% of women with severe obesity (BMI>40 kg/m²).[44]

ROLE OF IMAGING IN OBSTRUCTIVE SLEEP APNEA

Cephalometry and photographic craniofacial phenotyping are useful techniques to evaluate the craniofacial characteristics predisposing to OSA.[26,45] Although OSA is common in obese patients, leaner individuals with significantly abnormal craniofacial morphology in the form of inferior positioning of the hyoid bone, smaller maxilla, and retropositioned mandible may also have OSA.[46] Computed tomography and MRI are other useful imaging techniques that can detect upper airway narrowing in patients with OSA.[39]

CURRENT OBSTRUCTIVE SLEEP APNEA SCREENING METHODS

The 2 major considerations for choosing screening tests for OSA are feasibility and reliability.

Questionnaires and simple clinical models are the most feasible. Questionnaires are the most commonly used, with modest accuracy. Clinical models that incorporate simple clinical measurements are superior to questionnaires.

Only 4 screening questionnaires have been evaluated and validated in surgical populations: STOP-Bang (snoring, tiredness, observed apnea, high blood pressure [BP]), BMI, age, neck circumference, and male gender,[47] Berlin,[48] American Society of Anesthesiologists checklist,[48] and perioperative sleep apnea prediction.[49] The observational studies evaluating the screening questionnaires have reported sensitivity ranging from 36% to 86%, specificity from 72% to 96%, positive predictive values from 72% to 96%, and negative predictive values from 30% to 82%.[47–49] The inclusion of preoperative serum bicarbonate level may improve the predictive accuracy of the screening instrument.[50]

Overnight oximetry may play a role as a preoperative screening tool for OSA. Oxygen desaturation index has been found to have very good correlation with AHI in surgical patients.[51] Patients with preoperative mean overnight SpO_2 less than 93%, oxygen desaturation index greater than 29 events/h, or more than 7% of overnight duration of O_2 saturation less than 90% were shown to be at higher risk for postoperative adverse events.[52]

At present there is limited evidence to recommend in-laboratory PSG for diagnosing OSA in the preoperative period, but home sleep testing with a limited-channel portable PSG is evolving as a potential screening tool for OSA.[53] The American Academy of Sleep Medicine practice parameters for the use of portable monitoring devices in the investigation of suspected OSA in adults recommended that level 3 and 4 portable monitoring devices including nocturnal oximetry may be used to rule in or rule out diagnosis of OSA in patients without other comorbidities, provided that the proper standards for conducting the test are met and interpretation of results is performed by trained personnel.[54]

Between 10% and 20% of patients with OSA are known to have associated OHS. OHS is often unrecognized at the time of surgery. Serum bicarbonate is considered to be a surrogate marker for daytime hypercapnia and level greater than 27 mmol/L is more predictive of OHS.[55,56]

STOP-Bang QUESTIONNAIRE

The STOP-Bang questionnaire is the most validated screening tool to identify surgical patients at high risk of OSA.[47,57,58] It consists of 8 dichotomous (yes/no) items related to the clinical features of sleep apnea. The total score ranges from 0 to 8.

Patients can be classified for OSA risk based on their respective scores (**Box 1**).

Patient with STOP-Bang scores of 5 to 8 have a high probability of having moderate to severe OSA.[57] In contrast, patients with STOP-Bang scores of 0 to 2 are unlikely to have OSA. The sensitivity of STOP-Bang score greater than or equal to 3 is 93% and 100%, with a specificity of 43% and 37% at AHI cutoffs of 15 and 30, respectively.[47]

Several studies investigated the association of STOP-Bang scores with perioperative complications. Compared with surgical patients with STOP-Bang scores of 0 to 2 (low-risk OSA), those with STOP-Bang scores greater than or equal to 3 (high-risk OSA) had an increased rate of perioperative complications.[59] A recent prospective study of 3452 patients showed that patients identified as high risk for OSA by the STOP-Bang questionnaire had a higher rate of postoperative complications (9% vs 2%), difficult intubation (20% vs 9%), and difficult mask ventilation (23% vs 7%).[60] STOP-Bang scores of 3, 4, and 5 were associated with 2, 3, and 5 times increased odds of critical care admission respectively.[61] The STOP-Bang questionnaire can be used as a preoperative risk stratification tool to predict the risk of intraoperative and early postoperative adverse events.[59]

The major drawback of all screening tools is their modest specificity with a high false-positive rate. It is possible that patients identified as at risk for OSA may not have the disease. It is prudent to increase the diagnostic threshold of the screening questionnaire to improve the specificity in the preoperative setting. Overdiagnosing OSA could have negative consequences in terms of the cost of health insurance and the ability to continue to drive.

Improvements in the specificity of the STOP-Bang questionnaire can be made by considering the specific constellation of risk factors. For example, the specific combination of STOP (snoring, tiredness, observed apnea, high BP) score greater than or equal to 2 plus BMI greater than or equal to 35 kg/m^2 plus male gender showed a specificity of 97%.[62] A 2-step algorithm was developed for the STOP-Bang questionnaire to effectively identify patients with a high probability of moderate to severe sleep apnea (**Fig. 1**).[63] A higher STOP-Bang score yields a higher probability of moderate to severe OSA (**Fig. 2**).[62] The measures discussed earlier can help health care professionals to identify patients with a high probability of moderate to severe OSA.

Patients may be identified as having suspected OSA for the first time during their preoperative screening. They should be informed about the increased risk of perioperative complications associated with untreated OSA. The ultimate

---

Box 1
STOP-Bang questionnaire

STOP-Bang Scoring Model:

1. Snoring?

    Do you snore loudly (loud enough to be heard through closed doors or your bed-partner elbows you for snoring at night)?

    Yes/no

2. Tired?

    Do you often feel tired, fatigued, or sleepy during the daytime (such as falling asleep while driving or talking to someone)?

    Yes/no

3. Observed?

    Has anyone observed you stop breathing or choking/gasping during your sleep?

    Yes/no

4. Pressure?

    Do you have, or are you being treated for, high blood pressure?

    Yes/no

5. BMI more than 35 kg/m^2?

    Yes/no

6. Age more than 50 years?

    Yes/no

7. Neck size large (measured around Adam's apple)?

    For men, is your shirt collar 43 cm (17 in) or larger?

    For women, is your shirt collar 41 cm (16 in) or larger?

    Yes/no

8. Gender: male?

    Yes/no

Scoring criteria for general population:

Low risk of OSA: yes to 0 to 2 questions

Intermediate risk of OSA: yes to 3 to 4 questions

High risk of OSA: yes to 5 to 8 questions
or yes to 2 or more of 4 STOP questions, plus male gender
or yes to 2 or more of 4 STOP questions, plus BMI greater than 35 kg/m^2
or yes to 2 or more of 4 STOP questions, plus neck circumference (43 cm [17 in] in men, 41 cm [16 in] in women)

Courtesy of University Health Network, University of Toronto, Toronto, Ontario, Canada; and *Modified from* Refs.[47,57,63]

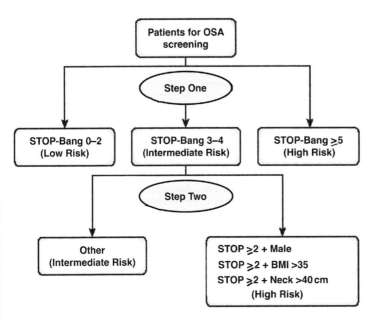

Fig. 1. Two-step strategy for using STOP-Bang questionnaire. (*From* Chung F, Abdullah HR, Liao P. STOP-Bang questionnaire: a practical approach to screen for obstructive sleep apnea. Chest 2016;149(3):635; with permission).

decision to proceed or refer patients for further work-up should be made on an individual basis in consultation with the surgeons and patients. The Society of Anesthesia and Sleep Medicine guidelines suggest that additional evaluation for preoperative cardiopulmonary optimization be considered in patients who have a high probability of OSA and for whom there is an indication of uncontrolled systemic conditions or additional problems with ventilation or gas exchange. These

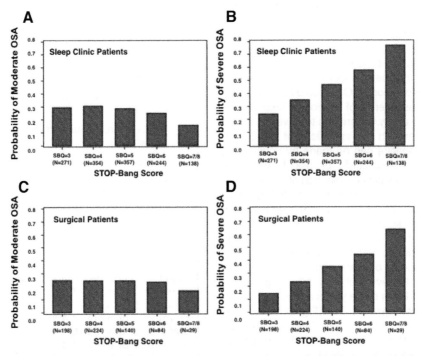

Fig. 2. Relationship between STOP-Bang score and the probability of OSA. (*A*) STOP-Bang score and probability of moderate OSA (AHI>15–30) in sleep clinic patients. (*B*) STOP-Bang score and probability of severe OSA (AHI>30) in sleep clinic patients. (*C*) STOP-Bang score and probability of moderate OSA (AHI>15–30) in surgical patients. (*D*) STOP-Bang score and probability of severe OSA (AHI>30) in surgical patients. SBQ, STOP-Bang questionnaire. (*From* Chung F, Abdullah HR, Liao P. STOP-Bang questionnaire: a practical approach to screen for obstructive sleep apnea. Chest 2016;149(3):634; with permission).

conditions include, but may not be limited to (1) hypoventilation syndromes, (2) severe pulmonary hypertension, and (3) resting hypoxemia not attributable to other cardiopulmonary disease.[13]

Patients who have suspected OSA, with no major comorbidities, are likely to have mild OSA and can proceed to surgery with necessary perioperative precautions.[64] Because OSA is associated with long-term cardiovascular and neurologic sequelae, it is beneficial to initiate long-term management in patients screened as high risk preoperatively. Hence patients should be advised to notify their primary medical providers, allowing appropriate referral for further evaluation.[13] **Fig. 3** shows the logical sequence of preoperative work-up for OSA. Further work is needed to define the optimal clinical pathways for surgical patients with suspected OSA.

SCREENING FOR OBSTRUCTIVE SLEEP APNEA IN SPECIAL POPULATIONS: OBSTRUCTIVE SLEEP APNEA IN PREGNANCY

The prevalence of OSA among women aged 30 to 39 years is estimated to be 5% to 6% but the exact prevalence of OSA among the pregnant population is not known.[65] Physiologic changes associated with pregnancy are known to predispose to OSA, but detection of OSA during pregnancy remains challenging. Sleep fragmentation and excessive daytime sleepiness are common in pregnant patients, making their correlation with OSA uncertain. These factors coupled with low awareness among physicians lead to delayed recognition and underdiagnoses of OSA in this population.

Lockhart and colleagues[66] compared 6 OSA screening tools in pregnant patients and concluded that the STOP-Bang questionnaire has the highest specificity (85%). The high negative predictive value may mitigate the need for PSG in patients with a score of 0 to 2. They also proposed that BMI greater than 35 kg/m^2, falling asleep while talking with someone, and history of treatment of hypertension were significant independent predictors of OSA in pregnant patients.[66] In-laboratory PSG is the gold standard for the diagnosis of OSA, but it is time consuming and expensive. Although portable home PSG can

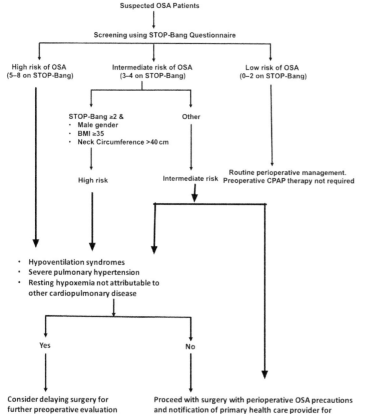

Fig. 3. Preoperative screening of patients for OSA in the anesthesia clinic.

facilitate rapid screening in pregnant women, further research is needed to confirm its validity in this population.[67]

A recent meta-analysis proved that SDB is associated with a 2-fold increase in preeclampsia in women.[68] A systematic review of 10,155 patients in 12 studies examining the maternal effects showed that moderate to severe SDB during pregnancy was associated with gestational diabetes mellitus (OR, 1.78; 95% confidence interval [CI], 1.29–2.46), pregnancy-related hypertension (OR, 2.38; 95% CI, 1.63–3.47), and preeclampsia (OR, 2.19; 95% CI, 1.71–2.80).[69] Adverse fetal outcomes, such as preterm delivery and low birth weight, are possible and may be secondary to worsening maternal health.[69,70]

CPAP treatment has been suggested to decrease BP and improve cardiac output in women with preeclampsia.[71] Positional therapy favoring lateral recumbent or head-elevated positions are preferable to the supine position, which generally worsens OSA. It may improve AHI and oxygenation in postpartum women with OSA.[72]

OBSTRUCTIVE SLEEP APNEA ASSOCIATED WITH OBESITY HYPOVENTILATION SYNDROME

OHS is characterized by the presence of obesity (BMI $\geq$ 30 kg/m^2), daytime hypoventilation (Paco$_2$ $\geq$45 mm Hg), hypoxemia (Pao$_2$ <70 mm Hg), and/or SDB.[73]

Patients with a BMI greater than 40 kg/m^2 have increased postoperative mortality and morbidity, which increases further with the presence of OSA.[74] Postoperative pulmonary complications are common in morbidly obese patients, increasing the LOS by approximately 8 days and the cost of surgery by 2-fold to 12-fold.[75] The STOP-Bang score has been validated in both obese and morbidly obese surgical patients. A STOP-Bang score of 4 has sensitivity of 88% and a score of 6 is more specific for identifying severe OSA in obese patients.[76] Screening for OSA in morbidly obese patients is a widely accepted practice before bariatric surgery.

Patients with a combination of OHS and OSA have a greater perioperative risk for cardiac and pulmonary complications, with higher rate of morbidity and mortality, than patients with OSA without OHS.[77] OHS was associated with 11 times increased odds for postoperative respiratory failure and ICU transfer. There was also an increased incidence of postoperative heart failure (OR, 5.4) and prolonged intubation (OR, 3.1). These patients also had a longer LOS compared with patients with only OSA (7.3 vs 2.8 days respectively).[77]

LONG-TERM ECONOMIC AND SOCIAL BENEFITS OF PREOPERATIVE OBSTRUCTIVE SLEEP APNEA SCREENING

An important public health implication of a preoperative OSA screening program is that it could improve the long-term health of patients through better OSA treatment. OSA is associated with an increased risk of other comorbidities, such as congestive heart failure, arrhythmias, coronary artery disease, stroke, diabetes mellitus, hypertension, metabolic syndrome, depression, cancer, and chronic renal failure.[4–6,78–80] There is overwhelming evidence from longitudinal community studies that untreated severe OSA is an independent predictor of mortality.[4,81] Preoperative diagnosis and treatment may yield similar benefits to those achieved by treatment of chronic diseases like hypertension, coronary artery disease, and diabetes mellitus.

Physician fees were higher by $149 ± $27 (95% CI, 95.12–202.10) in patients with OSA in the year before diagnosis, compared with the fifth year before diagnosis.[82] Two other case-controlled studies have shown that the overall health care costs are higher for patients with undiagnosed OSA. Increased health care expenditure to treat patients with undiagnosed OSA is estimated to be between $1950 and $3899 per patient per year. An estimate of the added burden on the health care system is between $34 billion and $69 billion annually.[83]

Patients with OSA experience daytime sleepiness and decreased cognitive function, and are at twice the risk for a road traffic accident.[84] The costs specifically related to OSA-related motor vehicle crashes are significant, amounting to $15.9 billion. Treating OSA with CPAP therapy and assuming 70% compliance would reduce motor vehicle crashes and the associated cost by roughly $11.1 billion.[85] Because a substantial proportion of patients with OSA participate in the workforce, subjective sleepiness influences job satisfaction, absenteeism, and productivity.[86] Thus, OSA imposes direct costs in the form of diagnosis and treatment of associated comorbidities as well as indirect costs from OSA-related road traffic collisions and other productivity losses.

Individuals with severe OSA report significantly poorer quality of life, and mild OSA is also associated with reduced vitality.[87] These effects are similar to those of other chronic diseases in the general population.

Health care costs decline considerably with prompt diagnosis and treatment of OSA with CPAP.[88] CPAP is the most effective and most widely used treatment modality. It reduces the nocturnal obstructive events and improves daytime sleepiness, cognitive function, and well-being.[89] It has also been shown to decrease BP in OSA patients with hypertension and improves glucose control in diabetic patients with OSA.[90,91] Prompt diagnosis of OSA and compliance with CPAP treatment have been shown to improve vitality and quality of life within 3 months of treatment.[92]

A 2-year follow-up study evaluated the long-term benefits of preoperative OSA screening, diagnosis, and CPAP therapy in terms of health and quality of life.[14] Treatment of OSA with CPAP therapy after subsequent diagnosis had health-related benefits. CPAP-compliant patients reported a 38% reduction in medication intake for comorbidities such as hypertension, diabetes, stroke, asthma, gastroesophageal reflux disease, and depression (**Fig. 4**). Also, more than 80% of CPAP-compliant patients showed improvements in fatigue, daytime sleepiness, and sleep quality (see **Fig. 4**).[14]

The consequences of sleep loss and sleep disorders are not restricted to the affected individuals; families and communities are also disrupted. The sleep quality and well-being of the family members can be affected. These adverse effects in turn can lead to severe family turmoil and divorce.[93] CPAP therapy was associated with subjective improvement in bed partners' sleep, although there was no objective improvement, as measured by PSG.[94]

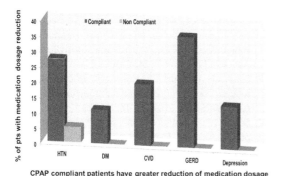

CPAP compliant patients have greater reduction of medication dosage

Fig. 4. Percentages of patients reporting reduction in medication after OSA treatment with CPAP. HTN, hypertension; CVD, coronary vascular disease; GERD, gastroesophageal reflux disease. (*From* Mehta V, Subramanyam R, Shapiro CM, et al. Health effects of identifying patients with undiagnosed obstructive sleep apnea in the preoperative clinic: a follow-up study. Can J Anaesth 2012;59(6):544–55.)

CURRENT TREATMENT OPTIONS FOR OBSTRUCTIVE SLEEP APNEA

The consequences of undiagnosed and untreated OSA are serious, and the associated health care costs are very high. Identification of patients with OSA and treating them is crucial. The current gold standard of treatment of OSA is CPAP therapy; however, adherence to CPAP remains poor. When a patient fails CPAP, alternate therapies need to be considered.

OSA is a heterogenous disorder with both anatomic and nonanatomic (physiologic) determinants. There is a potential to target treatment based on the underlying mechanism. For example, oral appliances and surgery in the form of uvulopalatopharyngoplasty is beneficial for patients with abnormal upper airway anatomy.[95] Similarly, stimulation of the hypoglossal nerve pharmacologically or by electrical stimulation could be beneficial for those patients with pharyngeal dilator muscle dysfunction.[96] Patients with unstable ventilatory control can benefit from oxygen and acetazolamide, which stabilize breathing.[97,98] Likewise patients with OSA with a low arousal threshold wake up prematurely and have inadequate time for the accumulation of respiratory stimuli to activate pharyngeal dilator muscles, leading to obstruction. Such patients may benefit from sedatives like trazodone and eszopiclone, which lower the arousal threshold.[99] One limitation of the personalized treatment approach for OSA has been the lack of simple, validated tests to identify the mechanism underlying OSA in each patient. Further work needs to be done in this area. The alternative treatment measures for OSA mentioned earlier have not been systematically studied in the perioperative setting, although patients using these as primary therapy for their OSA should be encouraged to continue their use in the perioperative period.

SUMMARY

OSA is highly prevalent in the surgical population. Perioperative screening using simple tools like questionnaires is reasonable to identify high-risk patients and institute appropriate precautions, risk mitigation, and monitoring. The decision of further referral and management before surgery should be individualized based on the associated comorbidities in the patient, nature and urgency of the procedure, postoperative requirement for opioids, and institutional capabilities and protocols. Routine screening for OSA increases the preparedness for effective perioperative management, ensuring that appropriate risk stratification strategy and monitoring are in place. Subsequent diagnosis and treatment of OSA are associated with long-term health benefits for patients with OSA and indirectly minimize the health care burden on the society.

REFERENCES

1. Peppard PE, Young T, Barnet JH, et al. Increased prevalence of sleep-disordered breathing in adults. Am J Epidemiol 2013;177(9):1006–14.

2. Frey WC, Pilcher J. Obstructive sleep-related breathing disorders in patients evaluated for bariatric surgery. Obes Surg 2003;13(5):676–83.

3. Singh M, Liao P, Kobah S, et al. Proportion of surgical patients with undiagnosed obstructive sleep apnoea. Br J Anaesth 2013;110:629–36.

4. Marin JM, Carrizo SJ, Vicente E, et al. Long-term cardiovascular outcomes in men with obstructive sleep apnoea-hypopnoea with or without treatment with continuous positive airway pressure: an observational study. Lancet 2005;365(9464):1046–53.

5. Mehra R, Benjamin EJ, Shahar E, et al. Association of nocturnal arrhythmias with sleep-disordered breathing: the Sleep Heart Health Study. Am J Respir Crit Care Med 2006;173(8):910–6.

6. Coughlin SR, Mawdsley L, Mugarza JA, et al. Obstructive sleep apnoea is independently associated with an increased prevalence of metabolic syndrome. Eur Heart J 2004;25(9):735–41.

7. Kaw R, Pasupuleti V, Walker E, et al. Postoperative complications in patients with obstructive sleep apnea. Chest 2012;141(2):436–41.

8. Hai F, Porhomayon J, Vermont L, et al. Postoperative complications in patients with obstructive sleep apnea: a meta-analysis. J Clin Anesth 2014;26(8): 591–600.

9. D'Apuzzo MR, Browne JA. Obstructive sleep apnea as a risk factor for postoperative complications after revision joint arthroplasty. J Arthroplasty 2012;27(8 Suppl):95–8.

10. Wong JK, Maxwell BG, Kushida CA, et al. Obstructive sleep apnea is an independent predictor of postoperative atrial fibrillation in cardiac surgery. J Cardiothorac Vasc Anesth 2015;29(5):1140–7.

11. Foldvary-Schaefer N, Kaw R, Collop N, et al. Prevalence of undetected sleep apnea in patients undergoing cardiovascular surgery and impact on postoperative outcomes. J Clin Sleep Med 2015; 11(10):1083–9.

12. American Society of Anesthesiologists Task Force on Perioperative Management of Patients with Obstructive Sleep Apnea. Practice guidelines for the perioperative management of patients with obstructive sleep apnea: an updated report by the American Society of Anesthesiologists Task Force on Perioperative Management of Patients with Obstructive Sleep Apnea. Anesthesiology 2014; 120:268–86.

13. Chung F, Memtsoudis S, Krishna Ramachandran S, et al. Society of Anesthesia and Sleep Medicine guideline on preoperative screening and assessment of patients with obstructive sleep apnea. Anesth Analg 2016;123:452–73.

14. Mehta V, Subramanyam R, Shapiro CM, et al. Health effects of identifying patients with undiagnosed obstructive sleep apnea in the preoperative clinic: a follow-up study. Can J Anaesth 2012;59(6): 544–55.

15. Debas HT. The emergence and future of global surgery in the United States. JAMA Surg 2015;150(9): 833–4.

16. Cordovani L, Chung F, Germain G, et al. Perioperative management of patients with obstructive sleep apnea: a survey of Canadian anesthesiologists. Can J Anaesth 2016;63(1):16–23.

17. Gali B, Whalen FX, Schroeder DR, et al. Identification of patients at risk for postoperative respiratory complications using a preoperative obstructive sleep apnea screening tool and postanesthesia care assessment. Anesthesiology 2009;110(4): 869–77.

18. Lynn LA, Curry JP. Patterns of unexpected in-hospital deaths: a root cause analysis. Patient Saf Surg 2011;5(1):1–24.

19. Weinger MB, Lee LA. No patient shall be harmed by opioid-induced respiratory depression. Indianapolis (IN): Anesthesia Patient Safety Foundation; 2011.

20. Memtsoudis SG, Stundner O, Rasul R, et al. Sleep apnea and total joint arthroplasty under various types of anesthesia: a population-based study of perioperative outcomes. Reg Anesth Pain Med 2013;38(4):274–81.

21. Reed K, May R. HealthGrades patient safety in american hospitals study. Denver (CO): Health Grades; 2011. Available at: https://www.hospitals. healthgrades.com/CPM/assets/File/HealthGrades PatientSafetyInAmericanHospitalsStudy2011.pdf. Accessed November 14, 2016.

22. Silber JH, Romano PS, Rosen AK, et al. Failure-to-rescue: comparing definitions to measure quality of care. Med Care 2007;45(10):918–25.

23. Smith GB, Prytherch DR, Meredith P, et al. The ability of the National Early Warning Score (NEWS) to discriminate patients at risk of early cardiac arrest, unanticipated intensive care unit admission, and death. Resuscitation 2013;84(4):465–70.

24. Opperer M, Cozowicz C, Bugada D, et al. Does obstructive sleep apnea influence perioperative outcome? A qualitative systematic review for the society of anesthesia and sleep medicine task force on preoperative preparation of patients with sleep-disordered breathing. Anesth Analg 2016;122(5): 1321–34.

25. Memtsoudis SG, Stundner O, Rasul R, et al. The impact of sleep apnea on postoperative utilization of resources and adverse outcomes. Anesth Analg 2014;118(2):407–18.

26. Khan NA, Quan H, Bugar JM, et al. Association of postoperative complications with hospital costs and length of stay in a tertiary care center. J Gen Intern Med 2006;21(2):177–80.

27. Dorman RB, Miller CJ, Leslie DB, et al. Risk for hospital readmission following bariatric surgery. PLoS One 2012;7(3):e32506.

28. Kaw R, Golish J, Ghamande S, et al. Incremental risk of obstructive sleep apnea on cardiac surgical outcomes. J Cardiovasc Surg (Torino) 2006;47(6): 683–9.

29. Mokhlesi B, Hovda MD, Vekhter B, et al. Sleep-disordered breathing and postoperative outcomes after elective surgery: analysis of the nationwide inpatient sample. Chest 2013;144(3):903–14.

30. Lockhart EM, Willingham MD, Ben AA, et al. Obstructive sleep apnea screening and postoperative mortality in a large surgical cohort. Sleep Med 2013;14(5): 407–15.

31. Liao P, Luo Q, Elsaid H, et al. Perioperative auto-titrated continuous positive airway pressure treatment in surgical patients with obstructive sleep apnea: a randomized controlled trial. Anesthesiology 2013;119(4):837–47.

32. Mutter TC, Chateau D, Moffatt M, et al. A matched cohort study of postoperative outcomes in obstructive sleep apnea: could preoperative diagnosis and treatment prevent complications? Anesthesiology 2014;121(4):707–18.

33. Abdelsattar ZM, Hendren S, Wong SL, et al. The impact of untreated obstructive sleep apnea on cardiopulmonary complications in general and vascular surgery: a cohort study. Sleep 2015; 38(8):1205–10.

34. Nagappa M, Mokhlesi B, Wong J, et al. The effects of continuous positive airway pressure on postoperative outcomes in obstructive sleep apnea patients undergoing surgery: a systematic review and meta-analysis. Anesth Analg 2015;120(5):1013–23.

35. Kain ZN, Vakharia S, Garson L, et al. The perioperative surgical home as a future perioperative practice model. Anesth Analg 2014;118(5):1126–30.

36. Trois MS, Capone GT, Lutz JA, et al. Obstructive sleep apnea in adults with down syndrome. J Clin Sleep Med 2009;5(4):317–23.

37. Hernández-Gordillo D, Ortega-Gómez MDR, Galicia-Polo L, et al. Sleep apnea in patients with acromegaly. Frequency, characterization and positive pressure titration. Open Respir Med J 2012;6:28–33.

38. Joosten SA, O'Driscoll DM, Berger PJ, et al. Supine position related obstructive sleep apnea in adults: pathogenesis and treatment. Sleep Med Rev 2014; 18(1):7–17.

39. Togeiro SM, Chaves CM Jr, Palombini L, et al. Evaluation of the upper airway in obstructive sleep apnoea. Indian J Med Res 2010;131:230–5.

40. Iida-Kondo C, Yoshino N, Kurabayashi T, et al. Comparison of tongue volume/oral cavity volume ratio between obstructive sleep apnea syndrome patients and normal adults using magnetic resonance imaging. J Med Dent Sci 2006;53(2):119–26.

41. Zonato AI, Bittencourt LR, Martinho FL, et al. Association of systematic head and neck physical examination with severity of obstructive sleep apnea-hypopnea syndrome. Laryngoscope 2003; 113(6):973–80.

42. Nuckton TJ, Glidden DV, Browner WS, et al. Physical examination: Mallampati score as an independent predictor of obstructive sleep apnea. Sleep 2006; 29(7):903–8.

43. Davies RJ, Stradling JR. The relationship between neck circumference, radiographic pharyngeal anatomy, and the obstructive sleep apnoea syndrome. Eur Respir J 1990;3(5):509–14.

44. Schwartz AR, Patil SP, Laffan AM, et al. Obesity and obstructive sleep apnea: pathogenic mechanisms and therapeutic approaches. Proc Am Thorac Soc 2008;5(2):185–92.

45. Lyberg T, Krogstad O, Djupesland G. Cephalometric analysis in patients with obstructive sleep apnoea syndrome. I. Skeletal morphology. J Laryngol Otol 1989;103(3):287–92.

46. Lee RW, Vasudavan S, Hui DS, et al. Differences in craniofacial structures and obesity in Caucasian and Chinese patients with obstructive sleep apnea. Sleep 2010;33(8):1075–80.

47. Chung F, Yegneswaran B, Liao P, et al. STOP questionnaire. Anesthesiology 2008;108(5):812–21.

48. Chung F, Yegneswaran B, Liao P, et al. Validation of the Berlin questionnaire and American Society of Anesthesiologists checklist as screening tools for obstructive sleep apnea in surgical patients. Anesthesiology 2008;108(5):822–30.

49. Ramachandran SK, Kheterpal S, Consens F, et al. Derivation and validation of a simple perioperative sleep apnea prediction score. Anesth Analg 2010; 110(4):1007–15.

50. Chung F, Chau E, Yang Y, et al. Serum bicarbonate level improves specificity of STOP-Bang screening for obstructive sleep apnea. Chest 2013;143(5): 1284–93.

51. Chung F, Liao P, Elsaid H, et al. Oxygen desaturation index from nocturnal oximetry: a sensitive and specific tool to detect sleep-disordered breathing in surgical patients. Anesth Analg 2012;114(5): 993–1000.

52. Chung F, Zhou L, Liao P. Parameters from preoperative overnight oximetry predict postoperative adverse events. Minerva Anestesiol 2014;80(10): 1084–95.

53. Chung F, Liao P, Sun Y, et al. Perioperative practical experiences in using a level 2 portable polysomnography. Sleep Breath 2011;15:367–75.

54. Chesson AL, Berry RB, Pack A. Practice parameters for the use of portable monitoring devices in the investigation of suspected obstructive sleep apnea in adults. Sleep 2003;26(7):907–13.

55. Mokhlesi B, Tulaimat A, Faibussowitsch I, et al. Obesity hypoventilation syndrome: prevalence and predictors in patients with obstructive sleep apnea. Sleep Breath 2007;11(2):117–24.

56. Chau EH, Mokhlesi B, Chung F. Obesity hypoventilation syndrome and anesthesia. Sleep Med Clin 2013;8(1):135–47.

57. Chung F, Subramanyam R, Liao P, et al. High STOP-Bang score indicates a high probability of obstructive sleep apnoea. Br J Anaesth 2012;108(5): 768–75.

58. Nagappa M, Liao P, Wong J, et al. Validation of the STOP-Bang questionnaire as a screening tool for obstructive sleep apnea among different populations: a systematic review and meta-analysis. PLoS One 2015;10(12):e0143697.

59. Seet E, Chua M, Liaw CM. High STOP-BANG questionnaire scores predict intraoperative and early postoperative adverse events. Singapore Med J 2015;56(4):212–6.

60. Corso RM, Petrini F, Buccioli M, et al. Clinical utility of preoperative screening with STOP-Bang questionnaire in elective surgery. Minerva Anestesiol 2014; 80(8):877–84.

61. Chia P, Seet E, Macachor JD, et al. The association of pre-operative STOP-BANG scores with postoperative critical care admission. Anaesthesia 2013; 68(9):950–2.

62. Chung F, Abdullah HR, Liao P. STOP-Bang questionnaire: a practical approach to screen for obstructive sleep apnea. Chest 2016;149(3):631–8.

63. Chung F, Yang Y, Brown R, et al. Alternative scoring models of STOP-bang questionnaire improve specificity to detect undiagnosed obstructive sleep apnea. J Clin Sleep Med 2014;10(9):951–8.

64. Seet E, Chung F. Obstructive sleep apnea: preoperative assessment. Anesthesiol Clin 2010;28(2): 199–215.

65. Young T, Palta M, Dempsey J, et al. The occurrence of sleep-disordered breathing among middle-aged adults. N Engl J Med 1993;328(17):1230–5.

66. Lockhart EM, Ben Abdallah A, Tuuli MG, et al. Obstructive sleep apnea in pregnancy: assessment of current screening tools. Obstet Gynecol 2015; 126(1):93–102.

67. Sharkey KM, Waters K, Millman RP, et al. Validation of the Apnea Risk Evaluation System (ARES) device against laboratory polysomnography in pregnant women at risk for obstructive sleep apnea syndrome. J Clin Sleep Med 2014;10(5):497–502.

68. Pamidi S, Pinto LM, Marc I, et al. Maternal sleep-disordered breathing and adverse pregnancy outcomes: a systematic review and metaanalysis. Am J Obstet Gynecol 2014;210(1):52.e1-14.

69. Ding X-X, Wu Y-L, Xu S-J, et al. A systematic review and quantitative assessment of sleep-disordered breathing during pregnancy and perinatal outcomes. Sleep Breath 2014;18(4):703–13.

70. Chen Y-H, Kang J-H, Lin C-C, et al. Obstructive sleep apnea and the risk of adverse pregnancy outcomes. Am J Obstet Gynecol 2012;206(2):136.e1-5.

71. Guilleminault C, Palombini L, Poyares D, et al. Pre-eclampsia and nasal CPAP: part 1. Early intervention with nasal CPAP in pregnant women with risk-factors for pre-eclampsia: preliminary findings. Sleep Med 2007;9(1):9–14.

72. Zaremba S, Mueller N, Heisig AM, et al. Elevated upper body position improves pregnancy-related OSA without impairing sleep quality or sleep architecture early after delivery. Chest 2015; 148(4):936–44.

73. Mokhlesi B. Obesity hypoventilation syndrome: a state-of-the-art review. Respir Care 2010;55(10): 1347–62.

74. Schumann R, Shikora SA, Sigl JC, et al. Association of metabolic syndrome and surgical factors with pulmonary adverse events, and longitudinal mortality in bariatric surgery. Br J Anaesth 2015;114(1):83–90.

75. Sabaté S, Mazo V, Canet J. Predicting postoperative pulmonary complications: implications for outcomes and costs. Curr Opin Anaesthesiol 2014;27(2): 201–9.

76. Chung F, Yang Y, Liao P. Predictive performance of the STOP-Bang score for identifying obstructive sleep apnea in obese patients. Obes Surg 2013; 23(12):2050–7.

77. Kaw R, Bhateja P, Paz Y, et al. Postoperative complications in patients with unrecognized obesity hypoventilation syndrome undergoing elective non-cardiac surgery. Chest 2016;149(1):84–91.

78. Arzt M, Young T, Finn L, et al. Association of sleep-disordered breathing and the occurrence of stroke. Am J Respir Crit Care Med 2005;172(11): 1447–51.

79. Elias RM, Bradley TD, Kasai T, et al. Rostral overnight fluid shift in end-stage renal disease: relationship with obstructive sleep apnea. Nephrol Dial Transplant 2012;27(4):1569–73.

80. Lavie P, Herer P, Hoffstein V. Obstructive sleep apnoea syndrome as a risk factor for hypertension: population study. BMJ 2000;320(7233):479–82.

81. Campos-Rodriguez F, Martinez-Garcia MA, de la Cruz-Moron I, et al. Cardiovascular mortality in women with obstructive sleep apnea with or without continuous positive airway pressure treatment: a cohort study. Ann Intern Med 2012; 156(2):115–22.

82. Albarrak M, Banno K, Sabbagh AA, et al. Utilization of healthcare resources in obstructive sleep apnea syndrome: a 5-year follow-up study in men using CPAP. Sleep 2005;28(10):1306–11.

83. Knauert M, Naik S, Gillespie MB, et al. Clinical consequences and economic costs of untreated obstructive sleep apnea syndrome. World J Otorhinolaryngol Head Neck Surg 2015;1(1):17–27.

84. Tregear S, Reston J, Schoelles K, et al. Obstructive sleep apnea and risk of motor vehicle crash: systematic review and meta-analysis. J Clin Sleep Med 2009;5(6):573–81.

85. Sassani A, Findley LJ, Kryger M, et al. Reducing motor-vehicle collisions, costs, and fatalities by treating obstructive sleep apnea syndrome. Sleep 2004;27(3):453–8.

86. Jurado-Gámez B, Guglielmi O, Gude F, et al. Workplace accidents, absenteeism and productivity in patients with sleep apnea. Arch Bronconeumol 2015;51(5):213–8.

87. Baldwin CM, Griffith KA, Nieto FJ, et al. The association of sleep-disordered breathing and sleep symptoms with quality of life in the Sleep Heart Health Study. Sleep 2001;24(1):96–105.

88. Tarasiuk A, Greenberg-Dotan S, Brin YS, et al. Determinants affecting health-care utilization in obstructive sleep apnea syndrome patients. Chest 2005;128(3):1310–4.

89. Montserrat JM, Ferrer M, Hernandez L, et al. Effectiveness of CPAP treatment in daytime function in sleep apnea syndrome: a randomized controlled study with an optimized placebo. Am J Respir Crit Care Med 2001;164(4):608–13.

90. Tun Y, Hida W, Okabe S, et al. Can nasal continuous positive airway pressure decrease clinic blood pressure in patients with obstructive sleep apnea? Tohoku J Exp Med 2003;201(3):181–90.

91. Hassaballa HA, Tulaimat A, Herdegen JJ, et al. The effect of continuous positive airway pressure on glucose control in diabetic patients with severe obstructive sleep apnea. Sleep Breath 2005;9(4): 176–80.

92. Antic NA, Catcheside P, Buchan C, et al. The effect of CPAP in normalizing daytime sleepiness, quality of life, and neurocognitive function in patients with moderate to severe OSA. Sleep 2011;34(1):111–9.

93. Breugelmans JG, Ford DE, Smith PL, et al. Differences in patient and bed partner-assessed quality of life in sleep-disordered breathing. Am J Respir Crit Care Med 2004;170(5):547–52.

94. McArdle N, Grove A, Devereux G, et al. Split-night versus full-night studies for sleep apnoea/hypopnoea syndrome. Eur Respir J 2000;15(4):670–5.

95. Sutherland K, Lee RW, Cistulli PA. Obesity and craniofacial structure as risk factors for obstructive sleep apnoea: impact of ethnicity. Respirology 2012;17(2):213–22.

96. Malhotra A. Hypoglossal-nerve stimulation for obstructive sleep apnea. N Engl J Med 2014; 370(2):170–1.

97. Wellman A, Malhotra A, Jordan AS, et al. Effect of oxygen in obstructive sleep apnea: role of loop gain. Respir Physiol Neurobiol 2008;162(2): 144–51.

98. Edwards BA, Sands SA, Eckert DJ, et al. Acetazolamide improves loop gain but not the other physiological traits causing obstructive sleep apnoea. J Physiol 2012;590(Pt 5):1199–211.

99. Heinzer RC, White DP, Jordan AS, et al. Trazodone increases arousal threshold in obstructive sleep apnoea. Eur Respir J 2008;31(6):1308–12.

Impact of Portable Sleep Testing

Vaishnavi Kundel, MD[a],*, Neomi Shah, MD, MPH[a,b],*

KEYWORDS

- Portable monitoring • OSA • Social and economic impact

KEY POINTS

- Portable testing (PT) is a reasonable alternative in patients with a high pretest probability of moderate-to-severe obstructive sleep apnea (OSA).
- PT should not be routinely ordered in those with coexisting sleep disorders, class 3 obesity, and severe cardiopulmonary disorders.
- A negative portable test should prompt an in-laboratory polysomnography.
- PT is cost-effective in a selected group of patients, mainly from the insurance-payer perspective, and cost-effectiveness can be enhanced when it is used in collaboration with a sleep center to ensure appropriate follow-up and adherence to treatment.
- Further research is needed to determine the utility of PT in diagnosing OSA among commercial motor vehicle operators.

INTRODUCTION

Obstructive sleep apnea (OSA) is a common condition affecting both children and adults, with an estimated prevalence of 1% to 5% in children, and 10% to 30% in adults.[1] It is characterized by recurrent obstruction in the upper airway during sleep, leading to arousals with fragmented sleep and intermittent hypoxemia, which can result in deleterious health effects, including neurocognitive problems and cardiovascular morbidity. Consequently, patients with untreated OSA present an increased use of health care resources, high socioeconomic costs, and increased overall mortality from all causes.[2]

In the past, the standard of care established by the American Academy of Sleep Medicine (AASM) was to diagnose OSA with in-laboratory polysomnography (PSG). PSG is accurate with a low failure rate because the study is attended by technical staff; however, it is considered relatively expensive and technically complex. Furthermore, access to in-laboratory sleep testing is limited because the prevalence and awareness of sleep disorders has grown in the past few decades. In preselected individuals, portable testing (PT) has been used as an alternative diagnostic test for OSA based in part on the premise that it is theoretically less expensive and quicker to deploy compared with in-laboratory PSG.[3] Portable sleep testing also alleviates the previously noted access issues by cutting back on the long wait times typically seen with in-laboratory testing.

CURRENT GUIDELINES FOR PORTABLE SLEEP TESTING

In 2007, the AASM appointed the Portable Monitoring Task Force to develop clinical guidelines for the use of PT in the diagnosis and management

Disclosure Statement: The authors have nothing to disclose.
a Division of Pulmonary, Critical Care, and Sleep Medicine, Icahn School of Medicine at Mount Sinai, Room 5-20, Annenberg Building 5th Floor, One Gustave L. Levy Place, New York, NY 10029, USA; b Department of Epidemiology and Population Health, Albert Einstein College of Medicine, 1300 Morris Park Avenue, Bronx, NY 10461, USA
* Corresponding author.
E-mail addresses: vaishnavi.kundel@mssm.edu; neomi.shah@mssm.edu

of OSA. The key features of the guidelines are as follows[3]:

- PT may be used as an alternative to PSG for the diagnosis of OSA in patients
  - With a high pretest probability of moderate-to-severe OSA
  - For whom in-laboratory PSG is not possible due to immobility or critical illness.
- PT is not appropriate for the diagnosis of OSA in patients
  - With significant comorbid medical conditions such as advanced cardiopulmonary disease that may degrade its accuracy
  - With evaluation showing suspected of having comorbid sleep disorders
  - With screening of belonging to an asymptomatic population.
- At a minimum, PT must record air flow, respiratory effort, and pulse oximetry.
- PT application, education, testing, scoring, and interpretation must be performed under an AASM-accredited comprehensive sleep medicine program.
- A negative or technically inadequate PT in patients with a high pretest probability of moderate-to-severe OSA should prompt in-laboratory PSG

PORTABLE MONITORING CLASSIFICATION SCHEME

The first widely used classification system for describing sleep testing devices was published by the AASM in 1994.[4] It placed available devices into 4 levels based on the number and type of leads used. **Table 1** provides details about this classification. It is important to note that level 3 and level 4 devices do not record signals to determine sleep staging or disruption.

However, with continued technological advances, many PT devices did not fit into these categories. Clinicians needed guidance to help decide which out-of-center (OOC) testing devices are appropriate for diagnosing OSA. In 2011, a new categorization scheme was developed, allowing easy classification of OOC devices based on the types of sensors that they use to aid in the diagnosis of OSA, including sleep, cardiac, oximetry, position, effort, and respiratory measures (SCOPER).[5] **Table 2** provides details about the new classification system for PT.

Table 1
Portable studies for sleep apnea evaluation: classification scheme (6-hour overnight recording minimum)

	Level 1: Standard PSG	Level 2: Comprehensive Portable PSG	Level 3: Modified Portable Apnea Testing	Level 4: Continuous Single or Dual Parameter Recording
Parameters	Minimum of 7: EEG, EOG, chin EMG, ECG, airflow, respiratory effort, oximetry	Minimum of 7: EEG, EOG, chin EMG, ECG or HR, airflow, respiratory effort, oximetry	Minimum of 4: ventilation (respiratory movement and airflow) HR or ECG, oximetry	Minimum of 1 (typically oximetry or airflow)
Body position	Documented or objectively measured	Can be objectively measured	Can be objectively measured	Not measured
Leg movement	EMG or motion sensor (optional)	EMG or motion sensor (optional)	May be recorded	Not recorded
Personnel attendance	Constant	None	None	None
Interventions Possible	Yes	No	No	No

Abbreviations: ECG, electrocardiogram; EEG, electroencephalogram; EMG, electromyogram; EOG, electrooculogram; HR, heart rate.

From Ferber R, Millman R, Coppola M, et al. Portable recording in the assessment of obstructive sleep apnea. ASDA standards of practice. Sleep 1994;17(4):378–92.

Table 2
Sleep, cardiac, oximetry, position, effort, and respiratory measures (SCOPER) categorization

Sleep	Cardiovascular	Oximetry	Position	Effort	Respiratory
S_1: 3 EEG channels, EOG, and chin EMG	C_1: >1 ECG lead, can derive events	O_1: Finger or ear oximetry with recommended sampling	P_1: Video or visual measurement	E_1: 2 RIP belts	R_1: Nasal pressure and thermal device
S_2: <3 EEG channels or without EOG or chin EMG	C_2: PAT	O_2: Finger or ear oximetry, without sampling	P_2: Nonvisual position measurement	E_2: 1 RIP belt	R_2: Nasal pressure
S_3: sleep surrogate (actigraphy)	C_3: 1 lead ECG	O_3: Oximetry, alternative site		E_3: Derived effort	R_3: Thermal device
S_4: Other sleep measure	C_4: Derived pulse (from oximetry)	O_4: Other oximetry		E_4: Other effort measure	R_4: $ETCO_2$

3 EEG channels defined as frontal, central, and occipital.

Abbreviations: ECG, electrocardiography; EEG, electroencephalography; EMG, electromyography; EOG, electrooculography; $ETCO_2$, end-tidal CO_2; PAT, peripheral arterial tone; RIP, respiratory inductance plethysmography.

From Collop NA, Tracy SL, Kapur V, et al. Obstructive sleep apnea devices for out-of-center (OOC) testing: technology evaluation. J Clin Sleep Med 2011;7(5):531–48.

OUTPATIENT VALIDATION FOR PORTABLE TESTING

There have been several trials validating the outpatient use of portable sleep tests in patients with a high pretest probability of OSA. Summarizing the evidence that PT is a reasonable substitute for in-laboratory PSG, a 2014 Cochrane meta-analysis of comparative studies to evaluate the accuracy of level 3 versus level 1 sleep tests in adults with suspected OSA confirmed that level 3 portable devices showed good diagnostic performance compared with level 1 sleep tests in adult patients with a high pretest probability of moderate-to-severe OSA.[6]

Several studies have found home diagnosis and treatment algorithms for OSA to be noninferior to traditional, attended, in-laboratory PSG studies. The protocol entails undergoing PT followed by autotitrating continuous positive airway pressure (CPAP) treatment.

A prospective, noninferiority, randomized trial published in 2011[7] showed that the home testing pathway was noninferior to the in-laboratory pathway in terms of CPAP adherence at 3 months, functional outcomes of sleepiness, and sleep-related quality of life.

Two major studies comparing outpatient initiation and titration of autotitrating PAP (APAP) versus in-laboratory CPAP titration showed that APAP-treated patients have a similar adherence to treatment compared with in-laboratory CPAP titration.[8,9] In the first study,[8] results showed that a home-based strategy for diagnosis and treatment OSA compared with a traditional, in-laboratory PSG was noninferior in terms of acceptance, treatment adherence, and functional outcomes. Additionally, CPAP adherence was higher at 3 months in the home testing and home titration group. **Fig. 1** provides contrasting information on the 2 models for sleep apnea diagnosis pathways.

Another study published in 2012[9] found that APAP-treated patients (compared with in-laboratory CPAP titration) had higher satisfaction with therapy, with no difference in positive airway pressure (PAP) adherence, residual apnea-hypopnea index (AHI), or functional outcomes. It is, however, important to highlight that an important feature of these trials was the degree of early and close follow-up provided to subjects after PAP initiation. Early, close follow-up in the diagnosis and treatment of OSA has been established to improve adherence.[10]

LIMITATIONS OF PORTABLE TESTING

Despite that portable monitoring studies and in-laboratory PSG have equivalent functional outcomes, they are not suitable for certain patient populations. Because most trials validating home sleep testing for OSA diagnosis excluded patients with comorbidities, such as chronic obstructive pulmonary disease and congestive heart failure,

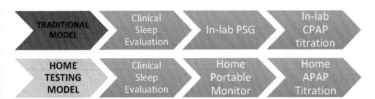

Fig. 1. Traditional in-laboratory and home PT pathways for the diagnosis of OSA, based on 90th percentile APAP pressure. (*Adapted from* Cooksey JA, Balachandran JS. Portable monitoring for the diagnosis of OSA. Chest 2016;149:1074–81.)

data regarding the use of home testing in patients with these medical comorbidities are limited.[10] No clear guidelines exist on using PT in patients with class 3 obesity (body mass index > 40) or elderly patients.

Therefore, in patients with significant medical comorbidities in high-risk populations (those with severe cardiovascular, pulmonary, or neuromuscular disease), concomitant sleep disorders despite effective PAP therapy, and a high pretest probability of OSA but negative portable study, there is a continuing role for in-laboratory PSG within the home testing algorithms (**Fig. 2**).[10]

DIRECT AND INDIRECT COSTS OF UNTREATED OBSTRUCTIVE SLEEP APNEA

Studies have shown that health care utilization and related costs are far higher for individuals with OSA compared with those without OSA. Although these costs are primarily due to OSA-related cardiovascular morbidities, this effect on cost may be independent of chronic disease burden. This is evidenced by the relationship between medical costs and OSA severity shifting from a linear relationship in mild-to-moderate OSA to a ceiling

effect in severe OSA.[11] A United States cross-sectional study from 1999 the found that untreated OSA may be responsible for up to $3.4 billion in additional medical costs (an average annual cost of $2720).[12]

Indirect costs pertain to losses in productivity and income as a consequence of disability related to the disease. In a Danish study comparing adults with OSA to healthy controls, untreated OSA was associated with higher direct and indirect costs, including significantly higher rates of health-related contact, medication use, and unemployment.[13] Additionally, employed adults with OSA had earnings (on average) one-third lower than their non-OSA counterparts, even after adjusting for the socioeconomic status of both cohorts.[11] This important study found a substantial association between OSA and socioeconomic costs and consequences for the individual patient and society.

THE TRANSITION FROM POLYSOMNOGRAPHY TO PORTABLE SLEEP TESTING

Given the socioeconomic impacts and costs of untreated OSA, an important challenge for the

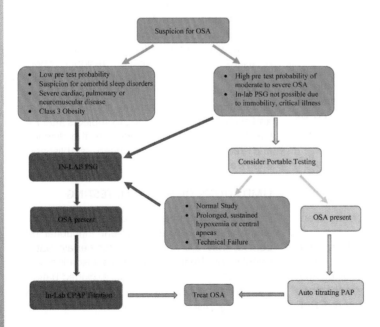

Fig. 2. Suggested algorithm for PT and indications for in-laboratory PSG versus PT. PT can be considered in patients with a high pretest probability of OSA; however, a normal study or technical failure must prompt an in-laboratory PSG. Patients with a low pretest probability for OSA, suspicion for comorbid sleep disorders, and severe comorbidities are not good candidates for PT, and must undergo monitored, in-laboratory PSG for evaluation of OSA.

clinician is understanding both the clinical effectiveness and cost-effectiveness of the available diagnostic and therapeutic strategies. Although in-laboratory PSG is the gold standard for diagnosis, it is often expensive, time-consuming, and frequently of limited availability. PT is now a part of routine care and an attractive alternative to diagnosing OSA in selected individuals.[11] Additionally, there are several socioeconomic advantages to PT, mainly related to its lower direct cost, increased accessibility, and convenience of testing for patients suspected to have OSA, resulting in an overall improvement of the diagnostic process. As the recognition and prevalence of OSA has increased, so has the demand for PT. In a recent 2013 survey of sleep centers, 64% of centers reported that they are offering PT for privately insured patients and 48% reported they were reducing their plans for expansion of laboratory beds as a result of home testing.[14]

Costs of Diagnostic and Therapeutic Strategies

The direct costs associated with different diagnostic and management strategies for OSA were published by the New England Comparative Effectiveness Public Advisory Council in 2013.[15] Cost-effectiveness was evaluated in a hypothetical cohort of 1000 Medicaid patients older than 16 years with suspected OSA. The comparator for all strategies was in-laboratory PSG. Outcomes evaluated included total cost, number of individuals diagnosed with OSA, number of false-negative results, and number of averted in-laboratory PSGs. Three distinct strategies were compared with PSG alone and conducted in all 1000 subjects, including screening with a symptom questionnaire plus PSG; morphometric examination plus PSG; and PT, in which patients were diagnosed based on PT findings alone and did not receive confirmatory PSG. Results showed that PT was the most cost-saving of all strategies, mainly driven by lower test costs in comparison with PSG alone (**Table 3**).

For the evaluation of the cost of diagnostic testing and CPAP titration, 3 test-and-treat strategies were analyzed, including (1) PT followed by autotitrating CPAP, (2) PT followed by split-night PSG for those who tested-positive with PT, and (3) these compared with the gold standard of in-laboratory PSG plus in-laboratory titration CPAP for all patients. Results showed that both PT plus autotitrating CPAP strategies were cost-saving relative to in-laboratory PSG plus CPAP titration, with the most substantial cost savings (more than $400,000) gained from the home

testing plus autotitrating CPAP strategy (see **Table 3**).[15]

Cost-Effectiveness of Polysomnography Versus Other Diagnostic Strategies

Although a PT may individually be less resource intensive than PSG with lower direct costs, clinical guidelines recommend that a diagnostic PSG be performed in patients with a high pretest probability of OSA who have a negative result on PT. This is due to concerns that PT may have lower sensitivity for diagnosing mild-to-moderate OSA. Thus, the PT strategy as a whole may not be cost-effective.[14]

Although comparing direct costs is informative, assessing the cost-effectiveness of various management strategies may be more revealing. Cost-effectiveness is assessed by the ratio of the incremental cost and change in quality-adjusted life years (QALYs) following the adoption of a treatment compared with no treatment.[16] This takes into account both added years of life by therapy and improvement in quality of life. An incremental cost-effectiveness ratio of less than $50,000 per QALY is often quoted as the threshold of cost-effectiveness.[17]

In 2006, one of the first analyses used 3 strategies: PT, split-night in-laboratory PSG (PSG followed by CPAP titration during the same night), and full-night in-laboratory PSG (a night of PSA followed by another night of CPAP titration) to compare their cost-effectiveness from a third-party payer perspective over a 5-year period.[18] Cost analysis was performed from the perspective of third-party payers and only direct health care costs were included in the analysis. Effectiveness was measured as QALYs, and costs were adjusted for variable CPAP compliance and dropouts. The study showed that PT was the most cost-effective alternative to split-night PSG and to full-night PSG but only at the lowest amounts of third-party willingness-to-pay. On the other hand, split-night PSG or full-night PSG were most cost-effective at higher amounts of third-party willingness-to-pay (**Fig. 3**). Therefore, third-party willingness-to-pay is an important consideration in choosing the most cost-effective approach.

Another study, published in 2011, was conducted to evaluate the cost-effectiveness of PT, split-night PSG, and full-night PSG in conjunction with CPAP therapy in subjects with moderate-to-severe OSA.[19] The study linked health-related quality of life to relevant outcomes observed in OSA by evaluating the impact of treatment on common negative outcomes associated with

Table 3
Outcomes and costs of different diagnostic and therapeutic strategies for obstructive sleep apnea among 1000 hypothetical Medicaid patients referred for testing and treated for 1 year if positive

Measure	Diagnostic Strategies		Diagnostic and Therapeutic Strategies		Test-and-Treat
	PSG (gold standard)	Type 3 monitor alone (PT)	PSG + fixed titration CPAP (gold standard)	Home monitor (PT) + autotitrating CPAP	Home monitor (PT): followed by split-night PSG, fixed titration CPAP if PT positive
Total cost ($)	652,830	200,700	1,244,905	811,129	1,112,731
Cost difference of PT vs PSG alone ($)	N/A	452,130	—	—	—
Cost differences of PT + APAP vs sleep laboratory strategy ($)	—	—	N/A	433,776	132,174

All numbers are for 1000 patients at high risk of OSA diagnosis. For the diagnostic testing, the cost-savings for the diagnosis of OSA using PT was $452,130 compared with PSG. For the test-and-treat strategies, cost savings for PT followed by auto-PAP compared with in-laboratory split-night PSG followed by CPAP titration was $433,776.

Abbreviation: N/A, not applicable.

From The New England Comparative Effectiveness Public Advisory Council. Diagnosis and treatment of obstructive sleep apnea in adults. 2013. Available at: https://icer-review.org/wp-content/uploads/2016/01/Final-Report_January20132.pdf. Accessed August 22, 2016.

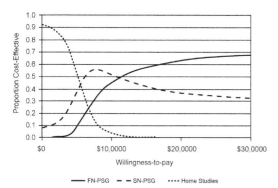

Fig. 3. Cost-effectiveness as influenced by third-party willingness-to-pay in 3 diagnostic and therapeutic strategies for OSA. Acceptability curves show the 3 pathways when the cost-effectiveness ratios are transformed to net benefits. Each curve represents the proportion of evaluations that are cost-effective for each pathway over a range of willingness-to-pay thresholds. Home studies is the pathway most frequently cost-effective when willingness-to-pay is less than $6500, as is split-night PSG when willingness-to-pay is between $6500 and $11,500, and full-night PSG willingness-to-pay is greater than $11,500. FN-PSG, full-night PSG; SN-PSG, split-night PSG. (*From* Deutsch PA, Simmons MS, Wallace JM. Cost-effectiveness of split-night polysomnography and home studies in the evaluation of obstructive sleep apnea syndrome. J Clin Sleep Med 2006;2(2):145–53.)

untreated OSA, including strokes, myocardial infarctions, and motor vehicle collisions (MVCs) due to excessive daytime sleepiness (EDS). Cost-effectiveness (assessed through incremental cost per QALY gained) of different diagnostic and therapeutic strategies were compared over a 10-year period and over the expected lifetime of a subjects, using a base-case of a 50-year-old man with a 50% pretest probability of OSA. Surprisingly, the results showed that full-night PSG was the preferred diagnostic strategy and the most cost-effective at any willingness-to-pay, owing to its superior diagnostic accuracy. In other words, PSG, although a more expensive test up front, ends up costing the health care system less over time by minimizing the number of patients with false-positive and negative tests, and results in more health benefits compared with PT. However, after closely examining the underlying assumptions of the model used in the study, a few things must be considered. The investigators' assumption that OSA treatment would dramatically reduce the risk of cardiovascular events (from 56% to 39%) with CPAP was extrapolated from observational studies rather than randomized controlled trials. This increases the economic impact of false-negative results in subjects in the

PT arm. Additionally, it was assumed that subjects incorrectly diagnosed with OSA versus PT would use CPAP long-term, magnifying the economic impact of false-positive PT. Lastly, it was assumed that 22% of subjects with a negative PT or technical failure would not return for a follow-up PSG, again increasing the economic impact of a false-negative test. As pointed out by the investigators, when it is assumed that all negative PTs will have a full PSG, and subjects with false-positive PTs who receive no benefit from CPAP are unlikely to use it long-term, PTs were more cost-effective compared with PSG.[17]

In contrast to this study, a more recent economic analysis of PT versus in-laboratory PSG for the diagnosis and management of OSA used data from the HomePAP study[8] (a randomized controlled trial that compared PT vs in-laboratory PSG for the diagnosis and management of OSA), with results analyzed in the context of both payer and provider perspective.[14] Results showed that, from the insurance-payer perspective, a home-based diagnostic pathway for OSA with adequate patient treatment was less costly, even after accounting for false-negative and technically inadequate PTs that prompted an in-laboratory PSG. For providers, there were no cost-savings for a PT approach and it even resulted in a negative operating margin.

Bottom Line: Is Polysomnography Cost-Effective?

Taken together, it can be concluded that in comparing direct costs associated with different diagnostic and management strategies for OSA, PT is the most cost-saving of all strategies, mainly driven by lower test costs in comparison with PSG. Additionally, a home testing plus autotitrating CPAP strategy has substantial cost savings compared with split-night PSG plus fixed CPAP titration and in-laboratory PSG with CPAP titration.

However, when taking into account cost-effectiveness of PT as defined by added years of life by therapy and improvement in quality of life (QALY), the economic models becomes more complex and a few things must be taken into consideration, including third-party willingness-to-pay, insurance-payer perspective, and provider perspective. PT seems to be the most cost-effective alternative at the lowest level of third-party willingness-to-pay, whereas split-night PSG or full-night PSG are most cost-effective at higher amounts of third-party willingness-to-pay. From the insurance-payer perspective, PT for the diagnosis of OSA is less costly; however, for providers this may result in a negative operating margin.

SOCIAL COSTS AND RISKS OF OBSTRUCTIVE SLEEP APNEA

EDS is a common and concerning symptom of OSA with several deep-rooted consequences. EDS is characterized by sleepiness that occurs in situations in which an individual is normally expected to be awake and alert. Up to 87% of adults with OSA may have EDS.[20]

EDS can impair functioning at both personal and social levels, leading to poor work-place performance, time-management skills, and personal interactions, all of which can be improved with treatment of OSA with CPAP.[21,22] A recent study found that individuals with OSA had an increased incidence of work-related absenteeism, lower work-related productivity, and a higher rate of psychological stress.[23] Taken together, OSA and EDS secondary to OSA seem to significantly affect daytime functioning and there is growing evidence regarding the repercussions of untreated OSA in terms of work-related productivity and accidents.

MVCs are another potential risk of EDS and impaired concentration in untreated OSA. Two studies, including a systemic review and a meta-analysis, showed that both noncommercial and commercial drivers with untreated sleep apnea are at a statistically significant increased risk of involvement in MVCs.[24,25] Notably, 1 of the investigators points out that the elevation in crash rate is comparable to drivers with moderate-to-severe dementia or with blood alcohol levels of 0.05 to 0.7 mg/dL. Successful treatment of sleep apnea improves driver performance with decreased MVC rates to a level comparable with the general population.[24]

Another recent study confirmed an increased risk of MVC among those with OSA compared with the general population and demonstrated that CPAP used 4 or more hours per night reduced MVC risk.[26]

Portable Sleep Testing in Commercial Motor Vehicle Operators

OSA has a high prevalence among commercial motor vehicle (CMV) operators and it is known to lead to fatigue and EDS, and to increase the risk of motor vehicle crashes. Unlike the typical setting in a sleep clinic where patients with undiagnosed OSA are actively seeking diagnosis and treatment of their symptoms, most CMV drivers are reluctant to carry a diagnosis of OSA because of its economic and occupational implications.[27] Most of those who are identified as high risk for OSA according to Joint Task Force criteria often either do not complete a full in-laboratory PSG due to lack of insurance or they go doctor shopping to seek an alternate commercial driver medical examiner who is not familiar with formal OSA screening recommendations or does not screen for OSA using objective criteria. This can lead to fraudulent certification. Those who undergo PSG are often lost to follow-up and a PSG diagnosis does not necessarily result in adequate treatment in this population. For this reason, there has been a growing demand to identify and develop alternative methods for diagnosing OSA in this high-risk population, such as PT.[27]

However, given these unique behaviors, diagnosis with PT is likely to be more challenging in this population, producing lower yield than among the general population. Because most PTs do not measure sleep or wake stages, the potential for sabotaging or falsifying the results remain a likely possibility. Although PT studies in the general population maybe more cost-effective than in-laboratory PSGs, CMV operators tested with PT may be more likely to require a follow-up in-laboratory PSG due to data loss and low sensitivity. In addition, some of the strategies being marketed to trucking companies lack sleep specialist involvement, potentially leaving the interpretation of PTs up to primary care providers who may be unaware of the technology's limitations. This decreases the likelihood that those drivers at high risk of OSA with negative PTs will be referred for a subsequent in-laboratory PSG.[27]

The only peer-reviewed, published study using PTs to diagnose OSA in the US CMV population used a type IV PT that measures airflow by a nasal cannula and estimates respiratory disturbance index.[28] Of those CMV operators who met criteria for high risk of OSA, 68 were randomly selected to use the PT device for 1 night at a certified community sleep center under the supervision of sleep physicians and undergo a subsequent formal PSG in the laboratory. Of those, 16% of drivers using the PTs produced invalid data, 22% were lost to follow-up, and 49% were noncompliant with physician recommendations and, therefore, not able to complete the subsequent PSG. These results predict that incidents of data loss and alteration, as well as loss to follow-up, will likely be higher when they are used on CMV operators in unsupervised home settings or on the road. These factors make it imprudent to directly extrapolate PT efficiency and cost-effectiveness assumptions from the general population to the professional driver population. Further research conducted in the trucking industry is needed to determine the utility of PT in diagnosing OSA among CMV operators.[27]

Portable Sleep Testing in an Urban Population

The advantages of home-based PT make it an especially attractive health service option for underserved, uninsured urban and rural populations with suspected OSA and limited access to fully equipped sleep laboratories. It is important to study the feasibility of home PT in these populations because home PT has a lower sensitivity and specificity, and is associated with false-negative and positive results, as well as technical failure, and may require follow-up by in-laboratory PSG. This may have a negative impact on cost-effectiveness of PT as a whole and potentially increase the gap in availability of health services for OSA in the urban population. One study examined the feasibility of home PT compared with in-laboratory PSG prospectively in an urban, largely under-served African American population, to determine the accuracy of a validated PT device, compare technical failure rates of home PT in this population, and understand patient preferences with respect to home versus in-laboratory PSG.[29] Approximately one-third did not have a high school diploma, more than half were unemployed, and 76% with annual household income less than $50,000. Technical failure rates were 5.3% for home versus 3.1% for in-laboratory PT. There was good agreement between AHI on PSG and AHI on home PT, and participants preferred home over in-laboratory testing. This study confirmed that home PT for diagnosis of OSA in a high-risk urban population is feasible, accurate, and preferred by patients. It is likely to improve access to care, and the cost-effectiveness of this diagnostic strategy for OSA should be examined in underserved urban and rural populations.

THE FUTURE FOR PORTABLE SLEEP TESTING

In the current health care delivery model, primary care providers are often not involved with subspecialists in a coordinated process, resulting in fragmented patient care, with increased health-delivery costs. The Affordable Care Act (ACA) is gearing toward the patient-centered medical home model, in which primary care physicians (PCPs) are at the heart of health care delivery and provide comprehensive, coordinated care.[30]

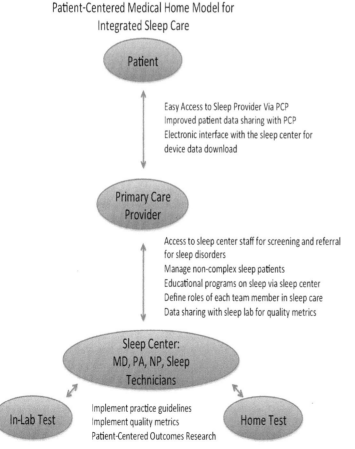

Fig. 4. Algorithm for primary care model of integrated sleep care and portable sleep testing. MD, Medical Doctor; PA, Physician Assistant; NP, Nurse Practitioner.

Patient-Centered Medical Home Model for Integrated Sleep Care

Patient

Easy Access to Sleep Provider Via PCP
Improved patient data sharing with PCP
Electronic interface with the sleep center for device data download

Primary Care Provider

Access to sleep center staff for screening and referral for sleep disorders
Manage non-complex sleep patients
Educational programs on sleep via sleep center
Define roles of each team member in sleep care
Data sharing with sleep lab for quality metrics

Sleep Center: MD, PA, NP, Sleep Technicians

In-Lab Test

Implement practice guidelines
Implement quality metrics
Patient-Centered Outcomes Research

Home Test

In this rapidly changing health care delivery model, the impact on sleep medicine delivery is substantial. The field has confronted implementation of sizable cuts in reimbursement rates for in-laboratory PSG and, as a result, use of PT has rapidly increased. In response, to comply with insurance company requirements, PCPs often refer patients needing evaluation for OSA for PT via an independent PT company that does not have a comprehensive sleep program. These patients are then prescribed automated treatment devices without appropriate education or access to follow-up with experienced sleep providers, subsequently resulting in poor compliance to treatment, and fragmented care.[31,32]

For PT to be cost-effective and beneficial within the provisions of the ACA, an integrated and collaborative sleep-care model is essential for meaningful improvements in the quality of sleep disorders care, with early, close follow-up for patients undergoing PT with APAP titration to improve adherence.[33] This can be executed via a PCP-based model, providing access to sleep providers and sleep testing, yet encouraging and educating the PCP to screen and treat noncomplex OSA in their own practices (**Fig. 4**).

SUMMARY

This article provides the current state of evidence on the socioeconomic impact of PT for sleep apnea. It seems that both models, the traditional in-laboratory and the newer home-based model for sleep apnea diagnosis, have a place in the current sleep medicine diagnostic algorithm. PT is an appropriate alternative to in-laboratory PSG, as long as the following criteria are carefully considered: (1) it needs to be targeted to the right patients (ie, those who have a high pretest probability of having sleep apnea and do not have coexisting sleep or cardiopulmonary disorders); (2) it needs to have an element of personalized medicine (ie, commercial drivers, urban population), and (3) it should be used as a part of an integrated and collaborative sleep-care delivery model to ensure appropriate follow-up and adherence to treatment. If these criteria are met, PT would be cost-effective in a selected group of patients.

REFERENCES

1. Franklin KA, Lindberg E. Obstructive sleep apnea is a common disorder in the population—a review on the epidemiology of sleep apnea. J Thorac Dis 2015;7(8):1311.
2. Chiner E, Andreu AL, Sancho-Chust JN, et al. The use of ambulatory strategies for the diagnosis and treatment of obstructive sleep apnea in adults. Expert Rev Respir Med 2013;7(3):259–73.
3. Collop NA, Anderson WM, Boehlecke B, et al. Clinical guidelines for the use of unattended portable monitors in the diagnosis of obstructive sleep apnea in adult patients. Portable Monitoring Task Force of the American Academy of Sleep Medicine. J Clin Sleep Med 2007;3(7):737–47.
4. Ferber R, Millman R, Coppola M, et al. Portable recording in the assessment of obstructive sleep apnea. ASDA standards of practice. Sleep 1994;17(4): 378–92.
5. Collop NA, Tracy SL, Kapur V, et al. Obstructive sleep apnea devices for out-of-center (OOC) testing: technology evaluation. J Clin Sleep Med 2011;7(5):531–48.
6. El Shayeb M, Topfer LA, Stafinski T, et al. Diagnostic accuracy of level 3 portable sleep tests versus level 1 polysomnography for sleep-disordered breathing: a systematic review and meta-analysis. CMAJ 2014; 186(1):E25–51.
7. Kuna ST, Gurubhagavatula I, Maislin G, et al. Noninferiority of functional outcome in ambulatory management of obstructive sleep apnea. Am J Respir Crit Care Med 2011;183(9):1238–44.
8. Rosen CL, Auckley D, Benca R, et al. A multisite randomized trial of portable sleep studies and positive airway pressure autotitration versus laboratory-based polysomnography for the diagnosis and treatment of obstructive sleep apnea: the HomePAP study. Sleep 2012;35(6):757–67.
9. Berry RB, Sriram P. Auto-adjusting positive airway pressure treatment for sleep apnea diagnosed by home sleep testing. J Clin Sleep Med 2014;10(12): 1269–75.
10. Cooksey JA, Balachandran JS. Portable monitoring for the diagnosis of OSA. Chest 2016;149(4):1074–81.
11. Ehsan Z, Ingram DG. Economic and social costs of sleep apnea. Curr Pulmonol Rep 2016;5:111–5.
12. Kapur V, Blough DK, Sandblom RE, et al. The medical cost of undiagnosed sleep apnea. Sleep 1999; 22(6):749–55.
13. Jennum P, Kjellberg J. Health, social and economical consequences of sleep-disordered breathing: a controlled national study. Thorax 2011;66(7): 560–6.
14. Kim RD, Kapur VK, Redline-Bruch J, et al. An economic evaluation of home versus laboratory-based diagnosis of obstructive sleep apnea. Sleep 2015; 38(7):1027–37.
15. The New England Comparative Effectiveness Public Advisory Council. Diagn Treat of Obstructive Sleep Apnea in Adults. 2013. Available at: https://icer-review.org/wp-content/uploads/2016/01/Final-Report_January20132.pdf. Accessed August 22, 2016.
16. Drummond M, Sculpher M, Torrance G, et al. Methods for the economic evaluation of health

care programmes. New York: Oxford University Press; 2005.

17. Ayas NT, Pack A, Marra C. The demise of portable monitoring to diagnose OSA? Not so fast! Sleep 2011;34(6):691–2.

18. Deutsch PA, Simmons MS, Wallace JM. Cost-effectiveness of split-night polysomnography and home studies in the evaluation of obstructive sleep apnea syndrome. J Clin Sleep Med 2006;2(2):145–53.

19. Pietzsch JB, Garner A, Cipriano LE, et al. An integrated health-economic analysis of diagnostic and therapeutic strategies in the treatment of moderate-to-severe obstructive sleep apnea. Sleep 2011;34(6):695–709.

20. Seneviratne U, Puvanendran K. Excessive daytime sleepiness in obstructive sleep apnea: prevalence, severity, and predictors. Sleep Med 2004;5(4):339–43.

21. Ulfberg J, Carter N, Talback M, et al. Excessive daytime sleepiness at work and subjective work performance in the general population and among heavy snorers and patients with obstructive sleep apnea. Chest 1996;110(3):659–63.

22. Mulgrew AT, Ryan CF, Fleetham JA, et al. The impact of obstructive sleep apnea and daytime sleepiness on work limitation. Sleep Med 2007;9(1):42–53.

23. Jurado-Gamez B, Guglielmi O, Gude F, et al. Workplace accidents, absenteeism and productivity in patients with sleep apnea. Arch Bronconeumol 2015;51(5):213–8.

24. Ellen R, Marshall SC, Palayew M, et al. Systematic review of motor vehicle crash risk in persons with sleep apnea. J Clin Sleep Med 2006;2(2):193–200.

25. Tregear S, Reston J, Schoelles K, et al. Obstructive sleep apnea and risk of motor vehicle crash: systematic review and meta-analysis. J Clin Sleep Med 2009;5(6):573–81.

26. Karimi M, Hedner J, Habel H, et al. Sleep apnea-related risk of motor vehicle accidents is reduced by continuous positive airway pressure: Swedish Traffic Accident Registry data. Sleep 2015;38(3):341–9.

27. Zhang C, Berger M, Malhotra A, et al. Portable diagnostic devices for identifying obstructive sleep apnea among commercial motor vehicle drivers: considerations and unanswered questions. Sleep 2012;35(11):1481–9.

28. Watkins MR, Talmage JB, Thiese MS, et al. Correlation between screening for obstructive sleep apnea using a portable device versus polysomnography testing in a commercial driving population. J Occup Environ Med 2009;51(10):1145–50.

29. Garg N, Rolle AJ, Lee TA, et al. Home-based diagnosis of obstructive sleep apnea in an urban population. J Clin Sleep Med 2014;10(8):879–85.

30. Davis K, Abrams M, Stremikis K. How the Affordable Care Act will strengthen the nation's primary care foundation. J Gen Intern Med 2011;26(10):1201–3.

31. Pack AI. POINT: does laboratory polysomnography yield better outcomes than home sleep testing? Yes. Chest 2015;148(2):306–8.

32. Kundel V, Shah N. Reforming the sleep apnea care delivery paradigm: sleep center and primary care integration. Chest Physician Newsletter 2016.

33. Edinger JD, Grubber J, Ulmer C, et al. A collaborative paradigm for improving management of sleep disorders in primary care: a randomized clinical trial. Sleep 2016;39(1):237–47.

Legal and Regulatory Aspects of Sleep Disorders

Saiprakash B. Venkateshiah, MD[a,1], Romy Hoque, MD[b],
Lourdes M. DelRosso, MD[c,d], Nancy A. Collop, MD[e,*]

KEYWORDS

- Sleep disorders • Legal aspects • Regulatory aspects • Obstructive sleep apnea • Parasomnia
- Sleep disparities

KEY POINTS

- There are multiple aspects of sleep disorders that may interact with the law making it important to increase awareness of such interactions among clinicians.
- Patients with excessive sleepiness may have civil (and in some states criminal) liability if they fall asleep at the wheel and cause a motor vehicle accident.
- An employer may be held "vicariously liable" for the acts of an employee performed as part of their duties if the employee driver falls asleep and injures a third party in a crash.
- Parasomnia-associated sleep-related violence represents potential medicolegal issues for clinicians, who may be called on to consider parasomnia as a contributing, mitigating, or exculpatory factor in criminal proceedings.
- Improving access to sleep medicine care in both pediatric and adult populations is an important aspect in reducing the adverse consequences of undiagnosed/untreated sleep disorders.

INTRODUCTION

Sleep disorders afflict a large proportion of the population and result in a high economic burden to society. Sleep disorders manifest in a variety of ways and are often not obvious to the individual who has the disorder. These complexities result in occasional entanglements with the legal system as we highlight in this article. We cover the most common interactions between sleep disorders and the law including the challenges of excessive sleepiness and driving including specifically sleepiness owing to obstructive sleep apnea (OSA); the legal ramifications of underdiagnosing or misdiagnosing OSA by physicians and employers; the liabilities associated with parasomnia disorder; and the ramifications of health disparities as they relate to sleep disorders.

LEGAL AND REGULATORY DIMENSIONS OF EXCESSIVE SLEEPINESS

Excessive daytime sleepiness can occur owing to a variety of causes, including sleep disorders such

Disclosure Statement: The authors have nothing to disclose. Dr N.A. Collop receives royalties from UpToDate and honoraria from Best doctors.
[a] Division of Pulmonary, Critical Care and Sleep Medicine, Department of Medicine, Emory University School of Medicine, 615 Michael Street, Suite 205, Atlanta, GA 30322, USA; [b] Department of Neurology, Emory Sleep Center, Emory University School of Medicine, 12 Executive Park Drive NE, Atlanta, GA 30329, USA; [c] Department of Pediatrics, University of California San Francisco, 747 52nd street, Oakland, CA 94609, USA; [d] Department of Pediatrics, UCSF Benioff Children's Hospital Oakland, 747 52nd Street, Oakland, CA 94609, USA; [e] Division of Pulmonary, Critical Care and Sleep Medicine, Department of Medicine, Emory Sleep Center, Emory University School of Medicine, 12 Executive Park Drive Northeast, Atlanta, GA 30329, USA
[1] Present address: 250 North Arcadia Avenue, RM 2D173, Decatur, GA 30030.
* Corresponding author.
E-mail address: nancy.collop@emory.edu

Sleep Med Clin 12 (2017) 149–160
http://dx.doi.org/10.1016/j.jsmc.2016.10.002
1556-407X/17/© 2016 Elsevier Inc. All rights reserved.

as OSA, narcolepsy, restless leg syndrome, insomnia, or from insufficient sleep syndrome, other medical disorders or medication induced sleepiness. OSA and insufficient sleep syndrome are the 2 common etiologies for excessive sleepiness. OSA is a very common condition, with a prevalence of around 5% in adults and 1% to 2% in children. OSA has wide-ranging complications, including an increase in motor vehicle crash risk in both general driving population and commercial drivers with many studies finding a 2- to 3-fold increased risk.[1–5]

Insufficient sleep syndrome is a chronic voluntary sleep restriction that is a widely prevalent cause of excessive daytime sleepiness and daytime fatigue. The Behavioral Risk Factor Surveillance System survey performed by the Centers for Disease Control and Prevention in 2009 included estimates of drowsy driving and unintentionally falling asleep during the day. In 74,571 adult respondents in 12 states, 35.3% reported fewer than 7 hours of sleep during a typical 24-hour period, with 37.9% reported unintentionally falling asleep during the day at least once in the preceding month, and 4.7% reported nodding off or falling asleep while driving at least once in the preceding month.[6] Clinicians, patients, and, in some cases, employers need to be aware of the legal and regulatory aspects that can impact the patients with sleep disorders. This is particularly important in patients working in safety-sensitive occupations, such as commercial trucking, aviation, railroads, and nuclear power plants.

The "blameworthiness" of an individual for a behavior is addressed by the legal issue of culpability. Anglo-American law discusses 2 components to crime: *actus rea*, the criminal act itself, and *mens rea*, criminal intent, both of which are required for criminal responsibility. The standard common law test of criminal liability is expressed by the Latin phrase "*actus non facit reum nisi mens sit rea*" (the act does not make a person guilty unless the mind is also guilty), wherein the guilty mental state must be present at the time of the action for criminal liability. This requires the act to have occurred in a conscious state, but in cases of sleepiness-related accidents, can be extended to include actions that begin in an unconscious state. Driving while drowsy is a decision made by the driver in a conscious state, but an accident may have occurred during sleep. Awareness before and during the sleepiness-related accident is often the central point when determining criminal liability. Herein we review relevant cases to point out how the law has decided in cases of "sleepy drivers."

LEGAL CASES INVOLVING SLEEPY DRIVERS

The Connecticut Supreme Court in 1925 addressed the driver's legal duty when possessed by sleep or other unconscious episode. In *Bushnell v Bushnell*, Mr and Mrs Bushnell drove from Connecticut to Rhode Island. On the return trip, Mr Bushnell dozed off at the wheel and crashed into a tree. Mrs Bushnell, who was a passenger in the car, was injured in the accident and sued her husband for negligence for failing to operate the car in a reasonable manner. Mr Bushnell argued that sleep occurs without warning. Hence, he was to be excused from his duty to maintain control of the car while asleep. The court challenged Mr Bushnell's explanation that he had no advance warning of sleep onset. The court reviewed medical evidence indicating that, unlike a sudden blackout, sleep displays routine and recognizable precursor conditions such as fatigue and dulling of the senses. Hence, the court ruled that Mr Bushnell knew, or should have known, that sleep was affecting his driving and that he should have pulled off the road. Because his sleep episode was foreseeable, the court found Mr Bushnell liable for the cost of his wife's injuries.[7,8]

This ruling did point out that an unforeseeable loss of consciousness (eg, sudden unexpected seizure or blackout) would excuse the driver's duty to exercise due care in driving. The "sudden blackout" defense is a legal protection for drivers who suffer from a sudden and unforeseen onset of sleep but may be difficult to establish if the patients has past experience of a tendency to fall asleep while driving. If one knew that he or she suffered from "sleep attacks" several times a day, it would be negligent for that individual to get behind the wheel of a car even if the "sleep attacks" were unexpected. This principle was reaffirmed in 2006 in Vermont, *State v Valyou*. In this instance, the defendant dozed off many times on the way to work but still continued to drive, ultimately colliding with another vehicle after falling asleep.[7,9]

These cases are not specific to a sleep disorder, but deal with excessive sleepiness and drowsy driving leading to motor vehicle crashes. The same legal principles would be applicable if patients have a motor vehicle crash owing to drowsy driving regardless of etiology of excessive sleepiness.

Some states have laws that can lead to criminal liability for drowsy driving. The states are New Jersey, through enactment of Maggie's Law in 2003, and, Arkansas, through enactment of Arkansas Act 1296 in 2013. Maggie's Law states that a sleep-deprived driver qualifies as a reckless driver who can be convicted of vehicular homicide. It is an evidentiary rule establishing that proof of driving after 24 hours of sleeplessness "shall give rise to an inference that the defendant was driving recklessly" to convict a defendant for vehicular homicide. The law also states that falling asleep while driving may infer recklessness without regard to sleeplessness. Proving reckless fatigue under Maggie's Law is difficult under the law's definition of sleeplessness (without sleep for a period in excess of 24 consecutive hours). Any evidence that the driver took a short nap of even a few minutes during the relevant 24-hour period can defeat inference of reckless driving owing to sleeplessness. If convicted, punishment may include up to 10 years in prison and a $100,000 fine.[7,10] Arkansas Act 1296 classifies "fatigued driving" as an offense under negligent homicide punishable when the driver involved in a fatal accident has been without sleep for 24 consecutive hours or is in the state of sleep after being without sleep for 24 consecutive hours. If convicted, punishment may include up to 1 year in prison, and/or a $2500 fine.[11]

Clinicians should inform patients with sleep disorders of the risks of driving or participating in safety-sensitive occupations while drowsy, especially when the patients are not following the treatment recommendations for their sleep disorders. In particular, clinicians should inform patients with the excessive daytime sleepiness that there may be civil and/or criminal liability if they fall asleep while driving or have cataplexy while driving. Such a discussion should be documented appropriately within the patient's electronic medical record. In certain states, the physician may be required to inform the department of motor vehicles that the patient is continuing to drive despite having excessive sleepiness due to their sleep disorder, thereby presenting a danger to the public. Each physician should be aware of the public safety disclosure laws of the state in which they practice.

LEGAL ISSUES FOR EMPLOYERS

The legal doctrine of *respondeat superior* (which means "let the master answer") provides that an employer may be held "vicariously liable" for the acts of an employee that are performed as part of the employee's duties. Therefore trucking companies, taxi cab companies, or even mail delivery services who employ drivers will be liable vicariously as employers if the driver falls asleep at the wheel and injures a third party in a crash while performing his or her job. The employers may also be held vicariously liable if they failed to screen for disorders that may impact their employees' ability to drive safely during the hiring process and continued employment.

One illustration of this principle is the case of *Dunlap v W.L. Logan Trucking Co*. Employee Norman Munnal fell asleep at the wheel of a tractor trailer and killed a woman. His employer invoked the "sudden blackout" doctrine by blaming the accident on Munnal's "sudden unconsciousness." In this case, Munnal testified that he had a propensity to fall asleep and that he had fallen asleep at the wheel at least once before. Further, Munnal was also diagnosed with severe OSA after a polysomnogram after the accident. The court found sufficient evidence that Munnal was aware of his excessive sleepiness. This and an expert's testimony documenting that Munnal probably fell asleep rather than suffering from a sudden blackout, concluded with the court finding Munnal negligent for failing to operate the truck in a safe manner and Logan Trucking Company was held liable vicariously because he had been operating the rig within the scope of his employment.[7,12]

There are lawsuits in which employees who fell asleep at the wheel after the end of a long work day and caused accidents, and then sued their employers holding them liable for scheduling excess work time. In general, courts have refused to hold employers liable for the "after work" actions of their employees, even if the employer's work conditions contributed to the employee's alleged fatigue. In the cases of *Black v William Insulation Co* and *Barclay v Briscoe*, the courts held the position that it is the employee's personal responsibility to ensure that he or she was capable of safely driving to and from work and an employer was not liable.[7,13,14]

LEGAL ISSUES REGARDING SURGICAL RISKS IN PATIENTS WITH OBSTRUCTIVE SLEEP APNEA

There is a paucity of data that specifically hold a health care provider liable for malpractice in the diagnosis or treatment of sleep disorders. Litigation related to OSA is frequently associated with perioperative complications more than nonoperative issues, such as a failure to diagnose OSA. Otolaryngologists and anesthesiologists were the most frequently named defendants in an analysis of a legal database of 54 cases. Eighty-seven percent of cases stemmed from OSA patients who underwent procedures with resultant perioperative adverse events. Common alleged factors included death (48.1%), permanent deficits (42.6%), intraoperative complications (35.2%), requiring additional surgery (25.9%), anoxic brain injury (24.1%), inadequate informed consent (24.1%), inappropriate medication administration (22.2%), and inadequate monitoring (20.4%).[15]

A retrospective review of 3 primary legal databases between 1991 and 2010 for cases involving adults with known or suspected OSA who underwent a surgical procedure associated with an adverse perioperative outcome revealed that the most common complications were respiratory arrest in an unmonitored setting and difficulty in airway management. Among 24 cases, the immediate adverse outcomes included death (45.6%), anoxic brain injury (45.6%), and upper airway complications (8%). The majority of the anoxic brain injury patients died, eventually giving an overall death rate of 71%. Verdicts favored the plaintiffs in 58% of cases and in cases favoring the plaintiff, the average financial penalty was $2.5 million (range, $650,000–$7,700,000). These data are likely underestimates given that most such cases are settled out of court and are not accounted for in the legal literature.[16]

Some specific examples include the following cases. In *Feitzinger v Simon*, the patient, Mr Feitzinger, was brought in for a routine hernia operation. In the preoperative evaluation, the anesthesiologist neglected to inquire about Mr Feitzinger's diagnosis of OSA and use of CPAP, which was not used during the postoperative period, in which the patient developed pneumonia and died of cardiac arrest 3 days after the hernia surgery. His estate sued for malpractice, claiming that had the anesthesiologist taken Mr Feitzinger's complete medical history, the anesthesiologist would have been aware of the patient's OSA and ordered CPAP during the postoperative period. According to expert testimony, CPAP use might have prevented the patient's pneumonia and eventual death. It was determined by the court that the anesthesiologist's failure to check for OSA established sufficient cause to take the trial to a jury.[7,17]

Another example is the case of *Cornett v State W.O. Moss Hospital* (Louisiana 1993), which emphasized the principle that a physician owes a duty of reasonable care to treat the patient's medical conditions and warn the patient of potentially fatal risks that may be associated with untreated OSA. In this case, the hospital treating Mr Cornett was found liable for his death after he suffered from cardiopulmonary arrest. Mr Cornett had complained to the hospital's physicians of sleep apnea symptoms, including his falling asleep at the wheel on multiple occasions. Mr Cornett was never tested or treated for OSA or warned of the risks posed by untreated sleep apnea, despite the hospital physicians knowing that OSA is a potentially fatal condition. Unfortunately, the hospital physicians had focused for the prior months on Mr Cornett's other medical conditions. It was determined,

based on expert witness testimony during trial, that Mr Cornett's death was likely caused by his untreated sleep apnea. Hence, the hospital and its physicians were liable for malpractice.[7,18]

The principle of informed consent mandates a physician who orders surgical treatment for OSA to inform the patient of surgical risks, benefits, and treatment alternatives such as CPAP. In *Russell v Brown*, the plaintiff visited an otolaryngologist with complaints of snoring and recurrent tonsillitis. The physician recommended a tonsillectomy for the tonsillitis and a uvulopharyngoplasty procedure for mild OSA. The patient suffered surgical complications and brought suit against the physician, claiming that the physician never informed the patient of the risks of surgery or the availability of nonsurgical alternatives such as CPAP or laser surgery. Medical experts testified that the physician's actions reasonably fell within the accepted standard of care and the patient had signed a broad consent form. In this case, the jury found in favor of the physician.[7,19] Regardless of the jury verdict in this case, it should be emphasized the established rule in informed consent cases is that patients must be informed of risks, benefits, and alternative methods of treatment.

EMPLOYMENT IN SAFETY-SENSITIVE POSITIONS

The negative consequences of having an accident in safety-sensitive positions such as commercial trucking, railroad, aviation, and nuclear power generator plants could potentially impact a large number of people and there is also concern for hazardous material exposure. Hence there is increasing awareness among the various regulatory agencies about the interplay between untreated OSA and excessive fatigue or sleepiness. Unfortunately, these varied regulatory agencies are not consistent in their approach to this population.

There are various recommendations that are published for commercial motor vehicle drivers, the details of which have been discussed in a recent review article.[20] A Joint Task Force of the American College of Chest Physicians, American College of Occupational and Environmental Medicine, and the National Sleep Foundation in 2006; the Medical Expert Panel of sleep experts commissioned by the Federal Motor Carrier Safety Administration (FMCSA) in 2008; the Motor Carrier Safety Advisory Committee-Medical Review Board in 2012; and the FMCSA again in 2012 have all published recommendations; the FMCSA 2012 recommendations were abruptly withdrawn shortly after release.[21–24] **Tables 1** and **2** summarize these varied recommendations.[20]

Table 1
Published recommendations for OSA risk assessment and screening

	JTF 2006	MEP 2008	MCSAC-MRB 2012	FMCSA 2012 (Withdrawn)
Sleepiness symptoms	• ESS >10 • Positive findings on alternative sleep questionnaires • Excessive sleepiness	• Daytime sleepiness • Excessive sleepiness while driving • BQ (OSA symptoms)	• Excessive sleepiness during major wake period, including while driving	• Excessive sleepiness during major wake period
Sleepiness observation	Observed sleepiness			
Accident history (subjective/objective)	Motor vehicle accident likely related to sleep disturbance or fatigue	Crash associated with falling asleep	• Crash associated with falling asleep or fatigue • Single vehicle crash	• Crash associated with falling asleep • Single vehicle crash
OSA symptoms (subjective)	• Snoring • Witnessed apneas • Excessive daytime somnolence	• Chronic loud snoring • Witnessed apneas or breathing pauses during sleep • Daytime sleepiness	• Loud snoring • Witnessed apneas • Sleepiness during major wake period	• Loud snoring • Witnessed apneas • Sleepiness during major wake period
OSA history assessment	Past OSA assess severity and treatment efficacy	Past OSA assess severity and treatment efficacy	Past OSA assess severity and treatment efficacy	Past OSA assess severity and treatment efficacy

OSA risk assessment by medical history[a]	• HTN
	  ◦ New or
	  ◦ Uncontrolled or
	  ◦ ≥2 medications
		• HTN
		• Diabetes type 2
		• Hypothyroidism (untreated)
		• Family history OSA
			• HTN
			• Diabetes type 2
			• Hypothyroidism (untreated)
			• Post-menopausal female
			• Family history OSA
				• HTN
				• Diabetes type 2
				• Hypothyroidism (untreated)
				• Postmenopausal female
				• Family history of OSA

OSA risk assessment by physical examination[a]	• BMI ≥35 kg/m²
	• Neck circumference
	  ◦ Male ≥17 inches
	  ◦ Female ≥16 inches
	• Enlarged tonsils or absence of uvula
		• BMI ≥33 kg/m²
		• Neck circumference
		  ◦ Male ≥17 inches
		  ◦ Female ≥15.5 inches
		• Small airway/jaw
		• Advancing age
		• BMI ≥28 kg/m² an additional risk factor
			• BMI ≥35 kg/m²
			• Neck circumference
			  ◦ Male ≥17 inches
			  ◦ Female ≥15.5 inches
			• Small airway (Mallampati 3 or 4)
			• Small or recessed jaw
			• Age ≥42 y
			• Male gender
			• BMI ≥28 kg/m² an additional risk factor
				• BMI ≥35 kg/m²
				• Neck circumference
				  ◦ Male ≥17 inches
				  ◦ Female ≥15.5 inches
				• Small airway (Mallampati 3 or 4)
				• Small or recessed jaw
				• Age ≥42 y
				• Male gender
				• BMI ≥28 kg/m² an additional risk factor

Abbreviations: BMI, body mass index; BQ, Berlin Questionnaire; ESS, Epworth Sleepiness Scale; FMCSA, Federal Motor Carrier Safety Administration; HTN, hypertension; JTF, joint task force; MCSAC-MRB, Motor Carrier Safety Advisory Committee-Medical Review Board; MEP, medical expert panel; Mallampati, Mallampati class score; OSA, obstructive sleep apnea.

[a] Referral recommended if there are 2 or more positive findings by blood pressure, BMI, or neck circumference criteria.

Reproduced from Colvin LJ, Collop NA. Commercial motor vehicle driver obstructive sleep apnea screening and treatment in the United States: an update and recommendation overview. J Clin Sleep Med 2016;12:117; with permission.

Table 2
Published recommendations for obstructive sleep apnea diagnosis and treatment

	JTF 2006	MEP 2008	MCSAC-MRB 2012	FMCSA 2012 (Withdrawn)

Testing	• PSG gold standard
	• HSAT not accepted
		• PSG gold standard
		• HSAT acceptable
		  ○ Oxygen saturation
		  ○ Nasal pressure
		  ○ Sleep/wake time
		  ○ 5-h recording
			• PSG more comprehensive
			• HSAT that is FDA approved with ensured chain of custody is also acceptable
			• Consider PSG if HSAT OSA severity underestimation is suspected
				• PSG more comprehensive
				• HSAT that is, FDA approved with ensured chain of custody is also acceptable
				• PSG if HSAT OSA severity underestimate suspected.

Treatment recommendation (for requiring therapy)	• AHI >30/h
	• AHI >5/h with
	  ○ EDS or
	  ○ MVA or
	  ○ HTN ≥2 medications
		• AHI >20/h
		• May be certified if
		  ○ AHI ≤20/h and no EDS or
		  ○ OSA effectively treated
			• AHI >20/h
			• May be certified if
			  ○ AHI ≤20/h and no EDS or
			  ○ OSA effectively treated
			• Treatment of AHI ≥5/h encouraged, particularly AHI ≥15/h
				• AHI >20/h
				• May be certified if
				  ○ AHI ≤20/h and no EDS or
				  ○ OSA effectively treated
				• Treatment of AHI ≥5/h encouraged, particularly AHI ≥15/h

AHI threshold	AHI >30/h	AHI >20/h	AHI >20/h	AHI >20/h
PAP usage	Minimum >4 h within each 24-h time period	• Minimum ≥4 h per night ≥70% of days • Minimum 1 wk • aPAP titration accepted	• Minimum ≥4 h per night ≥70% of nights • Minimum 1 wk adherence if disqualified • aPAP accepted	• Minimum ≥4 h per night ≥70% of nights • Minimum 1 wk minimum if disqualified

PAP objective efficacy assessment	• PSG CPAP titration
	  ○ AHI <5 ideal
	  ○ AHI <10 acceptable
		• AHI <5 ideal
		• AHI <10 acceptable
		• Documented by sleep study or PAP report
			Successful treatment efficacy is documented via PSG or aPAP	Successful treatment efficacy is documented via PSG or aPAP

Non-PAP therapy alternatives	• Weight loss • Airway surgery • Weight loss surgery • Oral appliance (AHI <30)	• Weight loss • Airway surgery • Weight loss surgery	• Weight loss • Airway surgery • Weight loss surgery	• Weight loss • Airway surgery • Weight loss surgery

Non-PAP therapy efficacy assessment	• Posttreatment sleep study assessment
	  ○ AHI <5 ideal
	  ○ AHI <10 acceptable
		• Posttreatment sleep study assessment
		  ○ ≥1 mo after airway surgery
		  ○ ≥6 mo after weight loss surgery
			• Posttreatment sleep study assessment
			  ○ ≥1 mo after airway surgery
			  ○ ≥6 mo after weight loss surgery
				• Posttreatment sleep study assessment
				  ○ ≥1 mo after airway surgery
				  ○ ≥6 mo after weight loss surgery

Abbreviations: AHI, apnea/hypopnea index; aPAP, auto positive airway pressure; CPAP, continuous positive airway pressure; EDS, excessive daytime sleepiness; FDA, Food and Drug Administration; FMCSA, Federal Motor Carrier Safety Administration; HSAT, home sleep apnea testing; HTN, hypertension; JTF, joint task force; MCSAC- MEP, medical expert panel; MRB, motor carrier safety advisory committee–medical review board; MVA, motor vehicle accident; PAP, positive airway pressure; PSG, polysomnography.

Reproduced from Colvin LJ, Collop NA. Commercial motor vehicle driver obstructive sleep apnea screening and treatment in the United States: an update and recommendation overview. J Clin Sleep Med 2016;12:118; with permission.

The Federal Railroad Administration does not have guidelines regarding OSA. In March 2016, the US Department of Transportation, the FMCSA, and the Federal Railroad Administration announced they were seeking public input on the impacts of screening, evaluating, and treating rail workers and commercial motor vehicle drivers for OSA.

The Federal Aviation Administration (FAA) has recognized that OSA is one of the factors causing pilot fatigue and OSA has been implicated in several aviation accidents. Aviation medical examiners are encouraged to ask about previous OSA diagnosis, and if not to evaluate if the pilot is (1) not at risk for OSA, (2) at risk for OSA, or (3) at extremely high risk for OSA. This determines the urgency and rapidity of workup with those in the extremely high risk of OSA category requiring immediate attention. Of note, the aviation medical examiner is not required to perform the assessment for OSA, but may perform the OSA assessment provided that it is in accordance with the clinical practice guidelines established by the American Academy of Sleep Medicine.[25] Pilots who are determined to be at risk for OSA will be issued a medical certificate and will then, shortly thereafter, receive a letter from the FAA's Federal Air Surgeon requesting that an OSA evaluation be completed within 90 days. If the evaluating physician determines that a sleep study is warranted, it should be done at that time. The pilot may continue flying during the evaluation period and initiation of treatment, if treatment is indicated. Pilots diagnosed with OSA and undergoing treatment must send documentation of effective treatment to the FAA to be considered for a special issuance medical certificate. In 2015, 4917 FAA-certificated pilots were being treated for sleep apnea and flying with a special issuance medical certificate. Untreated OSA always has been and will continue to be a generally disqualifying medical condition.[26,27]

Finally, the Nuclear Regulatory Commission has also taken notice and there is increased awareness to screen for OSA during medical assessments for nuclear power plant employees. The regulatory guide for medical assessment notes that operators with OSA may require a license restriction. There is also a requirement that, if during the term of the license, the licensee develops a condition such as OSA, the facility licensee shall notify the commission within 30 days, with the potential for stiff penalties if this reporting requirement is not met.[28]

LEGAL ASPECTS OF PARASOMNIA

Parasomnias are undesirable experiences that may occur during either non-REM (ie, confusional arousals, sleepwalking, sleep terrors), or REM sleep (ie, REM behavior disorder). Parasomnia-associated sleep-related violence (SRV) presents a potential medicolegal issue for sleep medicine physicians, because they may be called on to consider parasomnia as a possible contributing, mitigating, or exculpatory factor in criminal proceedings. Unfortunately, little research evidence and no consensus clinical guidelines are available to help guide sleep medicine physicians in this complicated task.

The prevalence of SRV in those with parasomnia is unknown, and may be underestimated given that most SRV is directed toward oneself. SRV directed at others, such as assault, homicide, sexual assault/rape, or motor vehicle related offenses, are the incidents that come to the attention of the criminal justice system, but may represent only a fraction of all SRV incidents.

LEGAL DEFINITIONS PERTAINING TO PARASOMNIAS

Legally, if an individual is neither awake nor able to make a decision to not act, such actions are termed "automatisms," which are divided into 2 categories: "sane automatisms" and "insane automatisms." Sane automatisms result from an external factor, for example, a blow to the head. Insane automatisms result from an internal factor, for example, a brain tumor or a psychological factor, and traditionally result in compulsory confinement in a psychiatric facility. Given that parasomnia is likely a neurologic disturbance, it falls into the category of insane automatism, and unfortunately may lead to institutionalization of those who are not mentally ill.

The legal concepts of *actus rea*, *mens rea*, sane automatisms, and insane automatism are all grounded in the philosophy of Cartesian dualism, where the mind and body are considered separate.[29] The current understanding of neurology, and of parasomnias in particular, has shown that motor function may be separate from cognitive awareness, which is requisite for criminal responsibility. As a result, the attempt to fit parasomnia behavior into the current Cartesian legal framework is fraught with difficulty and contradiction.

SLEEP-RELATED VIOLENCE DEFENDANT AND VICTIM CHARACTERISTICS

The most consistent risk factor for SRV is male gender. Moldofsky and colleagues[30] retrospectively assessed 64 adults with sleepwalking, or sleep terrors, and found that men with either sleepwalking or sleep terrors were more likely to commit violence against others if they experienced more stress, used caffeine excessively, or used illicit drugs. Young male exclusivity was found by Bonkalo[31] in a review of 20 homicide cases from 1791 to 1969. Ingravallo and colleagues[32] assessed case reports in the medical literature from 1980 to 2012 in which a sleep disorder was the defense during a criminal trial involving purported SRV or sexual behavior during sleep (SBS). Nine SRV and 9 SBS cases were included in the review, and in all cases the defendants were young men and all of the SBS victims were women, as were nearly all of the SBV victims. This finding is concerning, given the obvious incentive of men who commit violence against women to malinger, seeking parasomnia-related automatism as a legal defense. Nevertheless, the trial outcome in all of the SBS cases, and two-thirds of SRV cases, were favorable to the defendant.

MEDICATION-ASSOCIATED PARASOMNIA

Ingestion of benzodiazepines and nonbenzodiazepine benzodiazepine receptor agonists, have been associated with sleepwalking and other complex behaviors.[33] Poceta[34] assessed a case series of 8 clinical patients who presented with zolpidem associated sleepwalking, and 6 legal defendants prosecuted for driving under the influence of zolpidem. In these 14 cases, the clinical features of zolpidem associated complex behaviors included (1) poor motor control, dysarthria, and ataxia, (2) responsiveness to the environment, manifest as apparent wakefulness to observers, (3) confused ideation, and irrational speech, and (4) anterograde amnesia. Risk factors for zolpidem associated unusual behaviors are varied, and include (1) concomitant alcohol, or sedative medication use, (2) sleep fragmentation from sleep disordered breathing or periodic limb movements in sleep, (3) ingestion of zolpidem at times other than habitual bedtime, or when sleep deprived, and (4) poor management of pills resulting in accidental overdose.

THE SLEEP MEDICINE PHYSICIAN'S ROLE IN PARASOMNIA LEGAL CASES

In most SRV cases, sleepwalking is the purported defense. Consensus guidelines for the evaluation of SRV and/or SBS cases are lacking. Nevertheless, the clinical workup of such cases should include a complete history and physical, with special attention to acquiring historical details regarding habitual sleep–wake periods, prescribed medications (particularly hypnotics), illicit drug use, alcohol use, a personal history of prior parasomnia behaviors, and a family history of parasomnia behavior. Recollection of vivid, frightening dream imagery may suggest either sleep terrors or REM-associated nightmares. Although REM dream imagery may tend to have a more narrative sequence, it is often very difficult to distinguish clinically between sleep terrors and REM nightmares by dream recollection descriptions alone.

A critical historical detail is the proximity of the victim to attacker at the onset of the behaviors in question. According to the third edition of the *International Classification of Sleep Disorders*, the sleepwalker does not generally seek out the eventual victim.[35] More often, a person attempting to restrain, redirect, or awaken the sleepwalker during an episode is attacked unintentionally with primitive defensive aggression in the form of punching, kicking, and so on. If the victim is neither in proximity to the attacker nor provokes the attacker, these circumstances may cast doubt on a diagnosis of parasomnia-associated behavior.[36]

Electrophysiologic evaluation in SRV or SBS cases should include video polysomnography with surface electromyography assessment of all 4 extremities. Two groups of factors have been described as facilitating or precipitating sleepwalking in predisposed individuals: those that deepen sleep (eg, sleep deprivation) and factors that fragment sleep (eg, environmental noise, sleep-disordered breathing, periodic limb movements of sleep). A protocol using sleep deprivation combined with auditory stimuli has been shown to be effective in inducing parasomnia behavior in the sleep laboratory setting.[37] However, the limitation of video–polysomnography analysis should be clear, in that even if video polysomnography does not show evidence of parasomnia behavior, a parasomnia at the time of the incident cannot be excluded definitively. Ultimately, conviction or acquittal is based on the forensic evidence at the scene of the incident and, if available, eyewitness testimony.

LEGAL AND REGULATORY ASPECTS OF SLEEP DISPARITIES

Access to medical care is an important yet underappreciated legal and social justice issue in American society, affecting both children and adults, with widespread societal implications. In regard to pulmonary and sleep medicine, the American Thoracic Society defines health disparities as the differences in respiratory health that are associated with racial, social, economic, or environmental factors that adversely affect health, health care access, and health outcomes, and health care equality is defined as "the attainment of the highest level of respiratory care for all people."[38] The American Thoracic Society recommends advocacy, education, and public health policy as key factors toward achieving health equality (**Fig. 1**). A strategy to ensure sleep health equality must primarily involve ensuring equal health care access, broadening insurance coverage, and improving reimbursement to promote prompt and equal diagnosis and management of sleep disorders. The literature shows that African Americans, Latinos, and patients from low socioeconomic status have poorer sleep quality and an higher incidence of OSA than white patients and patients from higher socioeconomic status.[39,40] Access to health care for disadvantaged populations is often challenging and the diagnosis and management of sleep disorders is delayed.[41]

SLEEP MEDICINE HEALTH CARE DISPARITIES IN CHILDREN

The American Academy of Pediatrics estimates that 30 million children from low-income families are covered by Medicaid. Although Medicaid constitutes an important safety net for families with a low income, the reimbursement rates, qualification criteria, and number of providers that accept patients with Medicaid vary significantly among states. A study of access to specialty care for children with government issued insurance, including children referred to otolaryngology for surgical treatment of OSA, showed that 66% of children with government issued insurance were denied an appointment. Among the clinics that scheduled an appointment, the wait time for a child with government issued insurance was 42 days compared with 20 days for children with private-issued insurance.[42] Children with government-issued insurance had to wait 141 days to have a diagnostic polysomnogram, whereas children with private insurance only waited 49.9 days. Treatment of sleep-disordered breathing with adenotonsillectomy was also delayed in government-insured children (222.3 days) when compared with children with private insurance (95.3 days). Furthermore, children with government issued insurance were more likely to be lost to follow-up when compared with children with private insurance.[43] In addition, children with government-issued insurance have to travel longer distances owing to the limited number of providers accepting Medicaid. In a study comparing travel time for children referred to otolaryngology evaluation of sleep-disordered breathing, children with private insurance traveled an average of 9.86 miles, whereas those with public insurance traveled 18.05 miles to see a specialist.[44]

SLEEP MEDICINE HEALTH CARE DISPARITIES IN ADULTS

Access to health care has not been studied thoroughly in adult patients at risk of sleep disorders. One study compared referrals for polysomnography for adults at high risk of OSA. The study showed that primary care physicians referred more patients from low socioeconomic status for polysomnography than privately insured patients

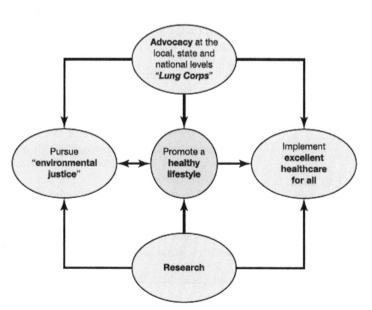

Fig. 1. Overview of the approach of the American Thoracic Society to help eliminate respiratory health care disparities, including sleep medicine health care disparities, through political and environmental advocacy, healthy lifestyle promotion, and improved access to high-quality health care. (*Reprinted with permission of* the American Thoracic Society. Copyright © 2014 American Thoracic Society. Celedon JC, Roman J, Schraufnagel DE, et al. Respiratory health equality in the United States. The American thoracic society perspective. Ann Am Thorac Soc 2014;11(4):473–79. The *Annals of the American Thoracic Society is* an official journal of the American Thoracic Society.)

with the same risk factors. There was no difference in referral for polysomnography among uninsured patients, patients with Medicaid, or those with Medicare.[45] However, even when patients from low socioeconomic status are referred for polysomnography, once the diagnosis is made, more patients are lost to follow-up or do not have the resources to obtain a positive airway pressure device. Comparisons between patients from a minority-serving institution and a middle class–serving hospital showed that 42% of patients diagnosed with OSA were lost to follow-up in the minority-serving institution compared with only 7% of patients in the middle class–serving hospital.[46] Even when CPAP devices were provided to patients at no cost, the time from diagnosis of OSA to CPAP procurement was an average of 62 days for uninsured patients compared with an average of 25 days for patients with Medicaid or Medicare.[47]

The socioeconomic-based differences in the diagnosis, management, and sequelae of OSA are known in both adult and pediatric patients. Despite efforts to improve accessibility to affordable health insurance and expansion in Medicaid programs for patients of low socioeconomic status, there remain significant and alarming differences in access to specialty clinics, diagnostic polysomnography, and treatment options with surgery or CPAP for uninsured or government insured patients when compared with patients with private insurance. Follow-up and positive airway pressure adherence also show significant disparities among patients from various socioeconomic statuses. Achieving a successful diagnosis and management of sleep disorders requires the elimination of health disparities. Research must continue to evaluate the myriad of factors that contribute to sleep health disparities in diagnosis, management, follow-up, adherence, and health outcomes. Research in combination with local, state, and national efforts to expand education to increase patient advocacy and health care policy should continue with the goal to close the existing gap in access to sleep health care.

SUMMARY

Sleep disorders and sleep deprivation can often lead to situations with legal and regulatory ramifications. As noted, these may vary from issues related to driving, employment, surgical procedures, and SRV. Clinicians must be aware of these issues and screen, treat and educate their patients. Improving patient access to treatment is also key to reducing the individual and societal burden of untreated sleep disorders.

REFERENCES

1. Ellen RL, Marshall SC, Palayew M, et al. Systematic review of motor vehicle crash risk in persons with sleep apnea. J Clin Sleep Med 2006;2:193–200.
2. Karimi M, Hedner J, Häbel H, et al. Sleep apnea-related risk of motor vehicle accidents is reduced by continuous positive airway pressure: Swedish traffic accident registry data. Sleep 2015;38:341–9.
3. Meuleners L, Fraser ML, Govorko MH, et al. Obstructive sleep apnea, health-related factors, and long distance heavy vehicle crashes in Western Australia: a case control study. J Clin Sleep Med 2015;11:413–8.
4. Tregear S, Reston J, Schoelles K, et al. Obstructive sleep apnea and risk of motor vehicle crash: systematic review and meta-analysis. J Clin Sleep Med 2009;5:573–81.
5. Tregear S, Reston J, Schoelles K, et al. Continuous positive airway pressure reduces risk of motor vehicle crash among drivers with obstructive sleep apnea: systematic review and meta-analysis. Sleep 2010;33:1373–80.
6. Morbidity and Mortality Weekly Report. Unhealthy sleep-related behaviors — 12 states, 2009. Atlanta (GA): Centers for Disease Control and Prevention; 2011. p. 233–68.
7. Brown D. Legal obligations of persons who have sleep disorders or who treat or hire them Elsevier. In: Kryger M, Roth T, Dement WC, editors. Principles and practice of sleep medicine. Philadelphia: Elsevier; 2016. p. 661–5.e3.
8. Bushnell v. Bushnell, 103 Conn. 583, 131 A. 432 (1925).
9. State v. Valyou, 910 A. 2d 922–924, 2006 VT 105 (2006).
10. N.J.S.A. § 2C:11-5(a).
11. Arkansas Code § 5-10-105.
12. Dunlap v. W.L. Logan Trucking Co., 161 Ohio App. 3d 51, 66; (2005).
13. Black v. William Insulation Co., 141 P.3d 123 (Wyo. Sup. Ct. 2006).
14. Barclay v. Briscoe, 47 A.3d 560, 427 Md. 270; (Md., 2012).
15. Svider PF, Pashkova AA, Folbe AJ, et al. Obstructive sleep apnea: strategies for minimizing liability and enhancing patient safety. Otolaryngol Head Neck Surg 2013;149:947–53.
16. Fouladpour N, Jesudoss R, Bolden N, et al. Perioperative complications in obstructive sleep apnea patients undergoing surgery: a review of the legal literature. Anesth Analg 2016;122:145–51.
17. Feitzinger v. Simon, 2009 NY Slip Op 31533 (N.Y. Sup. Ct. 2009).
18. Cornett v. State, W.O. Moss Hospital, 614 So.2d 189 (La. App. 3rd Cir. 1993).

19. Russell v. Brown, No. E2004-01855-COA-R3-CV 2005 WL 1991609 (Tenn. Ct. App.); (August 18, 2005).

20. Colvin LJ, Collop NA. Commercial motor vehicle driver obstructive sleep apnea screening and treatment in the United States: an update and recommendation overview. J Clin Sleep Med 2016;12: 113–25.

21. Hartenbaum N, Collop N, Rosen IM, et al. Sleep apnea and commercial motor vehicle operators: statement from the joint task force of the American College of Chest Physicians, American College of Occupational and Environmental Medicine, and the National Sleep Foundation. J Occup Environ Med 2006;48:S4–37.

22. Ancoli-Israel, S, Czeisler, CA, George, CFP, et al. Obstructive sleep apnea and commercial motor vehicle driver safety. Available at: http://www.fmcsa. dot.gov/sites/fmcsa.dot.gov/files/docs/Sleep-MEP-Panel-Recommendations-508.pdf. 2008. Accessed June 28 2016.

23. Parker D, Hoffman B. Motor carrier safety advisory committee and medical review board task force 11-05 report. 2012. Available at: http://mcsac.fmcsa. dot.gov/Reports.htm. Accessed June 28 2016.

24. U.S. Federal Register 77 FR 23794. Proposed recommendations on obstructive sleep apnea [Internet]. Washington, DC: U.S. Department of Transportation; Federal Motor Carriers Safety Administration; 2012. Available at: https://www.federalregister.gov/articles/2012/04/20/2012-9555/proposed-recommendations-on-obstructivesleep-apnea. Accessed June 28, 2016.

25. Epstein LJ, Kristo D, Strollo PJ Jr, et al. Clinical guideline for the evaluation, management and long-term care of obstructive sleep apnea in adults. J Clin Sleep Med 2009;5:263–76.

26. Fact Sheet – Sleep Apnea in Aviation. 2015. Available at: https://www.faa.gov/news/fact_sheets/news_story. cfm?newsId=18156. Accessed June 29 2016.

27. Guide for Aviation Medical Examiners. Available at: https://www.faa.gov/about/office_org/headquarters_offices/avs/offices/aam/ame/guide/. Accessed June 29 2016.

28. Medical Assessment Of Licensed Operators Or Applicants For Operator Licenses At Nuclear Power Plants. 2014. Available at: http://www.nrc.gov/docs/ML1418/ML14189A385.pdf. Accessed June 29 2016.

29. Popat S, Winslade W. While you were sleepwalking: science and neurobiology of sleep disorders & the enigma of legal responsibility of violence during parasomnia. Neuroethics 2015;8(2):203–14.

30. Moldofsky H, Gilbert R, Lue FA, et al. Sleep-related violence. Sleep 1995;18(9):731–9.

31. Bonkalo A. Impulsive acts and confusional states during incomplete arousal from sleep: crinimological and forensic implications. Psychiatr Q 1974;48(3): 400–9.

32. Ingravallo F, Poli F, Gilmore EV, et al. Sleep-related violence and sexual behavior in sleep: a systematic review of medical-legal case reports. J Clin Sleep Med 2014;10(8):927–35.

33. Hoque R, Chesson AL Jr. Zolpidem-induced sleepwalking, sleep related eating disorder, and sleep-driving: fluorine-18-flourodeoxyglucose positron emission tomography analysis, and a literature review of other unexpected clinical effects of zolpidem. J Clin Sleep Med 2009;5(5):471–6.

34. Poceta JS. Zolpidem ingestion, automatisms, and sleep driving: a clinical and legal case series. J Clin Sleep Med 2011;7(6):632–8.

35. American Academy of Sleep Medicine. International classification of sleep disorders; diagnostic and coding manual. 3rd edition. Darien (IL): American Academy of Sleep Medicine; 2014.

36. Morrison I, Rumbold JM, Riha RL. Medicolegal aspects of complex behaviours arising from the sleep period: a review and guide for the practising sleep physician. Sleep Med Rev 2014;18(3): 249–60.

37. Pilon M, Montplaisir J, Zadra A. Precipitating factors of somnambulism: impact of sleep deprivation and forced arousals. Neurology 2008;70(24): 2284–90.

38. Celedon JC, Roman J, Schraufnagel DE, et al. Respiratory health equality in the United States. The American Thoracic Society Perspective. Ann Am Thorac Soc 2014;11(4):473–9.

39. Patel NP, Grandner MA, Xie D, et al. "Sleep disparity" in the population: poor sleep quality is strongly associated with poverty and ethnicity. BMC Public Health 2010;10:475.

40. Punjabi NM. The epidemiology of adult obstructive sleep apnea. Proc Am Thorac Soc 2008;5(2):136–43.

41. Boss EF, Smith DF, Ishman SL. Racial/ethnic and socioeconomic disparities in the diagnosis and treatment of sleep-disordered breathing in children. Int J Pediatr Otorhinolaryngol 2011;75(3):299–307.

42. Bisgaier J, Rhodes KV. Auditing access to specialty care for children with public insurance. N Engl J Med 2011;364(24):2324–33.

43. Boss EF, Benke JR, Tunkel DE, et al. Public insurance and timing of polysomnography and surgical care for children with sleep-disordered breathing. JAMA Otolaryngol Head Neck Surg 2015;141(2): 106–11.

44. Penn EB Jr, French A, Bhushan B, et al. Access to care for children with symptoms of sleep disordered breathing. Int J Pediatr Otorhinolaryngol 2012; 76(11):1671–3.

45. Thornton JD, Chandriani K, Thornton JG, et al. Assessing the prioritization of primary care referrals for polysomnograms. Sleep 2010;33(9):1255–60.

46. Greenberg H, Fleischman J, Gouda HE, et al. Disparities in obstructive sleep apnea and its management between a minority-serving institution and a voluntary hospital. Sleep Breath 2004;8(4):185–92.

47. DelRosso LM, Hoque R, Chesson AL Jr. Continuous positive airway pressure device time to procurement in a disadvantaged population. Sleep Disord 2015;2015:747906.

Printed and bound by CPI Group (UK) Ltd, Croydon, CR0 4YY

03/10/2024

01040302-0013